A Clinical Guide to
Psychiatric Ethics

A Clinical Guide to
Psychiatric Ethics

Laura Weiss Roberts, M.D., M.A.

Chairman and Katharine Dexter McCormick and
Stanley McCormick Memorial Professor, Department of Psychiatry
and Behavioral Sciences, Stanford University School of Medicine,
Stanford, California

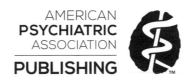

AMERICAN
PSYCHIATRIC
ASSOCIATION
PUBLISHING
TM

If you wish to buy 50 or more copies of the same title, please go to www.appi.org/specialdiscounts for more information.

Copyright © 2016 American Psychiatric Association Publishing

ALL RIGHTS RESERVED

Manufactured in the United States of America on acid-free paper

American Psychiatric Association Publishing
1000 Wilson Boulevard
Arlington, VA 22209-3901
www.appi.org

Library of Congress Cataloging-in-Publication Data
Names: Roberts, Laura Weiss, 1960– , author. | Roberts, Laura Weiss, 1960–
Concise guide to ethics in mental health care. Expanded version of (work):
| American Psychiatric Association Publishing, issuing body.
Title: A clinical guide to psychiatric ethics / Laura Weiss Roberts.
Description: Arlington, Virginia : American Psychiatric Association
Publishing, [2016] |
| Includes bibliographical references and index.
Identifiers: LCCN 2016007671 | ISBN 9781615370498 (alk. paper)
Subjects: | MESH: Psychotherapy—ethics | Professional-Patient
Relations—ethics
Classification: LCC RC455.2.E8 | NLM WM 21 | DDC 174.2/9689—dc23
LC record available at http://lccn.loc.gov/2016007671

British Library Cataloguing in Publication Data
A CIP record is available from the British Library.

For Eric

Contents

I
Fundamentals

II
Caring for Special Populations

III
Evolving Topics

Contributors

Jerald Belitz, Ph.D.
Professor of Psychiatry and Behavioral Sciences; Clinical Director, Children's Psychiatric Center/Outpatient Services; Training Director, Psychology Internship, University of New Mexico Health Sciences Center, Albuquerque, New Mexico

Michael P. Bogenschutz, M.D.
Professor of Psychiatry, New York University School of Medicine, New York, New York

Allen R. Dyer, M.D., Ph.D.
Professor of Psychiatry and Behavioral Sciences, The George Washington University, Washington, DC

Cynthia M.A. Geppert, M.D., M.A., M.P.H., M.S., D.P.S.
Professor of Psychiatry and Director of Ethics Education, University of New Mexico School of Medicine; Chief of Psychiatry and Ethics Consultation, New Mexico Veterans Affairs Health Care Systems, Albuquerque, New Mexico

Honor Hsin, M.D., Ph.D.
Resident, Department of Psychiatry and Behavioral Sciences, Stanford University School of Medicine, Stanford, California

Emily Yang Liu, B.A.
Medical Student, Stanford University School of Medicine, Stanford, California

Alan K. Louie, M.D.
Professor, Associate Chair, and Director of Education, Department of Psychiatry and Behavioral Sciences, Stanford University School of Medicine, Stanford, California

Lawrence M. McGlynn, M.D.
Clinical Professor, Department of Psychiatry and Behavioral Sciences, Stanford University School of Medicine, Stanford, California

Merry N. Miller, M.D.
Professor, Department of Psychiatry and Behavioral Sciences, Quillen College of Medicine, East Tennessee State University, Johnson City, Tennessee

Daryn Reicherter, M.D.
Clinical Associate Professor, Department of Psychiatry and Behavioral Sciences, Stanford University School of Medicine, Stanford, California

Laura Weiss Roberts, M.D., M.A.
Chairman and Katharine Dexter McCormick and Stanley McCormick Memorial Professor, Department of Psychiatry and Behavioral Sciences, Stanford University School of Medicine, Stanford, California

Tom Townsend, M.D.
Professor of Family Medicine and Director, Program in Clinical Ethics, Quillen College of Medicine, East Tennessee State University, Johnson City, Tennessee

Mickey Trockel, M.D.
Clinical Assistant Professor, Department of Psychiatry and Behavioral Sciences, Stanford University School of Medicine, Stanford, California

DISCLOSURES

The following contributors have stated that they have no competing interests during the year preceding manuscript submission:

Jerald Belitz, Ph.D.; Michael P. Bogenschutz, M.D.; Allen R. Dyer, M.D., Ph.D.; Cynthia M.A. Geppert, M.D., M.A., M.P.H., M.S., D.P.S.; Honor Hsin, M.D., Ph.D.; Emily Yang Liu, B.A.; Alan K. Louie, M.D.; Lawrence M. McGlynn, M.D.; Merry N. Miller, M.D.; Daryn Reicherter, M.D.; Laura Weiss Roberts, M.D., M.A.; Tom Townsend, M.D.; Mickey Trockel, M.D.

Preface

Providing ethical care is the aspiration of every dedicated psychiatrist and clinical trainee, yet fulfilling this ideal is not a simple matter of being—or trying to be—good. Each new day brings encounters with people with serious illnesses whose care presents new ethical questions and challenges. Each new clinical practice approach, each new technological development, and each new social policy creates complex, seemingly unprecedented, and irresolvable dilemmas. Traditions, codes, and legal rulings may provide little help and less comfort in these situations—situations that define the real meaning of professionalism in the care of human suffering.

A Clinical Guide to Psychiatric Ethics is about approaching the ethical aspects of mental health care—both subtle and dramatic—with clarity, coherence, and optimism. The text emphasizes real experience as opposed to remote theories involving concepts that may sound good but could cause harm when misapplied or are not attuned to clinical realities. As a result, this text does not offer simple answers. Rather, it seeks to provide guideposts, to impart information, to foster skill development, and to encourage openness, collaboration, and self-reflection. These elements, together with tenacious endeavors to be—and to try to be—good, represent a compass and a set of map-making tools for those traveling with their patients along the ethical frontier of mental illness.

This book is derived from the *Concise Guide to Ethics in Mental Health Care*, an earlier book that I wrote with colleagues and that was published in 2004 as part of American Psychiatric Publishing's Concise Guide series. This book has been revised, updated, and rewritten, with new chapters, new topics, and new data to help the interested reader. Framed in three sections, *A Clinical Guide to Psychiatric Ethics* covers fundamentals of psychiatric ethics, psychiatric ethics and caring for special populations, and evolving topics in psychiatric ethics. The chapters cover essential ethics principles and skills and address topics of special importance in mental health care, such as the ethical use of influence and role in high-risk situations, informed consent, and confidentiality. The book gives significant focus to the care of individuals who derive from distinct populations (e.g., children, veterans) and care occurring in unique contexts (e.g., small communities). Intended primarily as a clinical reference and an educational tool, the book contains case scenarios in each chapter that may be used in independent study or small-group discussions. At the back of the book are references and an appendix with more cases for discussion. The book does not seek to be wholly comprehensive, despite the wide coverage, but rather serves to illustrate principles and practices that may be applied by psychiatrists in the many roles and settings that they embrace.

Acknowledgments

I wish to thank all of the colleagues who have given so much to this book and its 2004 edition. Allen R. Dyer, M.D., Ph.D., receives my deepest thanks and appreciation, along with Jerald Belitz, Ph.D.; Michael P. Bogenschutz, M.D.; Cynthia M.A. Geppert, M.D., M.A., M.P.H., M.S., D.P.S.; Honor Hsin, M.D., Ph.D.; Emily Yang Liu; Alan K. Louie, M.D.; Lawrence M. McGlynn, M.D.; Merry N. Miller, M.D.; Daryn Reicherter, M.D.; Tom Townsend, M.D.; and Mickey Trockel, M.D., for their work on chapters and cases in this book.

I wish to acknowledge Allen R. Dyer, M.D., Ph.D., who wrote some chapters and cases with me for the *Concise Guide to Ethics in Mental Health Care* (Roberts and Dyer 2004), part of whose work was adapted in Chapters 1 and 12 of this volume. I thank Honor Hsin, M.D., Ph.D., for her assistance on Chapter 21.

Ann Tennier, ELS, my colleague, editorial savant, and sometimes personal savior, receives my heartfelt thanks for her help with this and every other project we have undertaken together. Katie Ryan, M.A., Jennifer Pearlstein, and Megan Cid provided invaluable assistance with this book, and I send my thanks to them as well. Debra J. Berman, Tammy J. Cordova, Catherine Fox, Patricia L. Freedman, and Susan Westrate all contributed their fine skills to the publication of this book.

My gratitude also goes to Robert E. Hales, M.D., John McDuffie, Ann M. Eng, Bessie Jones, and Rebecca Rinehart, who have been my wonderful friends and collaborators at American Psychiatric Association Publishing. It has been my privilege to develop scholarly works with you.

Disclaimer

The descriptions of people throughout this clinical guide—for example, in cases and vignettes—are hypothetical. Any resemblance to actual people is completely by chance, and names (if any) were chosen randomly. Some of these descriptions of people include interactions with a clinician and questions a clinician might ask. These described interactions are intended to be illustrative, and the descriptions are not of complete clinical interviews or analyses of cases.

The authors have attempted to ensure that all information is accurate at the time of writing and consistent with general psychiatric and medical standards. As medical research and practice continue to advance, however, information and standards may change. Specific situations may require a specific response not included in this manual. The authors cannot assume any legal liability for any mistakes of commission or omission in this manual. No information in this manual should be construed as providing treatment recommendations.

I

Fundamentals

1

Ethics Principles and Professionalism

Laura Weiss Roberts, M.D., M.A.

Ethics *refers to ways* of understanding and examining moral life to create a coherent sense of what is good and right in human experience. Ethics is an endeavor that requires sensitivity, knowledge, and skill. It is informed by scholarship and evidence and shaped by values and context. It is a branch of philosophy insofar as philosophy is the discipline involving rational thinking, but ethics is not just about thinking. It is also about feeling, observing, experiencing, and right action, and these involve all of life. In health care, the study of ethics has helped to develop principles and decision-making approaches that guide clinical practice. It also has helped to clarify how the health professions can best fulfill their responsibilities in serving patients, communities, and society.

Ethics in psychiatry, and in mental health care more broadly, is exceptionally complex, in part because of the nature of mental illnesses—which, by definition, affect an individual's most fundamental human capacities, relationships, and social roles. Mental illnesses affect aspects of life that we define as fundamental to being human, such as perceptions, feelings, relatedness, self-understanding, and choices. In addition, people who struggle with mental illness may be isolated, misunderstood, and stigmatized and have few resources to overcome barriers in their lives, including limited access to appropriate care. Moreover, the treatment of mental illness involves techniques that require exploration of intimate aspects of patients' lives and interventions that in some cases may limit the freedoms of patients who are at risk of harming themselves or others. People with mental illness may have exceptional strengths, but they also may have exceptional vulnerabilities. Ensuring the ethical use of the power entrusted to clinicians in these situations is very challenging. For these reasons, ethics lies at the very heart of psychiatry.

Skills that psychiatrists and other clinicians working in mental health care can bring to ethics are many. First, astute clinical care in this area requires attentiveness to the importance of human experience in relation to illness and suffering. Beyond eliciting symptoms, recognizing patterns, and treating disease, mental health care involves attention to a variety of patients' experiences—for example, the experience of losing their sense of being healthy and whole that accompanies a major depressive episode, the experience of perceiving voices that others do not hear in living with schizophrenia, the experience of surviving an event that forever changes their views of themselves and the world in posttraumatic stress disorder, and the experience of feeling their insight and abilities slip away in chronic progressive illnesses. Gaining an understanding of how these experiences intersect with the strengths, vulnerabilities, choices, hopes, development, and life history of the individual is essential to good clinical care. Awareness of such aspects of the illness experience requires sensitivity, attunement, and integration of diverse, dynamic influences, ranging from biological deficits to personal values. Paying attention to these elements of a patient's care prepares clinicians well for clarifying and addressing complex ethical considerations in serving the patient's overall well-being.

A second skill that psychiatrists and other clinicians working in mental health bring to ethics is a commitment to understanding how their own motivations, attitudes, values, life history, and behaviors may influence therapeutic interactions with patients. These insights bring with them a professional commitment to honest self-observation and to the habit of tracking internal responses (e.g., countertransference in the context of long-term therapy) to patients to discern biases and gaps in judgment. These "habits" of sound clinical practice in mental health care are extraordinarily important to ethical reflection and decision making as well.

A third, closely related skill is the recognition that excellence in the clinician's work is an ethical imperative and places requirements to continue to improve knowledge and expertise as a psychiatrist. Beyond this, however, the role in which the clinician serves often shapes the nature and limits of his or her professional obligations. For example, mental health clinicians function in a variety of roles, ranging from forensic consultant to school-based care provider, from emergency room clinician to psychotherapist, from psychopharmacological subspecialist to case manager. These roles carry with them diverse duties and, at times, divided loyalties. The psychiatrist performing fitness-for-duty evaluations of active-duty military personnel must share the findings with the commanding officer; a psychologist may need to disclose information on a student evaluation to the school where the psychologist works as a consultant; a case manager may need to report suspected child neglect or parole violation after a home visit. Given the significant, sensitive character of these activities in the realm of mental health, awareness of the special ethical commitments of each kind of role is particularly important for this field.

Other gifts that psychiatrists bring to ethics include attentiveness to processes of human interaction. Psychiatrists observe and reflect on the contribution of interpersonal conflict and unconscious elements in individual, dyadic, and group interactions. Psychiatrists working with people with mental illness will also recognize that there is more to ethics than rational thought. Unconscious motives, feelings, drives, and conflicts—both internal (indecision or guilt) and external (from argument to warfare)—both inform and are informed by ethics. Awareness of ethical tensions—sometimes between two competing "good" aims, such as respect for privacy and respect for the law—and articulating the impact of these tensions represent a natural role for psychiatrists in teams and in health organizations. To be useful, ethical analysis must offer help in resolving the conflicts that are central to human existence in communities. Mental health clinicians furthermore are accustomed to working with colleagues of different backgrounds and disciplines in the course of providing care to patients, and this interdependence is a valuable approach to identifying and resolving ethical problems that may be overlooked when clinicians practice in isolation.

This chapter describes the principles of traditional ethics as they have emerged and evolved within the clinical professions and lays out fundamentals of psychiatric ethics.

TRADITIONAL PRINCIPLES OF THE CLINICAL PROFESSIONS

Historically, Western medicine as a healing art traces its ethical foundations to the writings of Hippocrates, who lived in Greece from about 460–370 B.C. Hippocrates is considered the father of modern Western medicine because his approach was scientific—in that he tried to observe systematically the course of illnesses—yet he stood as a priest in the religious or shamanistic tradition. Hippocrates was both a naturalist and a spiritual healer. Confucian writings from around the same period speak of similar virtues: humanness, compassion, and filial piety. The writings of Maimonides and those from the various religious traditions more than 2,000 years ago likewise offer much inspiration, some guidance, and special demands for adherence to healers in all generations.

Over centuries, ethical schools have evolved and shaped aspects of modern Western medical practice. These ethical schools are quite different in their emphases and implications:

- The deontological school of Immanuel Kant gave primacy to the inherent worth of the individual person and the intention of each human being as a moral agent. His work focused not on consequences of actions, but on the rigor, rationality, and pure intention of the actions of a "good" person (e.g., "Act in such a way that you always treat humanity, whether in your own person or in the person of any other, never simply as a means").
- The utilitarian school of Jeremy Bentham and John Stuart Mill contrasts with deontological thinking in that it measures the morality of an action by its consequences, not its intent. In this view, "right action" is action that produces the greatest good for the greatest number of people. Actions occur in context, not in isolation, and unlike in the approach of Kant, a good person could "use" another person as a "means" to an end, if such use brings about benefit for multiple others.
- Beyond deontological and utilitarian schools, John Rawls articulated a system in which justice is the main objective and actions are "good" if they advance fairness and remediate disparities for individuals. Rawls emphasized the rights and well-being of each human being, rather than the good of entire groups, and in this sense his approach is often recognized as more similar to that of Kant than to that of Bentham and Mills. Rawls also focused on the intention of individual moral agents rather than the consequences of actions.
- Virtue-based theory has also greatly informed ethics concepts and the core ideals of professionalism. John Gregory and Thomas Percival, both physicians, elevated the importance of science and standards of competence in medicine. They spoke of empathy and compassion toward patients, the importance of self-sacrifice and humility of physicians, and the well-being and interests of patients and service to the public as the fundamental aims of medicine—not self-aggrandizement or financial

gain. They reflected on the moral obligation to advance science and training (at that time, training of apprentices in medicine) and to ensure the competence of colleagues.

- More recent ethicists have raised important new ideas that also have bearing on modern medicine. Feminist-ethicist Carol Gilligan (1993) has written about gender and ethical practices, advancing the idea that women seek to protect and preserve relationships as a moral "good," whereas men are more concerned with advancing rights-oriented, rationalistic, and justice-based approaches. She used the metaphor of masculine and feminine "voices" in ethical decision making. Interesting empirical work informed by this analysis has shown that medical practices are different depending on both the gender of the physician and that of the patient. Cross-cultural reflections and scholarship have fostered awareness of other schools of thought that are certain to have growing influence in the United States and its standards of medical ethics as the population becomes more diverse and its values more pluralistic (see Chapter 10, "People From Culturally Distinct Populations").

These schools of thought are not perfectly aligned, yet each has brought contributions to the modern Western view of ethics and ethical standards in medicine. These concepts underlying the ethics of healing have been reclaimed by modern physicians and other health professions: a band of healers, united by a shared commitment to articulated principles of ethics. *Beneficence*, for example, is one of the key principles of the Hippocratic tradition and is defined as the use of the physician's expertise exclusively to help the ill: "I will act only for the benefit of the patient." This idea is closely linked to the principle of *nonmaleficence*: "First, do no harm." The Latin version of this phrase, *Primum non nocere*, probably stems from nineteenth- and early twentieth-century British and American physicians, who studied Latin, used a Latin vocabulary for much of medicine, and wrote prescriptions in Latin. This early commitment to ethical principles gave medicine a touch of both mysticism and erudition, establishing the dual tradition so cherished by healers and sick alike: medicine can be viewed as both religious and scientific, as an art and as a science. These ethical principles, as described in Table 1–1, offer a useful point of departure for considering the dilemmas and conflicts that have emerged with the new technologies of modern medicine.

TABLE 1–1.   Ethical principles articulated in the Hippocratic writings

---

Beneficence ("I will come for the benefit of the sick")

Confidentiality ("What I see in the lives of men, I will not noise abroad")

Proscription against sex with patients ("I will not engage in mischief")

Proscription against euthanasia ("I will not give a deadly drug, nor suggest such a thing")

Proscription against abortion ("I will not give a woman an abortive remedy")

Practice within the limits of competence ("I will not…cut on the stone")

Hope and optimism ("[I will not] make gloomy prognostications")

Nonmaleficence ("First, do no harm")

Professional affiliations ("[I will] hold the one who has taught me this art as equal to my parents and live my life in partnership with him [or her]")

Source.   Adapted from Roberts LW, Dyer AR: *Concise Guide to Ethics in Mental Health Care.* Washington, DC, American Psychiatric Publishing, 2004, p. 5. Copyright © 2004 American Psychiatric Publishing. Used with permission.

PROFESSIONALISM AND THE EVOLUTION OF BIOETHICAL PRINCIPLES

A profession is entrusted with fulfilling special responsibilities in society. Medicine involves the use of specialized expertise and wisdom to enhance and preserve the lives of others, seeking to foster their health and well-being, to diminish their suffering, and to do so with honor, compassion, and respect. Six principles in particular have been identified as encompassing the basic ethical values on which complex, ethically important decisions may be made by health professionals:

- Beneficence
- Autonomy
- Nonmaleficence
- Justice
- Veracity
- Fidelity

The tensions and shifting emphases among these principles reveal much about social change and the place of medicine, especially during recent decades, in which technological developments have been extraordinary. They also set the stage for issues that health care, ethics, and society must address in the years ahead.

Beneficence, the duty to "do good," is intrinsically the subject matter of ethics. What does it mean to do good? From the standpoint of the moral agent—that is, the individual who is motivated to do good—it means to do right by others. For physicians since antiquity, beneficence has implied doing right by patients, a duty understood as a question for physicians to determine, although healers could hardly remain oblivious to the needs of those they cared for.

Autonomy, which can be understood simply as self-determination, is based in the fundamental imperative of *respect for persons*. It is linked with the concept of *privacy*, which in our society is understood as the individual's right to have the body or mind not intruded upon. It is also linked with the concept of *voluntarism*, which encompasses individuals' ability to act in accordance with their authentic sense of what is good, right, and best in light of their situation, values, and history. Voluntarism further entails the capacity to make this choice freely and in the absence of coercion. In this construction, beneficence is thus to be judged by the recipient, not just by the initiator. In legal terms, across society it is understood and accepted that individuals have a right to self-determination. Beneficence untempered by autonomy was and is often paternalistic, relying inordinately on the wisdom and conscience of the physician without sufficient regard for the perspective and values of the patient.

Since the 1960s, as medical technology came to offer more options for care and as society became more rights oriented, patients increasingly began to experience more authority in the process of making medical decisions. There has been a gradual and perceptible shift from beneficence as the keystone of medical ethics to autonomy as the dominant principle of bioethics in Western medicine.

Nonmaleficence is a word coined in the 1970s to express the concept "First, do no harm." In this phrase, harm is a key consideration in therapeutic interventions that may result in adverse effects or outcomes (e.g., medication for psychosis can cause tardive dyskinesia or increase the risk of bone marrow suppression or of developing metabolic syndrome). The principle of nonmaleficence is also critical in research, a venue that is dedicated not solely to patient benefit but constrained as a scientific task and involves a calculation of risk versus benefit.

The principle of *justice* brings equitable distribution of power and resources into ethical focus. On an individual level, the tensions between beneficence and autonomy assume a locus of decision making somewhere between the physician and patient. On a societal level, distributive-justice questions arise in regard to fair allocation of resources. What access to care, expertise, and other health resources might an individual patient reasonably expect in a just society? What obligations does a physician or health care provider owe a particular patient, and what roles can providers play in providing or limiting resources to particular individuals? How do providers understand their obligations to society as well as to those they serve directly? These questions might once have been perceived as beyond the scope of medicine and health care, understood either in technical or humanistic terms. Their resolution depends on an understanding of what constitutes a just society and the respective roles of the citizens, including clinicians, who play a direct role in allocation decisions. The major tensions in these debates center on concepts of social justice. Libertarian views hold that the highest political ideal is freedom; socialist views hold that equality is the highest distributive ideal. More practically nuanced views of justice derive from Immanuel Kant's views of welfare justice as elaborated by John Rawls, which hold that the ideal state is founded on a contract in which its members have the freedom to seek happiness up to the point that one person's pursuit of happiness does not limit another person's freedom to pursue happiness. Although these considerations seem abstract, their applications are quite practical.

The move from beneficence to autonomy as a dominant ethical principle was accompanied by a shift of the locus of decision making from the doctor to the patient or, more broadly, from professional to client (the very term *client* suggests a self-determining agent). The move to justice, seen in economic terms, removed the locus of decision making from the doctor and the patient (now considered "provider" and "consumer"); the consequence of this shift for health care professionals was that economic aspects of care began to intrude and to demand attention in ways that seemed novel and perplexing. Ethical principles must be understood within their social and economic contexts and cannot be separated from considerations of justice, which go beyond the doctor–patient (or professional–client) relationships.

Veracity is the principle of telling the truth. It is a positive duty to express the truth, but it also involves the obligation not to deceive through omission. *Fidelity* is the principle of serving faithfully—and often exclusively—a person or an explicit positive aim. These two principles have become very important in recent years in relation to conflicting roles and conflicts of interest (see Chapter 16, "Patient Care Ethics Committees and Consultation Services"). For example, disclosure (i.e., telling the truth) has become a primary safeguard surrounding conflicts of interest in clinical practice and human investigation, which can pose threats to exclusively serving the well-being of patients and research participants.

Modern formulations of these principles are being proposed and considered in relation to population health goals and broad systems of health care (see Chapter 21, "Population Health and Evolving Systems of Care"). As national health care strategies have evolved in the United States and throughout the world, new ethical challenges regarding resource distribution and individual physician responsibilities are being encountered each day. The professionalism charter consensus document of the American Board of Internal Medicine (ABIM Foundation et al. 2002) is one effort to address and resolve such challenges. In addition, Davidoff (2000) proposed seven key ethical principles for health care professionals: rights (to health and health care), balance (health of individuals and of populations), comprehensiveness (of care to encompass well-being and minimization of suffering and disability), cooperation (across segments and sectors of society), improvement (as a continuing responsibility), safety (avoidance of harm to patients), and openness (being honest and trustworthy).

The set of core competencies articulated by the Accreditation Council for Graduate Medical Education (2014) is a reflection of these evolving formulations of ethics in medicine. These competencies span patient care, medical knowledge, interpersonal and communication skills, professionalism, practice-based learning and improvement, and systems-based practice. In the competence domain of professionalism, residents in psychiatry, as elsewhere in medicine, must demonstrate a commitment to carrying out professional responsibilities and an adherence to ethical principles. Included are compassion, integrity, and respect for others; responsiveness to patient needs that supersedes self-interest; respect for patient privacy and autonomy; accountability to patients, society, and the profession; and sensitivity to a diverse patient population, including, but not limited to, diversity in gender, age, culture, race, religion, disabilities, and sexual orientation.

CONCLUSION

Schools of thought differ, principles differ, rules and regulations differ, accreditation standards differ, ethical and legal requirements differ, cultural values differ, peoples' strongly held views differ—and on and on, or so it seems. Finding one's way in the applied field of psychiatric ethics, as in other areas of clinical ethics in medicine, can be very difficult. But ethics is not completely subjective or unknowable, as one may worry. Ethics is simply complex and complicated, and it requires disciplined thought, careful analysis, knowledge, and practice. Ethics approaches are illustrated throughout this clinical manual, and the applications of ethics in clinical care generally and in caring for individuals who come from special populations are explored. Emerging topics in ethics, such as those that arise in clinical innovation and research, in conflict-of-interest issues, in ethics committee discussions, and in evolving health care systems, are also covered and show how even very difficult ethics issues can be resolved.

All of the approaches outlined in this chapter affirm the healing role and special duties of clinicians in caring for the sick and in seeking to promote the health and well-being of individual patients, vulnerable populations, and society broadly. The clinical professions carry the highest ideals: service, duty, honor, commitment to patients, self-sacrifice, and the doing and making of good. In essence, clinical work is not merely an occupation; it is a profession—and for some, perhaps, a vocation—and it is a privilege dedicated to the well-being of others. New conceptions of professionalism reclaim, reaffirm, and perhaps may redefine the ethical underpinnings of healing activity and emphasize the clinician's dual contract to patient and society (Table 1–2), as will be explored in this book.

TABLE 1–2.   Definitions of *professionalism*

Professionalism is the demonstration in practice of aptitudes, attributes, and attitudes to which practitioners lay claim and which might reasonably be demanded of them by those entrusted to their care, and by their colleagues "of good repute and competency." Its hallmark is commitment: (i) to the individual patient, requiring *professional courtesy*, continuing competence, personal *integrity*, and advocacy of the patient's interests; (ii) to the *health care system*, ensuring continuity of relevant care of the highest possible quality for all without discrimination; and (iii) to the profession, entailing active "allegiance to the bodies providing collective professional responsibility" (Boyd et al. 1997, p. 199).

Professionals are usually identified by their commitment to provide important services to clients or consumers and by their specialized training. Professions maintain self-regulating organizations that control entry into occupational roles by formally certifying that candidates have acquired the necessary knowledge and skills. The concept of a medical professional is closely tied to a background of distinctive education and skills that patients typically lack and that morally must be used to benefit patients. In learned professions, such as medicine, the background knowledge of the professional derives from closely supervised training, and the professional is one who provides a service to others (Beauchamp and Childress 2012).

A profession may be defined in terms of its knowledge, technology, or expertise, or it may be defined in terms of its ethics and values. A profession that understands itself in terms of its knowledge, technology, or expertise may be bartered in the marketplace (Dyer 1988).

TABLE 1–2.   Definitions of *professionalism (continued)*

"Being a professional is an ethical matter, entailing devotion to a way of life, in the service of others and of some higher good.... These special considerations imply specific and inherently medical obligations both of omission and commission, as well as appropriately reverential stance of the physician before his chosen profession" (Kass 1983, p. 1305).

Justice Louis Brandeis believed that a profession had three features: training that was intellectual and involved knowledge, as distinguished from skill; work that was pursued primarily for others and not for oneself; and success that was measured by more than the amount of financial return (Brandeis 2009).

The core of professionalism constitutes "those attitudes and behavior[s] that serve to maintain patient interest above physician self-interest. Accordingly, professionalism...aspires to altruism, accountability, excellence, duty, service, honor, integrity, and respect for others" (Stobo and Blank 1994, p. ii).

Source.   Adapted from Roberts LW, Dyer AR: *Concise Guide to Ethics in Mental Health Care.* Washington, DC, American Psychiatric Publishing, 2004, p. 15. Copyright © 2004 American Psychiatric Publishing. Used with permission.

CASE SCENARIOS

■ The housekeeper at a community health center stops one of the psychiatrists and asks him what to do about his sister, who has been severely depressed. The psychiatrist requests that the man bring his sister to the psychiatric emergency service and promises that he will arrange for her to be seen. The man shakes his head and says, "She will not come, because she does not have papers, and she is afraid of Immigration Services."

■ A 9-year-old child wishes to stop taking medications prescribed for his tic disorder because "other kids don't take pills at school."

■ A woman with bipolar disorder must ask permission of the leader of her religious community before she can consent to treatment with mood stabilizers.

■ A 43-year-old man with a personality disorder and alcohol dependence asks his physician not to tell him "anything" about a recommended sigmoidoscopy, because he "trusts" the doctor and does not want to know about "the specifics."

■ A woman with postpartum psychosis has intrusive thoughts of harming her new baby.

2

Clinical Decision-Making and Ethics Skills

Laura Weiss Roberts, M.D., M.A.

Psychiatrists are often well prepared to address ethical considerations that arise in the care of people living with mental illness. Mental health professionals attend to motivations that underlie choices and behaviors, and they sense the importance of insight, values, psychological development, and personal history in the lives of their patients, as individuals and moral persons in society. They understand self-observation and self-scrutiny to be essential habits to ensure clinical excellence. These characteristics help foster optimal ethical reflection and rigorous decision making in patient care, and often these qualities lead individuals to choose the field of psychiatry.

Beyond these personal qualities, the essential ethics skills listed in Table 2–1 should be in the tool kit of all clinical professionals working with people with mental illness. The clinician's repertoire should also include a specific, focused strategy for approaching ethical decisions in clinical care. One such strategy is described in this chapter, unifying four major elements: clinical indications, patient preferences, quality of life, and external considerations. These skills, taken together with this explicit ethical decision-making strategy, or other such strategies (Table 2–2), may be used in enacting ethically sound clinical behaviors and choices.

TABLE 2–1.   Essential ethics skills in clinical practice

1.   The ability to identify the ethical features of a patient's care

2.   The ability to see how one's life experiences, attitudes, and knowledge may influence one's care of a patient

3.   The ability to identify one's areas of clinical expertise (i.e., scope of clinical competence) and to work within those boundaries

4.   The ability to anticipate ethically risky or problematic situations

5.   The ability to gather additional information and to seek consultation and additional expertise in order to clarify and, ideally, resolve the conflict

6.   The ability to build additional ethical safeguards into the patient care situation

Source.   Reprinted from Roberts LW, Dyer AR: *Concise Guide to Ethics in Mental Health Care.* Washington, DC, American Psychiatric Publishing, 2004, p. 20. Copyright © 2004 American Psychiatric Publishing. Used with permission.

ETHICS SKILLS IN PSYCHIATRIC CARE

A first essential ethical skill is the ability to identify the ethical features of a patient's care. This capacity involves sensitivity and an ability to apply ethical principles such as respect for persons, beneficence, autonomy, nonmaleficence, justice, veracity, and fidelity. It involves an up-front appreciation for how the use of an alternative decision maker is different, for example, in arriving at a hospitalization decision for an elderly person with early Alzheimer's disease, an adult with bipolar disorder, a young adult with Down syndrome, or a child in need of an appendectomy (see Chapter 4, "Informed Consent and Decisional Capacity"). In providing psychiatric care, the clinician needs to discern how the patient's distinct cultural background, religious or spiritual beliefs, and personal history shape the values through which the patient understands the illness process and the decisions he or she may make (see Chapter 3, "The Tradition of the Psychotherapeutic Relationship," and Chapter 10, "People From Culturally Distinct Populations"). When intervening to help a person with an addiction disorder, for instance, the clinician must have a sense of the potential contribution of stigma, shame, symptoms, and compromised autonomy in managing not only the disease but also the psychosocial and ethical repercussions of the disease as experienced by the patient (see Chapter 14, "People Living With Addictions").

A second ethical skill is the ability to see how one's life experiences, attitudes, and knowledge may influence one's care of patients. What a prac-

TABLE 2–2. Models of ethical decision making

Author	Model	Ethical approach
Beauchamp and Childress (2012)	Balancing and specifying principles	Autonomy Beneficence Nonmaleficence Justice
Hundert (1987)	Theoretical framework for conceptualizing moral dilemmas	Lists of conflicting values (e.g., individual freedom vs. community safety)
Jonsen et al. (2015)	Clinical ethics	Clinical indications Patient preferences Quality of life Socioeconomic or external factors
Sadler and Hulgus (1992)	Clinical encounter within the biopsychosocial context	Knowledge Ethics Pragmatism

Source. Adapted from Roberts LW, Dyer AR: *Concise Guide to Ethics in Mental Health Care.* Washington, DC, American Psychiatric Publishing, 2004, p. 23. Copyright © 2004 American Psychiatric Publishing. Used with permission.

titioner assumes to be important regarding quality of life on the basis of his or her experiences as an athlete, for example, may affect his or her recommendations when consulting for the care of a person who has just survived a serious spinal injury. A corollary to this skill is the clinician's insight about what situations "feel" uncomfortable, which can signal potential conflicts and problems in patient care that may be ethical in nature. An example of this type of uncomfortable situation might be an interaction in which a colleague casually requests that the clinician write a prescription for an anxiolytic, wishing not to be seen formally as a patient because of concerns about stigma and being perceived as "weak" by coworkers.

A third ethical skill is the ability to identify one's areas of clinical expertise (i.e., scope of clinical competence) and to work within these boundaries. This is an ethical skill because clinicians working outside their expertise may not serve patients' best interests and may place patients in harm's way. The professional obligation in this situation is not to abandon the patient but instead to ensure that adequate expertise for the patient's care is obtained through consultation or referral. In certain situations, such as in frontier communities (see Chapter 8, "People in Small Communities"), emergencies, or training contexts (see Chapter 20, "Clinical Training"), clinicians may ethically perform care outside their scope of competence but only in response to imperatives to help patients and only with permission from those patients. A related concept is the ethical importance of continuing education so that the clinician's domains of competence remain within community standards and, preferably, the state of the art in broader communities. Another related concept is sensing the congruence between the clinician's role (e.g., psychotherapist vs. prison psychiatrist) and the scope and nature of his or her ethical obligations.

A fourth ethical skill is the ability to anticipate ethically risky or problematic situations. These situations usually pertain to the ethical use of power to ensure the safety of patients or others. Examples include reporting child abuse (see Chapter 7, "Children and Transitional Age Youth"), committing a patient to an inpatient unit involuntarily (see Chapter 5, "Ethical Use of Influence and the Role of Physician in High-Risk Situations"), diagnosing substance abuse in an airline pilot or a bus driver, caring for a public official with mental illness, or treating a patient with HIV who does not wish to inform previous sexual partners (see Chapter 11, "People Living With HIV/AIDS").

A fifth key ethics skill is the ability to gather additional information and seek consultation and additional expertise to clarify and, ideally, resolve the conflict. This skill may involve reading clinical practice and ethics guidelines, talking with a trusted supervisor, seeking advice from a colleague with specialized expertise, requesting an ethics or a legal consultation, and/or reviewing supplemental clinical data.

A final ethics skill is the ability to build additional ethical safeguards into the patient care situation. Appropriate use of alternative decision makers, treatment guardians, and advocates may be helpful in caring for an individual with serious mental illness, for example. Database security firewalls and password-protected computers may be necessary to protect sensitive patient information. Referring patients for confidential treatment off-site also may be necessary in certain circumstances in which dual roles and documentation safeguards may infringe upon optimal patient care (e.g., occupational health offices).

These skills represent the basis for ethical practice in psychiatric care and other clinical fields. They have behavioral components and therefore are observable and potentially measurable. They link directly with the ability to perform certain key activities, such as obtaining informed consent for HIV testing or speaking with a patient truthfully and responsibly about a medical error and its consequences. For these reasons, these skills will be incorporated increasingly into assessments of the professional and ethical competence of clinicians in coming years.

A STRATEGY FOR ETHICAL DECISION MAKING IN CLINICAL SETTINGS

Clinical ethics is the "identification, analysis, and resolution of moral problems that arise in the care of a particular patient" (Jonsen et al. 1998, p. 3). Clinical ethics centers on everyday choices of clinicians, whether dramatic and extraordinary or mild and mundane. Jonsen et al. (1998, 2015) present a strategy for approaching and making these sorts of clinical ethics decisions. As described in Figure 2–1, their model contains four major elements, in order of importance: 1) clinical indications, 2) preferences of patients, 3) quality of life, and 4) external considerations (see also Table 2–2). These elements are described in detail in the subsections that follow.

Other medical decision-making models have been proposed (see Table 2–2), although the development of such strategies for psychiatric decision making has been relatively neglected. Beauchamp and Childress (2012) based their model on specifying and balancing the four main ethical principles of nonmaleficence, beneficence, autonomy, and justice. Hundert (1987) proffered a technique for identifying lists of conflicting values (e.g., individual freedom vs. community safety) and then using those lists to analyze and resolve the conflicts. Sadler and Hulgus (1992) proposed a model

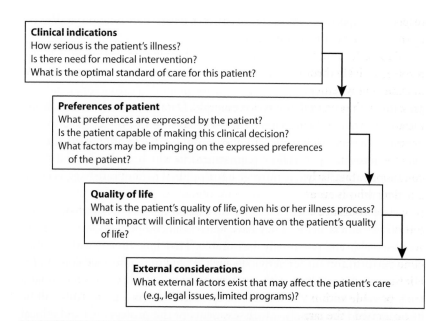

FIGURE 2–1.   A model for clinical ethical decision making.

Source.   Reprinted from Roberts LW, Dyer AR: *Concise Guide to Ethics in Mental Health Care.* Washington, DC, American Psychiatric Publishing, 2004, p. 307. Copyright © 2004 American Psychiatric Publishing. Used with permission.

in which the core aspects of the clinical encounter—encompassing knowledge, ethics, and pragmatism—are approached in a larger biopsychosocial context to recognize and process ethical dilemmas.

Clinical Indications

The first element in the widely applied clinical ethics model that Jonsen et al. (2015) proposed (sometimes called the "four box" model) is clinical indications. This element is grounded in the principle of seeking to help and to use all of the clinician's expertise—informed by the body of scientific and practical knowledge of medicine—to serve the well-being and best interests of a patient and to diminish his or her suffering. Clinicians have an obligation to diagnose a patient's condition, to inform and educate the patient about the illness process, to identify and ordinarily to recommend optimal options for treatment, and either to carry out those procedures themselves or to ensure that a competent colleague carries them out. This first element pertains to the notion of the clinician's accountability in fulfilling his or her responsibility by providing treatment that meets standards of care and is open to scrutiny of colleagues.

Many ethical problems arising in the care of individual patients can be resolved quickly through the application of this first element. For example, in exploring whether an actively suicidal person diagnosed with major depression with psychotic features requires electroconvulsive therapy, the clinician must first examine the severity of the symptoms, the patient's pattern of responsiveness to previous interventions, and the clinical treatment imperatives driven by optimal care standards within the local and national community. Similarly, in debating whether dialysis should be provided for a patient who is an undocumented immigrant or for a patient without appropriate insurance coverage, the first consideration is whether the medical intervention of dialysis is indicated on the basis of clinical knowledge and accepted standards of practice. For this element of ethical decision making, clinical indications for the individual patient have primacy. Seeking to benefit the individual patient is the imperative within the constraints of what is truly possible within the system of care available and the shared standards of care within the larger community.

Patient Preferences

In keeping with the principle of respect for persons, meaningfully incorporating the preferences of patients is the second element in Jonsen et al.'s (2015) decisional process. The importance of this consideration is self-evident, because it helps represent and express the enduring values, voluntarism, and "voice" of the patient. This element is certainly crucial to the therapeutic alliance and treatment adherence. Nevertheless, especially in the domain of mental illness, incorporating patient preferences can be very complicated. Affective, anxiety, psychotic, and personality disorders alike may be characterized by periods of uncertainty, psychological flux, and cognitive distortions, all of which may influence decisional capacity and the authenticity and stability of expressed choices. Similarly, end-of-life care preferences of patients with cancer or HIV may be determined more by the adequacy of treatment for pain and depression than by the seriousness or stage of the underlying disease. Cultural beliefs can add complexity; for example, a Native American man may decline a clinically indicated amputation not because he lacks an understanding or appreciation of the seriousness of the situation but rather because he is concerned that without the amputated tissue he will not be "whole" at the time of his death. In such cases, the clinician should explore the patient's objection and consider culturally sensitive interventions (e.g., inclusion of a native healer who can help find culturally and spiritually acceptable approaches; method for special preservation of the tissue).

Mental health professionals thus must view and interpret patient preferences within a clinical framework. In some cases, this consideration will allow the original therapeutic goal to be reached. In other cases, this approach will help the clinician to see how the patient's wishes may be adversely affected by illness states and to provide appropriate support and treatment. Through such approaches, it is sometimes possible to reach common ground, honoring all imperatives and values in the situation. As discussed in Chapter 13, "Difficult Patients," respecting the autonomy of patients and their wishes while also fulfilling the responsibilities of recognizing and responding to illness in a manner congruent with accepted standards of care can be quite challenging. Exercising beneficence—seeking to serve the well-being and best interests of patients—without acting paternalistically is very subtle work.

Quality of Life

Considering a patient's quality of life is the third element in the Jonsen et al. (2015) model of decision making. This element is considered after the clinical indication and patient preferences have been thoroughly evaluated. Although difficult to define, *quality of life* generally means the subjective sense of satisfaction an individual expresses and/or experiences regarding his or her physical, mental, and social situation. For this element, the clinician needs to use multiple forms of evidence and, to the greatest extent possible, direct information from the patient's perspective.

The problematic nature of this element stems from the fact that the clinician must rely on suppositions about how the ill individual feels and the experiences the individual has undergone. When disproportionately emphasized in decision making, quality of life may lead to inadequate treatment or nonbeneficent actions in clinical care. For example, studies of stroke patients and victims of accidents leading to paralysis suggest that individuals' perceptions of quality of life are determined not by physical deficits but other issues, such as level of pain or degree of disability in some, but not all, activities. Healthy individuals without such physical deficits may assess erroneously the patient's true quality of life, as perceived by the patient.

External Considerations

The fourth and final element in the Jonsen et al. (2015) model involves consideration of socioeconomic or external factors. These diverse factors include the interests of society, the role of family members, costs and limitations in access to care, and situational features (e.g., research or teaching settings). These features may not come into play in an ethically important decision because the three previous elements—considering clinical indications, patient preferences, and quality of life—may have already resolved the question at hand.

Socioeconomic or external factors may conflict with one another and with factors considered in the three previous elements. For example, the decision to hospitalize a patient may present a conflict between the imperative for acute medical intervention, the need to ensure safety for the patient and others, and the desire of a family to have respite and support, on the one hand, and by the patient's expressed desire not to be hospitalized, by lack of insurance, and by the limited number of inpatient beds in the region, on the other hand.

CONCLUSION

Conscientious psychiatrists who cultivate their ethics skills and employ a deliberate decision-making strategy—as well as carefully document their thoughts and actions—will do well by their patients and learn in the process. The disciplined effort to ensure opportunities for systematic reflection, especially in a fast-paced clinical setting in which many seriously ill patients receive care, is essential to prevent mistakes and enhance the likelihood of better outcomes in patient care. With use and adaptation, Jonsen et al.'s (2015) decision-making approach may become one of the clinical psychiatrist's most helpful and trustworthy tools.

CASE SCENARIOS

- A 23-year-old man with psychotic symptoms is arrested for shoplifting. The patient's family asks the clinical psychiatrist to explain his illness to the court and describe how his impulsivity is often driven by psychotic symptoms.

- A 32-year-old surgeon informs a consulting psychiatrist that he has chosen not to work up an abdominal mass found in a treatment-refractory patient with chronic schizophrenia because there are "no guarantees" that the mass can be resected or treated and the patient has a "terrible life.... If it is cancer, it will be a blessing."

- A 79-year-old man with early dementia refuses a preventive colonoscopy because he does not believe he could handle the surgery and adjunctive treatment. The resident treating the patient insists that the patient "must not" possess decisional capacity and suggests that an alternative decision maker be appointed to approve the procedure; however, the attending physician and the nurse caring for the patient believe that the patient's decision-making ability on this issue is intact.

- A 50-year-old patient with a history of alcohol dependence and bipolar II disorder is in psychotherapy. He has a history of repeated, near-lethal suicide attempts when severely depressed and intoxicated and refuses to admit himself voluntarily when his therapist calls him. The case manager states that she will check on him the next day. The psychotherapist arranges for an evaluation at the local psychiatric emergency room and completes the necessary paperwork to have the police transport the patient from his apartment.

- A 65-year-old woman with recurrent depression has tried many different antidepressants, with only partial response and numerous troubling side effects. After speaking with her psychiatrist, she decides to try electroconvulsive therapy. Her children become very upset and call the psychiatrist, telling him that their mother's decision must be a sign that she wants to die.

3

The Tradition of the Psychotherapeutic Relationship

Laura Weiss Roberts, M.D., M.A.

Allen R. Dyer, M.D., Ph.D.

Immanuel Kant once observed, "We are not gentleman volunteers; we are conscripts in the army of moral law" (Murdoch 1992, p. 35). Many individuals act primarily, perhaps exclusively, in self-interest, but Kant's observation that there is a moral imperative—what he called a "categorical imperative"—is compelling. Moral demands are placed on people by virtue of living in a social order.

Physicians and health professionals in particular live in a moral order, with incumbent obligations from the needs of those who seek their help. Some health professionals are motivated solely by self-interest rather than the service of others, but most health professionals properly fulfill the demands and specific moral obligations that their relationship with patients imposes on them. The clinician's promise and expertise to heal shape this relationship. The obligations that emerge from the imbalance that naturally exists between a person in need and a person who seeks to provide treatment, answers, and comfort in relation to that need have traditionally

25

defined this relationship as well. Whether the clinician understands these obligations as allegiance to conscience, allegiance to society, or a more direct allegiance to the patient, the obligations are present.

PROFESSIONALISM IN THE PSYCHOTHERAPEUTIC RELATIONSHIP

The tradition of the relationship between physician and patient is sometimes spoken of as a sacred trust. That bond deserves reflection and careful understanding. Law understands fiduciary relationships (i.e., relationships of trust) differently from medicine and other clinical fields. In law a fiduciary, or trustee, may act on behalf of a client. In the health professions, the trust derives from the clinician–patient relationship and must be earned repeatedly. The clinician acts with the patient in a true partnership characterized by genuineness, empathy, and positive regard.

When bioethics first began to emerge as a discipline distinct from medical ethics, the question was often posed, "Is there anything distinct about medical ethics, or is it just everyday ethics applied to medical situations?" (Clouser 1974). The more mature discipline of biomedical ethics recognizes multiple perspectives (e.g., those of the physician/professional, the patient/client, society) on what occurs in this very special and personal encounter. These diverse perspectives offer valuable insights into the relationship.

Since the early 1980s, many professionals have referred to this relationship with a client as representing a more explicit, business-oriented contract with a more or less coequal, autonomous person. Such a relationship implies more responsibility for the client, consistent with more contemporary notions of autonomy, but no less responsibility for the professional. Whereas physicians once understood their obligations almost exclusively in terms of beneficence, and still do, it would never be permissible to act with disregard for the patient's wishes and needs, although patient's wishes and needs may at times be in tension.

DECISION MAKING: A SHARED PROCESS

Since the 400s B.C., the Hippocratic writings (e.g., Oath, Corpus, Aphorisms) have placed special obligations on physicians that were not incumbent on members of society in general. For example, the proscription against sex with patients ("mischief") uniquely applied to physicians in ancient Greek society. As an itinerant healer, the physician might spend extended periods in a particular household. It would not be unusual in that society for the master of the house to provide sexual companions to a guest. Physicians who followed the Hippocratic Oath set themselves apart from this practice, no doubt with a sense that their function in the household was not as a recipient of hospitality and with recognition that indulging in their comforts would compromise their effectiveness.

Much of the understanding and misunderstanding about the therapeutic relationship has focused on an awareness of the intimacy that develops between therapist and patient. As in other areas of medicine, there is an accommodation between the physician and patient.

> The accommodation process depends on all of the particularities of the medical encounter. The nature of the patient involved—his personality, character, attitude, and values—and the factors which led him to seek a medical encounter with this particular physician are central components of the process. Similarly, the personality, character, attitude, values, and technical skills of the physician affect the accommodation. Further, the quality of the interaction between patient and physician—the chemistry of the interaction—modify the process. Of course, the nature of the medical problem, including its type, acuteness, gravity, and its potential for remediation, will be a major determinant of whether a physician–patient accommodation is achieved. (Siegler 1981, p. 62)

In the special situation of the therapist and patient, sometimes an intimacy may develop that reflects a sexual or sexualized tension between therapist and patient. Even though sex does not occur, there may be sexualized feelings and fantasies. Distinctions and subtleties are important. The clinician comes into contact with people at a time of vulnerability imposed by illness. For the clinician to understand the patient's illness, the patient must subject himself or herself to a degree of scrutiny not encountered elsewhere in life. The patient must be examined physically and psychologically—exposed, unclothed, naked, vulnerable. A person seeking care must disclose the most personal information imaginable—indeed, information that someone might not readily imagine as possible to discuss with another. Ancient traditions (Hippocrates as the most ready example) recognized the imperative that such information be kept confidential, private, and secret within the relationship ("not noised abroad"). Professionals have stood by this principle vigorously for millennia, holding that therapeutic work could not take place without the guarantee of that privacy. Certain situations are recognized in which it may be permissible or even mandatory to alter the expectation of complete privacy, such as when child abuse is suspected or the risk of violence is present. Even when such disclosures may be mandated by the state (i.e., government, court, or law), they are never made without re-gard for confidentiality—the confidence and trust of the patient.

Confidentiality, understood as trust, is gradually being eroded in modern health care. Medical information should be shared between practitioners only with the explicit consent of the patient. Insurance companies, how-ever, freely share pooled information about every claim, provider encoun-ter, diagnosis, and treatment, and signing up for electronic medical records is a prerequisite for care. Although consent is tacitly recognized in both cases, the patient has no choice. The patient cannot use insurance without giving consent for review of records and cannot receive care without inclu-sion in the electronic medical record. Perhaps most disturbing are guide-lines that eliminate formal requirements for patients to consent specifically and prospectively to the use of their medical information for many and di-verse purposes, far beyond the scope of the patient's direct care. Indeed, un-der the Health Insurance Portability and Accountability Act (HIPAA) of 1996, personal medical information no longer belongs to the patient. The ethical tradition of respect for confidentiality, the Hippocratic tradition, is more fundamental than governmental regulations of information privacy.

Psychotherapists, among all clinicians, are the first to sound the alarm, affirming the importance of confidentiality protections. True therapy can-not occur without the traditional assurance of privacy. A patient could not feel free to talk to a therapist (and certainly not about personal matters) if he or she knew or suspected that such information might be shared with others. Employers could misuse it, or it might be used at some future time to prevent employment or to discriminate against the patient—for exam-ple, in obtaining health insurance. Ethics in such considerations is not merely a matter of personal conscience for the provider; it is also a matter of social policy, law, and respect for and protection of individual rights.

The solely commercial understanding of the patient as a "consumer" undermines the understanding, professional relationship as an ethical com-mitment to the suffering person. Healing calls upon a more universal good. It invokes the sacred. It invokes the ability to appeal to another in a com-munity with the trust that such an appeal will bring needed help. The healer understands that appeal not just as a participant in a commercial transaction but also as a member of a caring community.

THE NATURE OF THE PSYCHOTHERAPEUTIC ENCOUNTER

In this modern, perhaps fundamentally transactional or commercial era, the therapeutic encounter is often thought of as an exchange of a commodity—a pill or a procedure. More basically, the therapeutic encounter encompasses all that transpires between doctor and patient (professional and client), including especially talking (e.g., the patient telling his or her story and medical history), listening, examining (often physically), evaluating, counseling, planning treatment, following up, reconsidering, recommending, and following up again. Many ancient and contemporary traditions view the medical practitioner as a shamanistic healer—someone who has magical powers to harmonize the spirits—the person to whom a sick person looks for help and who can be trusted because of the powers he or she possesses. These expectations are no different today, when the powers are understood to be medical technologies and complex information, much of which is arcane, most of which is believed and hoped to be useful.

The relationship between the "sick person" and the "healer" has received the most scrutiny in the psychoanalytic tradition—that is, in psychoanalysis and derivative psychotherapies. The therapeutic relationship is perhaps best understood in this more tightly defined encounter, which is essentially little different from the encounter with the stereotypical brusque surgeon or the mysterious shaman—except for the scrutiny given to the relationship itself.

Sigmund Freud's particular genius recognized that when two people spend time together, they develop feelings that derive from other significant relationships in their past experience. Significantly, the patient develops feelings for the physician that repeat feelings held for parents. Freud called this phenomenon *transference* and recognized that it could be a vehicle for understanding past experience. It is beyond the scope of this book to assess the place of Freudian theory in psychotherapy, but an appreciation of the concept of transference is essential for understanding the ethics of the therapeutic relationship.

Psychotherapists structure a frame within which the reflective process can occur. They agree to meet at a certain time, at a certain place, for a certain duration, at a certain frequency, for a certain purpose. These are the boundaries of the frame and the therapeutic relationship. Developing a therapeutic alliance is part of the therapy in which the patient connects with the clinician to get better. More specifically, the part of the patient that wants to get better allies with the therapist to understand the part of the patient that wants to repeat maladaptive behavior patterns. Maladaptive repetition is called *resistance*. In the early years of psychoanalysis, resistance was seen as an obstacle that needed to be overcome before analysis could be successful. Today, resistance is appreciated more sympathetically as part of a defense structure that must be accepted and understood. Disregarding boundaries compromises the therapist's opportunity to create a situation in which safe and supportive reflection can occur. The therapist walks a delicate tightrope, demonstrating concern and empathy yet insisting on scrutinizing what takes place between clinician and patient as a possible transference clue that needs to be understood.

CLINICAL CASES ILLUSTRATING PROFESSIONAL BOUNDARY TRANSGRESSIONS

The case examples that follow illustrate everyday dilemmas in matters of technique, judgment, and ethics.

Case Example 1

A woman approached therapy eagerly and with energy. She was polite, easygoing, and friendly. She was interested in the therapist, curious about his personal life, and in a social way asked ordinary but persistent questions, such as "Did you have a nice vacation? Where did you go?" The therapist recognized these questions as a departure from the therapeutic stance but believed that it would be too much work to keep inquiring about the curiosity behind the questions, when they seemed innocent enough.

This ordinary situation is one that every therapist encounters. How is the frame established? Should the therapeutic frame be set when the patient is met in the waiting room, when the door to the consulting room is closed, or when the patient settles down and begins to work? How should chance encounters be handled? What if patient and therapist are thrown together in some community activity, as is especially likely to happen in small communities? The Exploitation Index (Epstein and Simon 1990; Epstein et al. 1992) is an educational tool that asks therapists to self-rate their feelings, thoughts, and behaviors in situations they may encounter. Epstein and Simon developed the tool for examining therapeutic boundary issues, and it provides an opportunity to consider some of the situations in which boundary crossings or frank transgressions may be unrecognized.

Most therapists encounter such situations, which can be awkward and require discipline to remind the patient that therapy is different from a social relationship and to hold the therapeutic frame.

Case Example 2

A young woman consulted a psychiatrist for help with anxiety and disappointment in relationships with men. She was open, energetic, talkative, and highly successful in her profession. The psychiatrist considered himself a medical psychopharmacologist and prescribed an appropriate medication for her. He was skeptical of psychotherapeutic approaches to dealing with problems he knew could respond quickly to medication. He saw nothing wrong with an extraprofessional relationship that did not involve dating or physical intimacy, so he accepted the patient's invitations to her pool parties. Although he considered that he was just being sociable, the patient believed that more was involved and expected in their relationship.

Although this clinician had not crossed the boundary into a sexual relationship, he failed to appreciate the boundary that he should have recognized between a professional relationship and a social relationship.

Case Example 3

A young man sought therapy because of disappointments in his life. He believed that his therapist understood and cared for him, and he looked forward to their sessions. When he became particularly distressed, the therapist would schedule him as the last appointment of the day and sometimes extend the sessions. The therapist believed that supportive therapy was indicated and that the patient needed support to face the difficulties in his life. When the therapist later began to limit the time in the sessions, the patient became hurt and angry and decided to end the treatment because he believed that it was no longer working.

The preceding three cases share ordinariness; they are common situations in therapy that offer dilemmas and question values. They are matters involving technique and judgment. No deliberate harm was done, although opportunities for good might have been missed. Often, therapists will say that they do not deal with the transference, that it is an issue for psychoanalysis. As these mundane examples illustrate, however, feelings of transference can arise in all kinds of therapy. These cases illustrate professional boundary transgressions.

Clear boundary violations, such as sex with a patient or failure to maintain confidentiality, are obviously unethical and can be devastating for the patient because of the personal violation of trust. The proscription against sex with a patient is clear and unambiguous in the codes of ethics of all professions. The American Psychiatric Association's (2013b) *The Principles of Medical Ethics With Annotations Especially Applicable to Psychiatry* explicitly states that sexual activity with a patient is unethical.

Case Example 4

The dean of students threatened a medical student with expulsion from medical school when he learned that the student had engaged in sexual relations with a patient on the service where he had rotated the year before. The student stated in his defense that the sex was "consensual" and he had not realized there was anything wrong with it: "It didn't happen on the psychiatry rotation or anything like that."

Sexual relations with patients receive the closest scrutiny in psychiatry and in psychotherapeutic relations, but the same transferential concerns of trust, dependency, and idealization occur in other professional relationships as well.

What about sex with a former patient? Is that ever permissible? Are the expectations different for a relationship with a patient who is seen once on a consultative basis versus a patient who is involved in a psychotherapeutic relationship? Might it be possible after a specified period of time—perhaps 1 or 2 years—to engage in a personal, intimate, sexual relationship with a person who was formerly a patient? If so, how would the amount of time be determined? The American Psychiatric Association has taken an increasingly firm stance on this issue. The 1973 version of *The Principles of Medical Ethics* read, "Sex with a current patient is unethical. Sex with a former patient is almost always unethical." That annotation was revised in 1993, and in all iterations published since then, including the most recent 2013 edition, the statement is absolutely unequivocal: "Sexual activity with a current or former patient is unethical" (American Psychiatric Association 2013b, p. 4). This prohibition is based on awareness of the feelings that may develop in therapy and the need to understand them as developmental experiences relived in the present. The prohibition against sex with patients (and, of course, former patients, because transference endures in time) is crucial for psychotherapists. But the issues of trust and dependency are no less relevant for other professionals.

BOUNDARY VIOLATIONS

Boundary violations may be understood as breaches of trust primarily in the frame of the psychotherapeutic relationship. This description is the easiest way to grasp the concept of boundaries, but in fact boundaries are more complicated in everyday life. Boundaries in the modern world of social media and innovation are even more uncertain (see Chapter 19, "Innovation in Psychiatry"). The boundary that the therapist must respect is the boundary between self and other, between therapist and patient. That boundary is complicated because, like other relationships, it has a transference component.

The extent to which a patient may wish to please (or to rebel against) the therapist may be a repetition of feelings developed at an earlier point in his or her life in relation to significant others. For example, parents who use their children to gratify their wishes may leave those children vulnerable to exploitation by others. Such children are said to be narcissistic extensions of their parents. In the extreme form, the boundary between parent and child is not established, and the exploitation may be perverse. A child who becomes a successful student or athlete may work for the pride of his or her parent rather than personal accomplishment; a teacher or coach with the best of intentions might inadvertently exploit that pride. The effective and ethical therapist establishes and maintains a boundary that—despite often appearing artificial at first—eventually provides the emotional distance for the child to develop an autonomous sense of self. This sense of self expands the philosophical concept of autonomy that is important to bioethics.

With an appreciation of the transference dynamics of the boundary between therapist and patient (i.e., self and other) and the practical ethical consequences of this boundary's violation, it is possible to reexamine the question of a relationship with a former patient. From the standpoint of an enduring commitment, marriage might be the possible exception to the "never" rule. With the recognition of transference feelings, however, therapists must be aware that the partner may later claim that the feelings once understood as love were in actuality a transference that was exploited in therapy. It would be very difficult indeed to defend oneself against such a claim.

Sexual boundaries and boundary violations receive the most attention because they are the most devastating, but if the violations are understood to represent a transgression of self and other, other aspects of the relationship also can be transgressed—for example, business, financial, religious, political, and social.

BOUNDARY CROSSINGS

Sometimes therapists will experience internal discomfort at allowing themselves or their patients to cross a certain boundary. The transgressions may be minor self-disclosures (e.g., talking about a vacation or an aspect of personal life), extratherapeutic social encounters, or just a sense of not holding the therapeutic frame. Although unlikely to result in formal ethics complaints, such boundary crossings may undermine clinicians' ability to do effective therapy. Recognition of a boundary transgression should prompt therapists to seek consultation or supervision or reflect on their motives in personal therapy. If the therapist is a trainee, the supervisor's task is to create an environment in which such self-awareness can occur and to help the trainee reach an appropriate resolution. Sometimes boundary crossings can illuminate the transference-countertransference dynamic and thereby further therapeutic understanding.

Telepsychiatry, social media, and electronic medical records greatly expand ways people communicate beyond the private consulting room as well as the traditional understanding of "boundaries"—across countries and continents and even time. Patients or clients may have much easier access to information about their doctor from Internet searches. Issues of privacy, disclosure, and even security should be given careful attention in light of possible effects on patients and the treatment parameters.

DIVIDED LOYALTIES

Situations occur in therapy when the therapist experiences divided loyalties—allegiance to the patient and to some other interest. A physician or therapist is a dual agent, for example, if he or she owes an allegiance to an employer and to a patient. A classic example is the psychiatrist or psychologist working for the military or another governmental institution. Increasing numbers of physicians and other providers work for large organizations, such as health maintenance organizations or managed care companies, rather than independent practices. Subtler issues involving overlapping and divided loyalty arise for small-community clinicians, who must serve not only their patients but also their patients' families, who are neighbors and friends (see Chapter 8, "People in Small Communities"). More globally, clinicians increasingly recognize an allegiance to society, which makes it increasingly difficult to buffer concern for each patient.

Extreme cases put mundane cases into perspective. Psychiatrists in the former Soviet Union, Eastern European countries, and the People's Republic of China have come under scrutiny for hospitalizing political dissidents and labeling them mentally ill or psychiatrically impaired. Physicians in Latin American military governments and several African nations have cooperated with torture of political prisoners (perhaps under coercion). Nazi physicians conducted experiments in concentration camps, a situation that would previously have been unimaginable and that has given rise to many safeguards in human research, notably the emphasis on autonomy and the requirement of informed consent.

From a moral perspective, most dual-agent situations are best seen as cases of conflicting loyalty or clashing duties. The clinician must choose one duty over another. Perhaps most problematic are situations in which the patient assumes (because of the weight of the patient-centered ethic) that the clinician is working exclusively for the patient's best interests and well-being. Therefore, simply by projecting a trustworthy demeanor, a psychiatrist conducting a prearraignment examination might elicit more information than a police interrogator. If the message is not "I am here to help you," however, the purpose of the examination must be directly stated. A therapist conducting an administrative evaluation in a student health service should specify, "You are being evaluated at the request of the dean, who will receive a report of my findings." A mental health professional should not convey the impression that everything discussed will be confidential if that is not the case. In clinical research, the issue of dual agency (i.e., the therapeutic misconception) is a key ethical consideration (see Chapter 18, "Psychiatric Research").

Mental health professionals have a continuing obligation to review and examine dual-agent issues because such scrutiny is the only way to prevent these issues from disrupting the clinician–patient relationship. These issues often come before professional ethics committees and serve as reminders of the ethical principles kept alive through education, codes, and professional discipline (see Chapter 15, "Integrity and the Professional Roles of Psychiatrists").

CONCLUSION

The therapeutic relationship is fundamental to healing and to ethically sound clinical care. This relationship seeks to advance the well-being of the patient. Role conflicts or divided loyalties may threaten this foundation. When a conflict of interest arises, the health care professional should make his or her allegiance to the patient primary and fully inform the patient of the conflict. The goal of maintaining trust is essential to the therapeutic relationship, and anything that erodes that goal diminishes not only the therapy but also the therapist and the profession he or she represents.

CASE SCENARIOS

■ An intern completing a rotation in a rape crisis clinic notices a colleague from her training program in the waiting room; the colleague is there for a crisis evaluation and treatment after an assault.

■ A psychotherapist attending a small dinner party discovers that another dinner guest is a patient of his.

■ A psychiatrist routinely encounters one of his patients at a coffee shop near his office. The patient appears to be waiting for him there and often tries to engage in intensely personal conversations.

■ A young, married psychiatry resident begins treating a patient who has many sexual partners. He finds himself becoming very curious about the new sexual liaisons of the patient and very much looks forward to each session.

■ A consultation-liaison psychiatrist with duties at a community hospital receives a psychiatric referral for a patient who was recently diagnosed with testicular cancer. She has known the patient for several years, and they went on a casual date 4 years ago.

4

Informed Consent and Decisional Capacity

Laura Weiss Roberts, M.D., M.A.

Informed consent is a philosophical and legal doctrine that serves as the cornerstone of ethically sound clinical care. Informed consent requires that a patient truly understand and freely decide to undertake—or not—a proposed treatment approach in light of his or her health care goals. Informed consent emphasizes respect for the individual, and it is inherently relational—that is, it occurs in the context of a professional relationship. This chapter describes the core elements of informed consent in clinical care (Table 4–1) and surveys differing standards for consent, advance directives and surrogate decision making, and empirical studies related to consent; and in conclusion, discusses constructive approaches to the process of informed consent.

ELEMENTS OF INFORMED CONSENT

Consent occurs in a context, both institutional and interpersonal. Consent is obtained in jail psychiatric units, community clinics, and hospital wards by physicians, nurses, social workers, and other health professionals. In all these circumstances and relationships, fulfilling the concept of informed

TABLE 4–1.   Necessary elements of informed consent

1. **Information sharing**

    Dialogue/process

    Rationale

    Alternatives

    Risks/benefits and likelihood

    Future choices

2. **Decisional capacity**

    Communication

    Reasoning

    Understanding

    Appreciation

3. **Voluntarism**

    Developmental factors

    Illness-related issues

    Psychological history/cultural values

    Contextual factors

Source.   Copyright © 2015 Laura Weiss Roberts, M.D., M.A. Used with permission.

consent in clinical care means that concern for promoting the health and alleviating the suffering of the individual patient will be the absolute basis of any recommended treatment. In clinical consent, dedication to the patient's well-being is primary, regardless of whether the relationship involves a brief encounter to refill a patient's medications in a busy walk-in clinic, a problem-focused consultation by a specialist on a hospital ward, or intensive therapy sessions over many years.

The clinician's focus on the health, well-being, and best interests of the patient is embodied in the therapeutic relationship. It emphasizes the patient's personal values and overall goals for care. Informed consent should occur in a context characterized by compassion, trust, and honesty. In research settings, these qualities continue to characterize the relationship, but there is a balance between the needs of the patient and the scientific endeavor (see Chapter 18, "Psychiatric Research").

Information Sharing

Sharing appropriate information is the second core element of informed consent. Clinicians should provide patients with accurate and balanced information regarding the anticipated risks and benefits of a given treatment, as well as alternatives and expected outcomes. Alternatives may include implementing another treatment or additional treatment or providing no intervention in the course of illness.

To obtain informed consent for treatment of mild depression, for example, the psychiatrist needs to discuss the variable course of depressive illnesses, including the potential for symptom resolution in the absence of treatment. In this discussion, the clinician should review the rationale for a proposed intervention, such as an antidepressant agent or a specific form of psychotherapy, given the specific patient's symptoms (e.g., obsessionality, psychotic features, insomnia, agitation) and the patient's attitudes and values (e.g., fears about being "dependent" on a medication, concerns related to sexual functioning or weight gain, individual preferences for psychosocial treatments, culturally influenced interpretations of personal symptoms). In regard to psychopharmacological treatment, the discussion should cover the medication's possible side effects, potential adverse effects, and the relative likelihood of these effects. Alternative approaches to treatment should also be reviewed in light of their merit for a patient. Topics that may arise in this discussion include insight-oriented, interpersonal, and supportive therapies; electroconvulsive therapy (ECT); light therapy; "natural" approaches (e.g., herbal remedies, St. John's wort, vitamins); placebo effects; and no treatment.

Determining how much detail to offer about a specific treatment approach and its alternatives can sometimes be difficult. It is good to start with a "reasonable person" standard—that is, explaining what a reasonable person would need to know to make this decision. For instance, in obtaining consent to initiate a psychotropic medication, such as carbamazepine, it is important to explain the utility of serum levels and the potential effects of the medication on the patient's liver and bone marrow. Decreased white blood cell counts and increased vulnerability to infection are not so rare that they should be omitted, and the predictable hepatic metabolism changes should be explained so that the patient can anticipate and understand necessary adjustments in other medications. Such information may need to be offered in increments, and additional information about the specific treatment rationale may be appropriate for some patients. In some cases, less information may be necessary, but in no case should the aim in omitting data be to deceive or mislead the patient so that he or she will accept the offered treatment.

Decisional Capacity

Decisional capacity, the third element of informed consent, represents a sophisticated clinical assessment of an individual's global and specific cognitive abilities within a particular context. Such an assessment can be a very subtle and complex exercise. Decisional capacity must be understood according to the type of decision to be made; the enduring, emerging, and fluctuating attributes of the individual; the nature and severity of the person's symptoms; the precise nature of the patient's situation; the individual's prior experiences, personal values, psychological defenses, and coping style; and other factors.

The presence of a serious symptom (e.g., delusions, memory loss, suicidal ideation, diminished cognitive functioning) or a serious diagnosis (e.g., schizophrenia, dementia, major depression, developmental disability) does not mean that an individual, by definition, lacks decisional capacity. Similarly, being a young child or a very elderly person does not preclude someone from being decisionally capable (see Chapter 7, "Children and Transitional Age Youth"). Decisional capacity is a clinical assessment. It is distinct from competence, which is a legal determination—that is, a formal assessment by a judge or other officer of the court regarding a person's ability to function within a particular domain of life (e.g., financial or treatment decisions).

Decisional capacity has four principal components (Appelbaum and Grisso 1988), each of which should be viewed on a continuum, not as an "all-or-none" phenomenon.

1. The individual's ability to **express a preference** (i.e., *capacity for expression of choice or for communication*). On the extreme end of the continuum, for instance, are patients with severe psychiatric illness who are mute or catatonic or manifest complete language and thought disorganization (e.g., word salad) and therefore are incapable of communication. In the medical context, a patient who is comatose due to metabolic disturbances, aphasic secondary to a stroke, or unconscious after a head injury will also lack this first, most fundamental ability. Individuals who have periods of altered consciousness in delirium may be intermittently incapable of communication. Patients with depression who are so severely ill that they do not speak or care for themselves often may be deemed decisionally incapable simply because they do not make their preferences clear, either through language or action. At times this component of decisional capacity is very difficult to assess, such as in a patient with spinal cord injury who can communicate only through eye blinks or a stroke patient with Broca's aphasia who is overwhelmed and frustrated

by the process of generating words. For these reasons, although the ability to express a preference is often obvious, in many situations this assessment will require careful interactions with patients and astute observational and listening skills on the part of the clinician.

2. The individual's ability to **think through the choice at hand in a way that is rational and deliberate** (i.e., *capacity for reasoning or rational thinking*). This component of decisional capacity relates to the person's analytical abilities when given a specific set of facts or data. For instance, with all other factors being equal, the rational person will consistently choose a medication that has a 75% likelihood of treating the illness effectively over one that has a 50% likelihood of treatment efficacy. Similarly, the rational person will consistently choose the medication that poses the fewest risks and promises the fewest adverse side effects. In essence, this dimension of decisional capacity is the ability to use information in an objective manner. This aspect of decisional capacity does not mean, however, that the individual must actually and in fact choose the "rational thing" when making a treatment decision; rather, it relates to the person's ability to see the reasons for and against a given option in the larger setting of his or her life.

3. The individual's ability to **understand relevant information** (i.e., *capacity for comprehension*). In talking with the clinician, the patient with this ability will be able to take in factual information regarding the nature of the illness, the need for intervention, the kinds of treatments under consideration, their relative risks and benefits, and the possible consequences of not intervening with treatment. Depending on the patient's illness, comorbid conditions, potential therapeutic options, and educational level, this information may be relatively straightforward or highly complicated. For the clinician to assess this element of decisional capacity, it is critical that the patient state his or her understanding of the situation and the choices at hand in his or her words. Otherwise, it is difficult to know whether the patient is using the clinician's terms and phrases without truly understanding their meaning and implications.

4. Often most important, the person's ability to **make meaning of the decision and its consequences** within the context of his or her history, values, emotions, and life situation (i.e., *capacity for appreciation*). Deeply dependent on psychological insight, this component is the most sophisticated element of decisional capacity and can be very difficult to assess clinically. For instance, some individuals with early dementia have relatively intact social and cognitive skills, yet are unable to think through the meaning of an important treatment decision and its repercussions. Similarly, for certain patients with mental disorders, the negative cog-

nitive distortions caused by the illness may interfere with their ability to interpret information within a personal context. Ganzini et al. (1994) found that the end-of-life care preferences of inpatients with severe depression may be shaped by their negative expectations of the future, guilt, self-blame, and dysphoria, all of which are attributable to their mental illness, not to their authentic and stable beliefs and values. After treatment, these same individuals made significantly more positive care choices when they envisioned the future (e.g., desire for life-preserving interventions, predictions of likely outcomes of these interventions).

Consider two contrasting examples related to the decision to amputate an infected foot.

Case Example 1

A patient with insulin-dependent diabetes mellitus, a seriously infected lesion on the sole of his foot, and multi-infarct dementia was seen on the consultation-liaison psychiatry service because of concerns for his ability to make a decision about possible amputation. He could state the reasons for the recommended procedure, and he appeared to agree with the amputation. With careful inquiry, however, the clinician determined that the patient did not really understand that amputation meant he would lose his foot permanently, require a prosthesis in his shoe, and receive physical therapy. The patient also did not understand that the surgery might not successfully contain the infection and that he might need another surgery to preserve the functioning of his leg. Furthermore, he did not understand that he could die if the infection progressed and were not treated aggressively. The issue was not simply insufficient communication, inadequate information, or poor understanding of factual information; different individuals on various occasions had explained all these things to him and discussed multiple scenarios for treatment outcomes with him. He had listened attentively, and he could repeat the information and apparently state the rational implications of this information to his clinicians. Nevertheless, he could not apply the meaning of the surgery to his life situation, present or future.

Case Example 2

The consultation-liaison service evaluated a Navajo man with diabetes and an infected foot who refused amputation. The treatment team believed that he was being irrational because of the possibility of becoming septic and facing a life-threatening health situation. The patient was able to communicate and understand the need for the procedure and the full ramifications of declining it and still elected to continue with antibiotic therapies, which previously had met with little success. In this case, the patient was a very traditional Navajo man, and he was able to clearly state his thoughts that the amputation was too dangerous spiritually and psychologically in the absence of a native healer. His desire was to delay the procedure, not refuse it altogether, because he appreciated what the true effect of the decision would be for him if the amputation were performed in a manner incongruent with his culture.

Ganzini et al. (2004) described "myths" about decisional capacity. For example, decisional capacity and competency are not the same; decisional capacity is a clinical assessment, whereas competency is a formal legal determination. Decisional capacity may evolve and is not a fixed attribute. Very importantly, the presence of a psychiatric disorder does not mean the absence of decisional ability. Moreover, perhaps counterintuitively, being involuntarily committed does not mean that an individual, by definition, lacks decision-making ability. Finally, lack of decision-making capacity cannot be presumed simply because cognitive impairments exist or patients decline recommendations of their doctors.

In sum, appreciation is the dimension of decisional capacity that integrates personal values with expressive, factual, and rational data and processes within the context of the patient's life. Clarifying the strengths and potential threats to decisional capacity may require persistent and sensitive evaluations.

Voluntarism

Beyond the therapeutic relationship, information sharing, and decisional capacity, the final element of informed consent is the capacity for voluntarism, which encompasses the individual's ability to act in accord with his or her authentic sense of what is good, right, and best in light of his or her situation, values, and history. Voluntarism further entails the capacity to make this choice freely and in the absence of coercion. Deliberateness, purposefulness of intent, clarity, genuineness, and coherence with previous life decisions are important to voluntarism.

Voluntarism thus manifests the autonomous, authentic preferences of the individual. Social and cultural expectations and psychological history may deeply influence autonomous wishes. For instance, a patient with military experience may be oriented to hierarchical power relationships and view a clinician's recommendation as an order to obey. Similarly, a patient who has been a victim of violence may see herself as relatively powerless, and a patient who has been institutionalized involuntarily in the past may see himself as no longer possessing the right to his views. In sum, voluntary preferences may be tempered by the realities of the situation (e.g., the presence of a serious diagnosis, the lack of "curative" treatments for many mental illnesses) but should reflect the person's genuine wishes in the absence of external coercion (e.g., pressure by an employer not to seek mental health care).

Voluntarism is influenced in four areas: 1) developmental factors, 2) illness-related considerations, 3) psychological issues and cultural and religious values, and 4) contextual factors.

1. A person's development in cognitive abilities, emotional maturity, and moral character will affect capacity for voluntarism. As a simple illustration, a child is less capable of deliberate, voluntary choice than is an adolescent or an adult.
2. Illness-related considerations influence the capacity for voluntarism, such as diminished concentration, poor energy, and indecisiveness—as seen, for example, in some people with major depression—or apathy, cognitive deficits, alexithymia, and ambivalence—as seen, for example, in some people with schizophrenia. These illness manifestations may vary, with more symptoms at some times and fewer at others. Illness-related considerations can prevent individuals from collecting their thoughts, feelings, and personal values to make a coherent and enduring choice.
3. Psychological factors and cultural and religious values influence voluntarism. These issues and values may contribute in a manner that enhances the person's sense of individual autonomy and empowerment. Alternatively, these influences may diminish voluntarism or simply render as less relevant various factors associated with voluntarism. Even seeing one's ideal self as a separate, autonomous individual—as an agent able to decide and act—is a perspective that some have characterized as distinctly Western, culture-bound, and masculine in its approach to decision making.
4. Contextual factors potently influence voluntarism. An individual who is physically dependent on others or who has limited activities due to living in an institutional setting is less able to exercise voluntary choices. For example, a nursing home resident may be so dependent on her clinicians that she may feel she has little voice in a new treatment decision. Similarly, a patient who is admitted involuntarily to a psychiatric unit can, by law, refuse medication and other treatments but may feel coerced by his context to accept these interventions.

DIFFERING STANDARDS FOR CONSENT

Sometimes the most critical task for a clinician is to assess what kind of decision a person is truly capable of making: Can the ill individual make part of the decision, select someone to make the decision, or identify someone to describe his or her values to help influence the ultimate decision? For instance, although a woman with mild to moderate dementia may be incapable of making a choice about use of a new medication or a sophisticated imaging study, she may be capable of deciding which person knows her best and can represent her views in making such a choice. Although patients may not be capable of making decisions about clinical treatment, they may well be capable of deciding who loves them and can be trusted to make that decision. It also may be possible to break down clinical decisions into component parts and to introduce each element incrementally to patients, later pulling together the whole set in a manner that makes sense and is understandable. In other words, decisional capacity must be examined in relation to the nature of the decision. It may be that a different decision, or set of decisions, will be possible for a given individual.

In general, the level of risk and the overall risk-to-benefit ratio that accompany the choice drive the stringency of the standard for consent or refusal of recommended treatment (Drane 1984). If acceptance of a recommended treatment has few and less serious risks, the standard is relatively low. If, however, refusing a recommended treatment is likely to have many or more severe risks, the standard's stringency is relatively high (Figure 4–1). The rationale for this variation within the standard is not arbitrariness or paternalism but rather follows the duty to act faithfully with beneficence and nonmaleficence as guideposts and to ensure that an illness-related condition is not interfering with the judgment of patients who are making a choice that may put them in harm's way.

Emergency or Acute Care

To a large extent, the clinical situation determines the standard for informed consent in emergent or acute care. There may be little time for information sharing and mutual decision making. Acting beneficently—that is, with a view toward saving the life or preserving the health of the patient—is the clinician's duty in such circumstances. This action on behalf of the patient is ethically and legally justifiable; it is presumed that in emergencies the patient wishes to be helped in the best manner known to the clinician and the clinician has permission to act with the patient's well-being and best interests at heart. Often the patient, if alert and conscious, will explicitly assent to treatment (i.e., voluntarily accept the choice proffered by the clinician at the time). If the patient is unconscious or unable to communicate, the clinician acts with the implied or presumed consent of the patient.

When the patient refuses treatment in an emergent situation, however, a very rigorous standard for consent must be applied, for two reasons: the

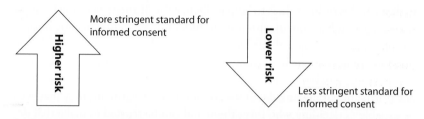

FIGURE 4–1.   Stringency of standard for informed consent linked with risk associated with the decision.

Informed consent decisions posing higher risk or representing a less favorable risk-to-benefit ratio must fulfill a more stringent standard for information sharing, decisional capacity, and voluntarism. Informed consent decisions posing lower risk or representing a more favorable risk-to-benefit ratio must fulfill a fundamental standard for sharing information, decisional capacity, and voluntarism but may meet a less stringent standard.

Source.   Copyright © 2015 Laura Weiss Roberts, M.D., M.A. Used with permission.

anticipated likelihood of an adverse outcome and the possibility that clinical factors may be adversely affecting the patient's judgment. Undiagnosed delirium, delusional thinking, severe physical pain, emotional distress, and interpersonal pressure may undermine a patient's ability to make a fully informed, autonomous choice in an acute situation. When a patient refuses treatment, the clinician should take into consideration that focusing too much on the patient's philosophical and legal right to self-determination may obscure the presence of a significant clinical issue that requires attention. Clarification of underlying clinical considerations in such circumstances is the clinician's primary responsibility, grounded in the bioethics principles of respect for persons, clinical standards of care, fidelity, and beneficence. The intention here is not to undermine the patient's autonomy but rather to empower the clinician to help advance the health and well-being of the patient and ensure that the patient is optimally able to express his or her true wishes to accept or decline a given therapeutic approach.

In sum, in situations in which clinical decisions may have very serious or irreversible health consequences, including death, informed refusal of treatment must fulfill the most stringent standards. The clinician must be certain that medical and psychiatric issues are carefully assessed for their contribution to the patient's choice (e.g., insufficient pain treatment in a patient who has cancer and requests that life-saving treatment be discontinued). The patient must clearly demonstrate knowledge, understanding, and appreciation of the ramifications of the decision to refuse care. The patient must indicate that this choice is consistent with his or her life patterns and personal values (e.g., past refusal of certain treatments). External coercive forces (e.g., a family member who pushes the patient to refuse care because of religious beliefs or financial concerns) must be eliminated as much as possible. In alignment with the duties of beneficence, fidelity, and clinical competence, keeping a patient alive and safe, to whatever extent possible, is essential in any situation in which the individual's wishes are unclear, inconsistent, or compromised by clinical symptoms.

Care for Chronic Illness

The context of care for chronic illness may fulfill more clearly the goal of informed, voluntary decision making. Over the course of time, the clinician may come to know a specific patient—his symptoms, values and concerns, responsiveness to treatment interventions, and personal supports. In turn, the patient may acquire a greater sense of trust, express himself with greater openness, and gather more complete information about the illness and potential therapeutic interventions over time. A patient with a chronic illness also lives out the consequences of side effects, adverse reactions, and benefits of treatments differently than a patient with a time-limited health problem. She may appreciate better how her illness and treatment affect other aspects of her life, and the clinician may come to know the patient's preferences and concerns with greater certainty. Expressing autonomous wishes and deciding on specific treatment approaches and the overall goals of therapy through mutual understanding and dialogue are intrinsically more possible in the context of chronic illness. Consequently, the standard for consent in chronic illness is very rigorous in attempting to increase the patient's level of information, seeking opportunities to enhance decision making, and creating the circumstances in which patients may indicate their wishes and hopes.

The following case illustrates how a consent discussion can facilitate the aims of the therapeutic relationship in chronic care.

> A patient with recurrent, very severe depression who is unresponsive to medications and psychotherapy previously had experienced relatively rapid recovery with ECT. Clarification of outcomes associated with these dramatically different treatment approaches provides an occasion for the clinician to understand ethically relevant factors in the patient's treatment choices. The patient expresses interest in trying one of the newly released antidepressant medications but states that she is willing to undergo ECT again "if it will help more."

With this patient, clarification of what the patient means by "help more" is important. For example, does she mean help with severity of symptoms right now, help with functioning while waiting for the worst of the symptoms to go away, help with removing most of the symptoms as quickly as possible, or help with preventing future periods of depression? Symptom severity, ability to cope while depressed, length of time until improvement, and prevention of future episodes are quite different outcome dimensions in the experience of the depressed patient, and different therapies may have different strengths in these dimensions. An intensive course of ECT may help address very severe depressive symptoms quickly but not facilitate social role functioning during the treatment. Alternatively, psychosocial interventions may assist the patient to perform critical work activities while waiting for antidepressant medications to improve symptoms. A consent dialogue focused on outcomes thus integrates clinical knowledge of potential treatments with the patient's concerns, duties, and values.

Routine or Preventive Care

Routine or preventive care that focuses on the patient's benefit and presents little risk entails a less rigorous level of consent. Examples include drawing a serum lithium level or performing thyroid and renal function tests. Patients presumably understand that such tests are clinically valuable and associated with relatively few risks and harms. Clinicians should review the need for the information from these tests, but formal, detailed consent procedures are not necessary. Neuroimaging or neuropsychiatric assessments, though common diagnostic procedures, represent greater biological and psychosocial risks to patients and, for this reason, require a more systematic and intensive approach to consent.

ADVANCE DIRECTIVES AND SURROGATE DECISION MAKING

Through advance directives, patients articulate their preferences for future care. Advance directives often are formal written papers that the patient creates and signs; they may also consist of a body of documentation that the patient, family members, and clinicians develop to articulate the patient's wishes and values regarding health care. Ideally, they will document the person's values and pattern of life choices as they relate to possible future decisions that are carefully described and envisioned.

Advance directives are most helpful when they have ecological validity—that is, when they have enough depth and texture to be applied meaningfully. A bald statement such as "I do not want machines" or "I do not want to be in the hospital" does not convey enough and can cause more harm than good in honoring an individual's stated preferences. Documents that characterize the thinking and the values shaping the stated choices, in light of multiple different scenarios, are of greatest assistance to clinicians and families. Published materials such as the Values History Form (University of New Mexico Health Sciences Center Institute for Ethics 2015) and Five Wishes (Aging with Dignity 2011) are excellent tools to facilitate discussions of personal values and preferences with patients or within families for many medical decisions, especially end-of-life care.

Recent scholarship has elevated the idea of a "patient preference predictor" (Rid and Wendler 2014), extrapolating optimal choices on the basis of a patient's characteristics and past decision making. It is argued that this methodology would be more faithful to the patient's actual preferences than would an alternative decision maker. Considerable evidence is needed to validate this claim, although with rigorous new analytic techniques and the existence of "big data" regarding individuals and their life patterns, values, and choices, the notion of a patient preference predictor is becoming more likely.

Advance directives are useful in two important ways:

1. They serve as a reference for the clinician if the patient becomes decisionally incapable or compromised. For example, a patient with bipolar disorder knows that he has a pattern of very compromised judgment during periods of mania and completes an advance directive requesting that treatment be instituted despite his (anticipated) protests.
2. Advance directives provide evidence of the patient's past health care preferences that may result in controversial clinical decisions. For instance, advance directives may become critical when patients refuse treatment on the basis of deeply and consistently held personal convictions (e.g., refusal of blood transfusions by a patient who is a Jehovah's Witness).

Ideally, these issues will not be addressed for the first time in a moment of great crisis but will be anticipated, discussed, and documented carefully beforehand.

Advance directives do not *ever* replace the wishes expressed by a patient who is decisionally capable. Moreover, there should be opportunities to adapt, or even reverse, earlier decisions, because patients cannot always predict how they will feel in a crisis. For these reasons, advance directives may guide but should never supplant prudent, reflective clinical decision making.

In surrogate decision making, also referred to as proxy or substitute decision making, another person makes health care choices for the decisionally impaired patient. This person may be a spouse, sibling, adult child, friend, or court-appointed guardian. The surrogate decision maker has a large responsibility: he or she must serve the best interests and well-being of the patient (the best-interests standard) while making decisions that are faithful to the values and prior wishes of the patient (substituted-judgment standard). Fulfilling this responsibility can be extremely difficult. In some situations, the best-interests and substituted-judgment standards do not yield the same result, in which case the surrogate decision maker must abide by legal statutes operative in the state. In other circumstances, the patient's values and wishes are not known. A patient may be too young or cognitively compromised to have demonstrated personal values and wishes, for example. In yet other situations, the patient's values and wishes are known but conflict with the values and wishes of the surrogate decision maker—or with accepted standards of clinical care.

Consequently, in working with surrogate decision makers, clinicians must clarify the goals and values governing the choices made on behalf of the patient. The clinician must assess the patient's decisional capacity accurately and, in most circumstances, treat the patient's symptoms aggressively so that he or she can contribute to the choices made to whatever extent possible. In contrast with many medical situations, in which the patient's decisional ability diminishes over time, such efforts are especially important in the context of psychiatric illness, in which patients' decisional abilities may fluctuate.

EXAMPLES OF EMPIRICAL STUDIES RELATED TO CONSENT

Evidence gathered since the 1950s suggests that informed consent is an ideal that is often difficult to achieve in clinical care, perhaps particularly with mentally ill populations (Sugarman et al. 1999). A full overview of the broad empirical literature on consent is beyond the scope of this text. Studies of individuals living with psychotic, affective, and dementia disorders have shown both strengths and potential vulnerabilities to bring to the process of informed consent.

Several studies have revealed that symptoms of mental illness may adversely influence information-based or more strictly cognitive aspects of consent. For example, Appelbaum and Grisso, in their classic MacArthur Treatment Competence Study (Appelbaum and Grisso 1995; Grisso and Appelbaum 1995; Grisso et al. 1995), assessed the decisional abilities of patients with schizophrenia or major depression, patients with ischemic heart disease, and nonpatient community volunteers. When acutely ill, the psychiatric patients had greater difficulties with decision making on several formal cognitive measures than did the medically ill patients and the nonpatient community participants. The problems were more severe for individuals with psychotic symptoms than for individuals with depression. Constructively, clinical treatment led to significant improvement of these deficits, resulting in closer resemblances across the three groups assessed. Marson et al. (1995) used a clinical vignette–based instrument to measure the level of competency exhibited in medical treatment decisions by individuals with dementia and healthy comparison subjects. Their findings revealed that greater severity of cognitive impairment in dementia correlated with diminished ability to formulate logical reasons for treatment choice (i.e., addressing the "rational reasons" dimension of decisional capacity) and that global measures of dementia severity did not predict clinical decision-making capacity and therefore should not be considered alone in the assessment of decisional capacity.

Problems arise with informed consent in medically ill populations as well. In an early, elegant study of 200 cancer patients who had consented the previous day to chemotherapy, radiation therapy, or surgical interventions (Cassileth et al. 1991), the majority of patients (75%) reported that the explanations offered during the consent process had helped them to decide about their care. When questioned closely, however, only 60% actually understood the nature and purpose of the procedure and only 55% correctly identified a single risk of the proposed treatment to which they had consented. A survey study comparing patients with breast cancer in clinical trials and healthy control subjects showed that the cancer patients retained less but, importantly, were provided with less information (e.g., written descriptions, expected physical discomforts, side effects) during the consent process of research protocols (Tomamichel et al. 1995). A study of 861 people living with HIV-related illness revealed that whereas all had clear wishes regarding their care, only 35.8% had spoken with their physician about their preferred care (Mouton et al. 1997). Barriers to informed consent identified in an observation and structured interview study on a surgical ward and a medical ward included patient and physician attitudes that minimized the importance of consent processes, the "general passivity" of inpatients and acutely ill individuals, the complexity of the medical system, and the sheer number of decisions that needed to be made during the course of a given patient's treatment (Lidz et al. 1983).

Studies of advance directives and surrogate decision making have important clinical implications. Numerous surveys and interview-based projects have revealed that advance directives are underutilized and that patient preferences are rarely identified prospectively (Bradley et al. 1998; Sharp et al. 2013). Many studies have shown that most elderly patients would prefer that a family member (e.g., a spouse or an adult child) serve as an alternative decision maker (High 1990, 1994). In a study I recently conducted with colleagues, we found that preferred alternative decision makers of people living with schizophrenia are highly accurate in predicting the preferences and values of the ill individuals but unexpectedly showed greater accuracy in research-related decision making than in clinical treatment–related decision making (Roberts and Kim 2015a). The dyads of preferred decision makers and ill individuals in this study were very close and had frequent contact. Other studies of hypothetical decision making by proxies, however, suggest that such individuals may not assess patients' wishes accurately. Sachs et al. (1994) studied 42 decisionally capable dementia patients, 64 proxy decision makers, and 60 well elderly individuals and found that the decision makers' predictions of patient preferences were overall discordant with the patients' stated wishes. Similarly, Warren et al. (1986) studied participation choices made by proxy decision makers and 168 decisionally capable nursing home patients for hypothetical, minimal-risk research projects. The surrogate decision makers used criteria other than the patients' predicted preferences (e.g., attitudes toward research) in making these choices.

Fortunately, evidence is emerging that the deficits and barriers that hamper the consent process for mentally and physically ill patients may be amenable to intervention. Interventions in which information is presented verbally and in writing, using clear and understandable language, improve patients' understanding of consent decisions (Carpenter et al. 2000; Flory and Emanuel 2004; Ruiz-Casares 2014). The timing of consent information—for instance, providing information in a relaxed manner or on repeated occasions—is important to patients' abilities to integrate and apply these data. Treatment of symptoms, ranging from hallucinations to physical pain, also can improve the quality of patients' decision making. Finally, patients and surrogate decision makers value clinician behaviors that demonstrate respect for and commitment to the consent process (e.g., devoting ample time to the consent dialogue). The observation that educational efforts, symptom treatment, and attitudinal obstacles can be addressed suggests a number of constructive approaches to consent in the context of clinical care.

Issues regarding informed consent in novel situations arise every day for psychiatrists—such as the challenges associated with consent and return of results in translational genomic studies or with innovative treatments, such as deep brain stimulation or text-based psychotherapies. In thinking about consent for genetic innovation, physician-scientists and regulators are struggling with how best to describe anticipated genetic findings, interpret their meaning, determine which results to share and when, decide how to handle future risk and discoveries, and evaluate what data should be entered into the formal medical record (Henderson et al. 2014). In considering informed consent for deep brain stimulation, which the U.S. Food and Drug Administration has approved for certain psychiatric conditions and not others, psychiatrists are confronted with many challenges related to the quality of evidence, the problems of predicted outcomes, and the impact of stigma, while they also reflect on the terrible abuses of psychosurgery in the past. The widespread use of technology in clinical settings similarly raises new questions about treatments that lack an evidence base, that may introduce direct risk or displace treatments with known value for patients, and that may present greater opportunities for patients' personal information to be breached. Informed consent for clinical research raises many intriguing questions (see Chapter 18, "Psychiatric Research"), particularly as forms of research expand to encompass basic, translational, clinical, community-based, and population and global methodologies (Roberts et al. 2014). Policy makers, opinion leaders, and practitioners find themselves working through these complex ethical issues without empirical evidence and clear conceptual guidance or benchmarks, as society and the practice of medicine change rapidly. For these reasons, evidence-based ethics studies to address emerging issues around consent are essential to develop data-driven, best-practice approaches.

CONCLUSION

Informed consent is not reducible to a piece of paper. A signature on even the most thoughtfully crafted consent form is meaningless if the patient was poorly informed or did not understand the choice at hand or the decision was coerced. Informed consent is thus a process that hinges on the clinician's professional integrity and attunement. It requires sensitivity. It entails dialogue. It takes time. It involves posing the right questions for consideration. Clinicians may take several constructive steps to support the process of consent.

A sound informed consent process requires that clinicians closely attend to information sharing, decision-making abilities, and voluntarism issues (Table 4–2). The process of imparting consent information, for instance, requires attention to the patient's interpersonal cues and communication style. The information should be provided at the right educational level to foster understanding, and optimally the clinician will incorporate both verbal and written materials. Moreover, the process requires a sense of timing and context so that patients can absorb the information they will need to make the choices they must without feeling confused or overwhelmed with facts that have no real personal relevance.

TABLE 4–2. Strategies for enhancing the effectiveness of informed consent interactions

1. Information sharing

Pay attention to the patient's interpersonal cues and communication style.

Avoid technical jargon and provide information at the right level to foster understanding.

Involve translators if necessary.

Offer both verbal and written material whenever possible.

Be aware of timing and context of information sharing so that patients do not experience an information overload devoid of personal meaning.

Encourage the patient to seek advice from loved ones.

Create opportunities for questions and dialogue.

2. Decisional capacity

Assess the patient for deficits in decisional capacity.

Provide emotional support and reassurance.

For patients with decisional capacity deficits, approach things in a stepwise fashion—seek consent for beginning treatment, and as the patient's symptoms and functioning improve, approach the patient for the larger decisions.

If the patient is not capable of providing consent at all, designate an appropriate family member as an alternative decision maker.

3. Voluntarism

Establish a trusting relationship.

Seek to understand the values and choices of the patient now and in the past.

Address symptoms and illness phenomena (e.g., negative cognitive distortions, compromised insight) to whatever extent possible.

Avoid pressuring the patient for a quick decision unless absolutely necessary; reduce pressures in the environment when possible.

Source. Adapted from Roberts LW, Dyer AR: *Concise Guide to Ethics in Mental Health Care.* Washington, DC, American Psychiatric Publishing, 2004, p. 70. Copyright © 2004 American Psychiatric Publishing. Used with permission.

With respect to decisional capacity, the process of informed consent should enhance the patient's ability to make choices to whatever extent possible. The involvement of patient advocates, family members, or social workers and case managers and the use of medications, supportive therapy, partial hospitalization, and other interventions may help provide emotional support and diminish illness symptoms so that patients are able to make the necessary decisions. Use of written documents such as advance directives, the Values History Form (University of New Mexico Health Sciences Center Institute for Ethics 2015), and Five Wishes (Aging with Dignity 2011) can help encourage patients and families to talk about their health care preferences. It is also essential that the process of consent foster autonomy through repeated efforts to clarify the individual's wishes, past choices, relevant experiences, and symptoms.

On one hand, the process of exploring a patient's wishes can be very challenging, because psychological defenses and illness phenomena such as compromised insight may greatly influence the individual's ability to be fully autonomous. Similarly, prior experiences of involuntary treatment may profoundly undermine a patient's sense of self-efficacy and interpersonal power. On the other hand, the informed consent dialogue can strengthen the depth, trust, attunement, and understanding that exist between a psychiatrist and patient. Iterative conversations about the goals of treatment, strategies for care, and the patient's hopes and concerns can establish a more robust therapeutic relationship and thereby foster better patient outcomes.

CASE SCENARIOS

- A 68-year-old woman with early Alzheimer's disease is asked to consent to treatment for acute pneumonia.

- After a difficult encounter with an assaultive, intoxicated patient, the multidisciplinary care team serving a psychiatric emergency room wishes to adopt a policy that all individuals seeking acute care services will have substance and HIV testing as a requirement for clinical care without explicit written consent.

- A 56-year-old man who has major depression with psychotic features initially rejects ECT and then refuses antipsychotic treatment because he does not like the side effects of the medication.

- On his eighteenth birthday, a young man with intellectual disabilities and generalized anxiety wishes to decline treatment that previously had been arranged through parental consent.

- A 36-year-old living in a rural community seeks transgender surgery at the nearest urban academic center and is referred to a psychiatrist for an assessment of depression. The patient is willing to be psychiatrically evaluated for depression but does not consent to a comprehensive evaluation related to identity and gender, which may have bearing on the surgeon's willingness to perform surgery.

5

Ethical Use of Influence and the Role of Physician in High-Risk Situations

Laura Weiss Roberts, M.D., M.A.

Providing mental health care involves ethical use of influence and the role of physician—that is, influence that exists within the healing relationship and the role that the physician is entrusted to play in society. Influence, in this context, inversely relates to the vulnerability and the emotional and physical risk present in a situation. The *ethical* use of influence and role is a fairly elusive concept. It is characterized by the *intent* (i.e., seeking to do good and to minimize harm to individuals and affected others) and the *outcome* (i.e., whether in fact there has been minimized suffering, preserved life, ensured safety, or enhanced well-being) of the clinician's actions. Ethical use of influence and role is expressed in diverse ways, ranging from offering a subtle interpretation in the course of intensive psychotherapy with a traumatized person to administering emergency medications and committing a person with serious mental illness involuntarily to ensure patient safety. Both actions may be undertaken with integrity and faithful intent to help a suffering person and to protect others from harm—or not. And both actions may—or may not—result in good outcomes for individuals and affected members of society irrespective of original intent.

This chapter begins with a brief discussion of the special ethical nature of the therapeutic relationship and the ethical use of influence and role in different therapeutic activities inherent to mental health care. That topic is followed by a discussion of imperatives and safeguards in the use of power in high-risk (e.g., dangerous, suicidal, homicidal) situations and ethically complex situations that may precipitate the specific therapeutic uses of power (e.g., treatment refusal by individuals who are ill or decisionally compromised). Many of these issues are also addressed in other chapters, such as in Chapter 3, "The Tradition of the Psychotherapeutic Relationship," and Chapter 4, "Informed Consent and Decisional Capacity." The chapter concludes with suggestions for the ethical use of influence and role of the psychiatrist as physician in serving to promote mental health and the well-being of patients in need.

NOTIONS OF STRENGTH AND VULNERABILITY IN THERAPEUTIC WORK

Central to the field of mental health care is the ability to heal. This ability derives from the strengths of the patient and the expertise of the clinician. With special training, knowledge, and experience, the clinician is able to alleviate, or at times lift completely, the burden of suffering associated with mental illness. For example, patients and families know that it is the psychiatrist who can prescribe potent medications to manage symptoms, offer reassurance, arrange hospitalization for safety and stabilization, and mobilize beneficial services. Interestingly, the ability to heal in therapeutic work also derives from the interpersonal process between patient and clinician, which can be among the more intimate of all human relationships. In the context of psychotherapeutic work, patients share their life stories, innermost concerns, disquieting fantasies and fears, and loves and losses. This openness and transparency make patients vulnerable, thus testing the limits of trust and interpersonal reliance.

The pairings of strength and vulnerability and of trust and dependence allow therapeutic healing to occur in the face of tragedy and serious suffering. This vulnerability, however, gives clinicians the power to harm, reject, misunderstand, or exploit patients who struggle with the experience of mental illness, which itself may generate helplessness, despair, distress, and exceptional dependence on the clinician. For these reasons, it is incumbent upon the clinician to treat every interaction with the patient as having the potential to help or harm and as being very significant in the life of the patient.

ETHICAL CONSIDERATIONS IN HIGH-RISK SITUATIONS

High-risk situations heighten the obligations of clinicians to use power responsibly to help ill individuals and protect both them and others from harm. These are situations in which dangerous behaviors, threats of suicide or homicide, and grave passive neglect due to mental illness become evident.

Insufficient information often characterizes high-risk situations in psychiatry. For instance, a patient with serious mental illness with severe symptoms and erratic, impulsive behavior, who has recently arrived by bus from another town, is brought to the community mental health center for evaluation. Under such a circumstance, the psychiatrist may make mistakes with serious consequences. For example, the clinician may underestimate the seriousness of a situation, thereby failing to intervene to protect the well-being and safety of the individual and others involved. It is also possible for the psychiatrist to overinterpret and overreact to a situation, moving quickly to more aggressive interventions than may be necessary to fully discharge obligations to the patient and society.

In addition to the challenges of clinical assessment and insufficient information in high-risk situations, judgment errors may occur. Clinicians may overvalue independence and autonomy to the point of permitting decisionally compromised patients to act in ways that are dangerous to themselves or others. Overvaluing safety, however, may cause clinicians to usurp the rights of individuals who might be cared for adequately under less restrictive means. In a different scenario, psychiatrists who do not understand key issues at the interface of clinical medicine, ethics, and law or who do not recognize key countertransference issues may inadvertently shield individuals who are engaging in dangerous behavior not attributable to mental illness. This quiet, often unrecognized form of collusion may lead to diminished accountability of individuals and greater overall societal harm. In all of these cases, psychiatrists and other mental health professionals find themselves in binds, vulnerable to the risk of not adhering to appropriate standards for clinically and ethically sound care, just as their patients are at risk for harms ranging from having their rights violated to losing their lives.

Consideration of these difficult issues inherent to high-risk situations reveals tensions across the competing values within society. The profession of law, for instance, places primacy on autonomy and privacy, which translates in mental health care to "freedom from" involuntary commitment, treatment against the patient's will, overriding of confidentiality, or external control of finances. The profession of medicine, however, places primacy on preserving life, alleviating suffering, and improving functioning and quality of everyday life. Clinicians thus may understand freedom as "freedom to" think clearly, form relationships of care and concern, not be overwhelmed by negative emotions or lack of emotion, work meaningfully, and enjoy simple pleasures. Legal imperatives in a high-risk situation may pertain to accountability in behavior, whereas ethical imperatives may relate more to explaining behavior and sharing responsibility in minimizing danger. Beyond these differences in emphasis of values shaping perspectives, duties, and decisions are differences in approaches to complexity. For example, whereas legal and political systems may engage in adversarial processes that rely on argument and debate, modern practices in mental health care and clinical ethics may involve processes that seek common ground and build consensus. Both approaches are necessary to enable people living with mental illness to receive treatment that is humane and just, but in many high-risk situations societal imperatives may contradict each other.

SUICIDE, VIOLENT BEHAVIOR, AND MENTAL ILLNESS

Suicide represents a serious public health burden, disproportionately affecting persons with mental illness. Suicide is consistently among the top 10 causes of death in the United States. In the past decade, hundreds of thousands of individuals have committed suicide, and millions have received emergency treatment for serious attempts. Most of those who commit suicide have a diagnosable mental disorder, most commonly depression, often complicated by comorbid substance abuse. Mentally ill ethnic minority youth, elderly white men, and other specific subgroups (e.g., indebted farmers) are at particularly high risk. Suicide risk is linked with enduring attributes, such as gender, and acute factors that work in concert to produce devastating outcomes, including access to means, immediate and severe distress, and a feeling of thwarted belongingness or loss (Cornette et al. 2009; Hill and Pettit 2014).

Unlike suicidality and mental illness, violent behavior and mental illness are not tightly linked (Swanson et al. 1997, 2015). People living with mental illness are more likely to be victims of violent crimes than perpetrators of violence (Hiroeh et al. 2001; Maniglio 2009). Historically, findings of the Epidemiologic Catchment Area study indicated, for example, that 90% of persons with mental illness were nonviolent (Swanson et al. 1990).

Publicized cases of individuals with mental illness who perform violent acts, though perhaps rare statistically, cause great concern, however. Shootings at schools and churches, hotels, and places of business, where a person sought to cause great harm, have been highly visible in recent media stories. The number of people living with mental illness who are incarcerated or kept in forensic facilities has attained a historical high (Fuller Torrey et al. 2010). Escalating media coverage, new legislation, new empirical work, and broad dialogue represent only a few indicators of the importance of these issues in society.

The Epidemiologic Catchment Area study also found that among violent individuals with mental illness, a feeling of being threatened or of losing internal control; agitation; substance abuse; and lack of treatment were all related to violent actions (Swanson et al. 1997). Other past research has revealed that it is not the presence of delusions or hallucinations per se but rather of command voices and beliefs that the individual is being controlled or threatened that precipitate violence in people with psychotic disorders (Harris and Rice 1997). A highly publicized early case of violence by a person with mental illness led to the death of Kendra Webdale in 1999. Ms. Webdale was pushed under the wheels of an oncoming subway train by Andrew Goldstein, a patient with schizophrenia who had undergone multiple psychiatric admissions. Mr. Goldstein had been released after a 22-day hospitalization a few weeks before the murder. He told police that a spirit or ghost had entered his body and told him to push the woman under a train. Reports at trial indicated that when taking medications, Mr. Goldstein was functional and nonviolent. This incident provided much of the impetus for the passage of outpatient commitment laws in New York and other states. In March 2015, Andreas Lubitz piloted a Germanwings jetliner with 149 others on board. Midflight, he locked the copilot out of the cockpit and intentionally crashed the plane into the French Alps, killing himself and all the passengers. It was later learned that he had suppressed and misrepresented information to his employer regarding his diagnosis of a serious mental disorder. This tragedy, in which victims from more than a dozen countries perished, has led to international discussions of fitness-for-duty regulations and the adequacy of approaches to public safety.

Devastating stories such as these must be put in the context of evidence pertaining to violence and stigma. In a survey of 1,444 people by Link et al. (1999), 87% believed that violence was likely in an individual who showed symptoms of illegal drug abuse, 61% thought it likely in someone with schizophrenia, and 33% believed it likely in a person with depression. Two-thirds of respondents said they would use legal means to force people with substance abuse into treatment, and half reported that they would use similar interventions for treating people with schizophrenia. Ninety percent believed that those who were dangerous to themselves or others should be forcibly treated.

Ironically, as noted earlier in this section, people living with mental illness are far more likely to be the victims of violent crime than to act as perpetrators. Hiday et al. (1999) investigated 331 involuntarily hospitalized psychiatric patients who were court-ordered to outpatient commitment after discharge. The rate of criminal victimization of these more seriously mentally ill individuals was 2.5 times that of the general population. Interestingly, the patients' recognition of being vulnerable to crime was low—only 16.3% were concerned about their safety. Factors that contributed to victimization were substance use, urban dwelling, unstable housing, and personality disorder. A subsequent study demonstrated that outpatient commitment reduced the rate of criminal victimization, substance abuse, and violent incidents (Hiday et al. 2002).

Psychiatrists often have to make sense of these very difficult issues, serving as advocates for people with mental illness while at the same time communicating the importance of protecting the safety and well-being of all—including people with mental illness who may be misjudged or prejudicially treated. Psychiatrists and other mental health professionals, moreover, are commonly stigmatized along with the people for whom they seek to provide clinical care.

ETHICAL USE OF INFLUENCE AND ROLE IN SITUATIONS INVOLVING POTENTIAL FOR HARM

I wish to highlight four central issues surrounding ethical use of influence and the role of physician in relation to high-risk situations involving the potential for suicidal and violent behavior: prediction, duty to intervene, duty to warn and duty to protect, and strengths and accountability of people with mental illness. Table 5–1 provides examples of questions to consider in high-risk situations.

Prediction

The first consideration pertains to the challenges of predicting suicidal and violent behavior. It is widely understood that accurate prediction of self-harm and violent behavior is extraordinarily difficult. With respect to suicide and parasuicidal behavior, the clinician can be guided by past patterns of behavior and a constellation of traditionally recognized risk factors (e.g., male gender, being unmarried and without children) and risk factors more recently recognized for their potency (e.g., extreme anxiety, agitation, hope-

TABLE 5–1.   Questions to consider in high-risk situations

What clinical illness factors are driving the situation?

What are the ethical and legal mandates governing the situation?

What additional clinical information must you obtain to understand the situation more fully? What collateral sources of information (e.g., from medical records, family, police) have you reviewed?

Who can you include in this decision-making process to double-check yourself, your facts, and your judgment?

Does your patient agree with and accept the recommended treatment? Is the patient capable of this decision? Why or why not?

What is the least intrusive, least restrictive intervention to ensure the safety of the patient? An intended or threatened victim? The community at large?

Have you documented your reasoning and the disposition of the case in terms of risk, your approach, and necessary treatment? Are your rationale and approach adherent to appropriate clinical and legal standards of care?

Source.   Adapted from Roberts LW, Dyer AR: *Concise Guide to Ethics in Mental Health Care.* Washington, DC, American Psychiatric Publishing, 2004, p. 83. Copyright © 2004 American Psychiatric Publishing. Used with permission.

lessness) (Fawcett 2001; Simon and Hales 2012). Hall et al. (1999) reviewed risk factors for 100 patients who made severe suicide attempts. Factors predictive of suicidal behavior included severe anxiety; panic attacks; depressed mood; major affective disorder; loss of a relationship; recent alcohol or drug use; feelings of helplessness, hopelessness, and worthlessness; insomnia; anhedonia; inability to hold a job; and recent onset of impulsive behavior. Presence of a suicide note was not an accurate indicator in this study. In a comprehensive review of risk appraisal and management of violent behavior, Harris and Rice (1997) found that the factors most consistently associated with violence were male gender, youth, past antisocial and violent conduct, psychopathy, substance abuse, and aggression as a child. Major mental disorder or other psychiatric distress was a poor predictor of violence.

Thus, prediction of these high-risk behaviors is partly an issue of clinical acumen and awareness of patient risk factors and certainly also a matter of curiosity, intuition, and diligence in evaluating patients, gathering additional data, and reviewing collateral materials. However, risk assessment is inherently probabilistic, which means that expertise will never fully eliminate uncertainty. This fact is cold comfort after an at-risk patient takes a self-harmful step or acts violently. Studies of suicidality related to returning veterans have shown that access to means, acute distress, and the experience of loss, primarily of social role or relationships, may drive a suicidal or self-harmful act in these and other at-risk populations (Simon and Hales 2012). For many reasons, ranging from ethical ideals to pragmatic parameters, the clinician simply cannot hospitalize all individuals merely on the basis of risk of possible suicide or violence at some point in the future. Consequently, the clinician has the difficult task of balancing many complex factors in fulfilling the duty of caring for mentally ill individuals who have the potential for enacting self-harmful and violent wishes and behaviors. Evaluating access to means, acute stressors, and threats to the sense of belonging and well-being is important, as is building appropriate safeguards for individuals who appear to be at immediate risk.

Duty to Intervene

The second consideration pertains to the professional obligation to intervene therapeutically in the context of severe illness. This obligation represents the confluence of a medical ethical duty to help and a legal duty to act to protect vulnerable or endangered members of society. The ethics concept related to this obligation is beneficence. The legal concept is *parens patriae*—literally, the "parental" responsibility to seek to keep an individual from harming himself or herself through active or passive means, invoking the power of the state to act.

The duty to intervene therapeutically becomes ethically complex particularly when the ill individual wishes to decline care. In such situations, an intentional process to preserve the rights of the ill individual is enacted. This usually involves placing a patient on an involuntary hold for a time period specified by state law (e.g., 24 hours in some states, up to 7 days in others), during which the physician assumes responsibility for keeping the patient safe and administers only those treatments to which the patient consents or that are absolutely necessary for safety. This process seeks to ensure that the patient's autonomy is encroached upon only as much as is necessary to keep him or her safe and to allow for a formal determination of appropriate treatment in the context of a legal hearing. Given that even voluntarily admitted patients to psychiatric units feel some degree of coercion, as evidenced in a study by O'Donoghue et al. (2014), it is difficult to ensure that patients feel supported in their autonomous decision making to the full extent possible, in light of the specific circumstances of each case.

Criteria for retaining a person against his or her wishes for reasons of mental illness fall under the jurisdiction of each state and, accordingly, may vary considerably. Such criteria ordinarily relate to two core elements, which must coexist: 1) mental illness is present, causing an individual to be at risk for imminent harm to self and/or others, by either active or passive means, and 2) the proposed intervention is believed to be beneficial and effective and is the least restrictive means of keeping the individual, or others, safe from harm. These criteria help prevent abuses of power, such as detaining a person without mental illness for inappropriate reasons or placing individuals with mental illness in more restrictive settings than are absolutely necessary. The emphasis on the least restrictive means has led to the option of mandatory or involuntary outpatient commitment for treatment of some disorders, and this approach has met with initial success in the treatment of addiction and comorbid conditions. These criteria also help distinguish duties to intervene for reasons of mental illness from duties to intervene for other reasons. For example, if a person without mental illness is purposely violent, society mandates that he or she should not be shielded by a mental health code but rather should fall under the purview of the laws governing criminal behavior. The same is true for a person with mental illness who commits a violent act if it is determined that the mental illness was incidental to, not causal of, the behavior.

Empirical research on involuntary treatment has yielded interesting insights into the ethical acceptability of such treatment. Some studies suggest, for example, that the experience of coercion is not related to efforts to persuade or the presence of incentives but rather is associated with perceptions of threat, either physical or psychosocial in nature. Lorem et al. (2015) recently found that patients who undergo involuntary treatment respond with acceptance, fighting, or a sense of personal resignation. Lidz et al. (1995) found that patients who reported that they were listened to, validated, given a choice in the way the commitment was handled, and treated with dignity and justice had far fewer feelings of coercion despite the involuntary status (Owen et al. 2009). Schwartz et al. (1988) examined 24 involuntarily medicated patients; at discharge, 17 patients (70%) reported that their treatment refusal had been appropriately overridden and that they wished to be treated involuntarily again if a similar situation arose. Those who persisted in refusing treatment were highly grandiose and psychotic and had not responded to intervention.

Empirical work is just starting to be published on newer approaches, such as psychiatric advance directives, to determine their effectiveness in minimizing the experience of coercion and enhancing the rights of people with mental illness. It is important to note that much of this empirical work is taking place in high-income countries where values and systems of care are, arguably, not comparable with those throughout most of the world. For this reason, key leaders have called for more international studies and dialogue to explore coercive treatment and its implications (Molodynski et al. 2014).

Interesting recent empirical work has examined the psychological impact on mental health professionals of implementing involuntary treatments. Many communities and prominent opinion leaders across the mental health professions find themselves in disagreement about coercive interventions, even when patient and community safety is at stake. Hem et al. (2014) conducted seven focus groups in three mental health institutions in Norway and found that coercive treatment has many ramifications for staff who feel great responsibility for resolving ethical challenges faced in the respectful, albeit involuntary, care of their patients. The issues encountered relate to patient dignity and respect balanced against the safety—and the very lives—of these same patients. These authors recommend that a common language for understanding ethical conflicts, more explicit opportunities to reflect on practices and the impact of implementing certain practices, and more evidence-based ethics studies are needed to improve the quality of mental health care.

Duty to Warn and Duty to Protect

The third consideration pertains to confidentiality and the obligation to help others who may be in danger. These issues tragically collided in the *Tarasoff v. Regents of the University of California* case (see discussion of this case in Chapter 6, "Confidentiality and Truth Telling"). The 1974 and 1976 *Tarasoff* rulings in California changed the climate of psychiatric practice, mandating a duty both to warn and to protect individuals who are endangered by a potentially violent person with mental illness. In such situations, the patient's privilege of confidentiality is overridden by the imperative to seek to preserve others' safety. The standard of care in these emergency situations is to inform the endangered individual of a threat and try to ensure his or her safety. Obtaining collateral information from police officers, family members, friends, or staff of other health care and social service agencies is essential. Although clinicians clearly should make every effort to obtain the patient's permission for these contacts, if such permission is not granted, they must proceed to comply with their ethical and legal obligations (Layde 2015).

A post-*Tarasoff* study found that 14% of psychiatrists in the United States had warned a potential third-party victim in the year preceding the survey. Forty-five percent of those who chose to report did so against their best clinical judgment, and this figure was much higher than the percentage who had performed mandatory reporting for other reasons, such as child abuse (Givelber et al. 1984). The few studies that have investigated the impact of reporting on the therapeutic alliance have not substantiated the widespread concern that the ruling would have detrimental effects on the therapeutic relationship (Anfang and Appelbaum 1996). Of the 3,000 mental health professionals studied by Givelber et al. (1984) in the immediate post-*Tarasoff* period, 70%–80% believed that an ethical duty to override confidentiality and to take action to protect a potential victim from a dangerous patient had existed before the *Tarasoff* rulings.

The duty to warn and protect has found an unexpected application in treating patients with HIV/AIDS who engage in unprotected sexual activity and refuse to inform their sexual partners. The clinician's legal obligation varies by state, but the ethical conflicts and tensions inherent to this situation do not. Most ethical standards indicate that clinicians should make every effort to convince or assist the patient to inform his or her partners and to act in conformity with local law (see Chapter 11, "People Living With HIV/AIDS").

Strengths and Accountability of People With Mental Illness

In discussions of influence and role in the therapeutic relationship, it is natural to emphasize the potential vulnerability of the ill person. However, doing so may leave the impression that people with mental illness are so powerless and dependent that they have no responsibility for their actions or treatment. On one hand, psychiatric patients often have several overlapping vulnerabilities—such as minority status, poverty, gender, homelessness, lack of education, and medical illnesses—that expand and augment the power of psychiatrists, psychologists, physicians, and mental health clinicians in subtle, complex, and often culturally determined ways. On the other hand, persons with mental illness have equal rights and responsibilities in society, although they do have some additional protections as well. Furthermore, psychiatrists with extensive clinical experience will attest to the heroic and virtuous individuals who, day in and day out, live through the reality of the most severe and devastating forms of mental illness. These individuals fully understand what it means to be responsible, to be good citizens, to be compassionate, and to endure a very unfair "deal" in life with great dignity. A paternalistic approach that further stigmatizes people with mental illness and inadvertently denies them equal human and moral standing in this world is fundamentally unjust and certainly unkind. In situations with potential for harm, the psychiatrist has a duty to use influence and the role as physician to assist individuals with mental illness in a manner that demonstrates respect, fosters health, and protects against adverse outcomes but also encroaches as little as possible upon patient strengths and their accountability in society.

ETHICAL USE OF INFLUENCE AND ROLE IN THE CONTEXT OF TREATMENT REFUSAL

Refusal of psychiatric treatment, particularly medication, has unique clinical and ethical aspects in comparison with treatment refusal in medical or surgical settings. The most important consideration is the decisional capacity of the patient, because this capacity may be a direct manifestation of the illness process itself. When an elderly woman with depression rejects antidepressants, for example, her refusal may well be an expression of the despair and negative cognitive distortions that are characteristic of the disorder. Early empirical work suggests that denial (often of delusional proportions), mistrust, and thought disorder may be powerful inducers of treatment refusal (Appelbaum and Gutheil 1980; Marder et al. 1983). By current professional and clinical standards, the more grave the consequences of refusal, the more strongly the clinician is ethically required to override the patient's refusal. If, on the day of admission, a patient experiencing an exacerbation of posttraumatic stress disorder symptoms refuses to sit with his back to the door in a group meeting, it is probably not worth contesting. However, if a patient with schizophrenia admitted for chest pain after a cocaine binge will not allow an electrocardiogram because he believes he will be electrocuted, the conscientious clinician will address the voiced objection therapeutically, if possible, with the engagement and agreement of the patient. When the patient's life is endangered, however, the obligation to protect the patient's health and safety in the emergency situation overrides other concerns.

Treatment refusal by a decisionally capable person who understands and appreciates the consequences of the decision and whose choice is shaped by deeply held and enduring personal values should simply be honored. Treatment refusal is not pathognomonic of decisional incapacity, as noted in Chapter 4, "Informed Consent and Decisional Capacity." This said, often simply listening to patients, allowing them to express their fears, and providing choices and reassurance in a manner that is genuine may resolve the issue. Enlisting family members, case managers, friends, or other nursing and support staff often can help address a patient's fears and objections. Finally, attention to the very real and terrifying side effects of psychiatric treatment may be important in obtaining patients' authentic acceptance of treatment.

There will of course be times when all efforts to obtain consent for treatment fail, generally because the patient is too ill or symptomatic and lacking insight into the need for treatment. In these cases, clinicians must have recourse to whatever judicial options are available in their state and institution. Most states allow treatment on an emergency basis or permit expedited medication reviews, although locales vary in how strictly to interpret the duration of an emergency even in crisis situations. When a patient is truly decisionally incapable and is not likely to regain this capacity without medication, a mental health court or judge can appoint a treatment guardian to act as a surrogate decision maker. Courts vary on whether they use a best-interests or substituted-judgment standard for the guardian. In cases where the court appoints a surrogate decision maker, the adversarial nature of the court proceeding can be mitigated if the physician presents only the facts necessary to establish the case, treats the patient with respect and kindness, and makes every effort to explain to the patient that he or she is acting out of concern for the patient's well-being. On occasion, treatment guardians will not follow the medication recommendations of the treatment team, but clinicians can employ the same diplomatic techniques and interpersonal sensitivity used with patients in working toward a solution with the appointed guardian.

ETHICAL USE OF COERCIVE PRESSURE IN MENTAL HEALTH CARE

Intervention affecting the thoughts, feelings, relationships, and sometimes the liberties of people with mental illness is considered a necessary part of psychiatric treatment because of the nature of mental disorders. Ethical principles govern such intervention, however, such as seeking to help, avoid harm, and minimize encroachment on a person's personal rights. Intervention should never occur solely for the gratification or convenience of the clinician.

It is important to acknowledge differing perspectives about coercive pressure in mental health care. On one side of the debate are civil rights advocates, some consumer movements, and a number of psychiatrists, such as expressed in the work of the late Thomas Szasz (1976), who claim that any effort to treat a patient against his or her will is always coercion and inherently unethical. Proponents of this position disagree about whether a patient's violence toward self or others is a valid criterion for involuntary psychiatric admission or whether community sanctions and the criminal justice system should address these threats. Many who oppose involuntary commitment and forced treatment are protesting against the excesses of the past (e.g., when patients were warehoused for decades without due process) and present (e.g., some countries institutionalize individuals on the grounds of mental illness merely because they hold nonconforming political beliefs). On the other side of the debate are organizations advocating for patients, such as the National Alliance on Mental Illness, and the majority of psychiatrists and physicians, who believe that schizophrenia, bipolar disorder, and depression are neurobiological disorders that affect cognition and the expressed preferences of ill individuals. From this perspective, mental illness merits intensive treatment as matters of beneficence and justice. Most proponents of commitment and forced treatment acknowledge the violation of rights that occurred in the past and the corresponding duty to protect the liberty of patients to the fullest extent possible. In all cases, these groups affirm that ill individuals must be treated with dignity and respect.

There is also, unfortunately, a darker side to the use of commitment, forced medication, restraint, and seclusion that is ethically unacceptable to all involved in this discussion: the abuse of power in treatment settings to demean or punish individuals with mental illness. In the rarest of cases, sociopathic clinicians may seek out roles that place them in control of vulnerable individuals (Epstein and Simon 1990; Gabbard et al. 2012). More commonly, poorly screened and trained staff or exhausted and demoralized clinicians may use their power inappropriately against patients with chronic suicidality, personality disorders, psychopathy, or cognitive impairment. Clinicians who view treatment refusal as a challenge to their power may be more apt to react with anger. Realizing that patients are expressing themselves in one of the only ways left open to them in their virtually powerless situation can go a long way toward eliminating the physicians' wish to punish or abandon them. In sum, the best clinicians will manage their occasional feelings of antipathy toward patients through vigorous and honest self-scrutiny, teamwork, consultation, and proper self-care if they are to engage in ethical treatment of vulnerable patients with mental illness.

CONCLUSION

Ethical use of influence and role in high-risk situations rests on several pillars. First, the principles of respect for persons, autonomy, beneficence, nonmaleficence, and justice together suggest the importance of economical and judicious use of power in high-risk situations. The clinician must act in a manner that involves the minimal exertion of power in achieving a necessary aim, such as safety, so that the rights of the individual with mental illness are minimally encroached upon.

Second, mental health clinicians have complex obligations—therapeutically, ethically, and legally. Given the high stakes, clinicians in high-risk situations should never be completely alone in making tough decisions. They should seek consultation, gather advice from multidisciplinary colleagues, and intensively pursue additional information from multiple

TABLE 5–2.   Working therapeutically in the ethical use of influence

Understand treatment refusal as a possible expression of distress.

Ascertain the reasons for refusal.

Allow the patient to discuss his or her preferences and fears.

Explain the reason for the intervention in simple language.

Offer options for the disposition of treatment.

Appropriately enlist the assistance of family and friends.

Request support from nursing and support staff.

Assess decisional capacity and if necessary have recourse to the judicial system.

Attend to side effects—both long and short term, serious and bothersome.

Employ emergency treatment options where available.

Work to preserve the therapeutic alliance.

Engage treatment guardians where appropriate.

Source.   Adapted from Roberts LW, Dyer AR: *Concise Guide to Ethics in Mental Health Care.* Washington, DC, American Psychiatric Publishing, 2004, p. 93. Copyright © 2004 American Psychiatric Publishing. Used with permission.

sources, including recent and nontraditional sources of information that may reflect evolving societal mores. These clinicians must be extraordinarily attentive to countertransference feelings and extraordinarily diligent in seeking, synthesizing, and documenting information and making clinical judgments. Knowing the legal and policy requirements of the state and the setting is imperative. In the current care environment, legal and economic considerations may too often determine clinical care practices. Clinicians who place the safety and well-being of patients and the community as their highest priority and exemplify this advocacy in their therapeutic relationships are actually less likely than practitioners who are less cognizant of these issues to be the objects of legal actions or institutional censure (Hickson et al. 2002). This finding must be tempered by the humbling realities of the difficulty in predicting harmful behavior. These recommendations obviously cannot guarantee a beneficial clinical outcome, but they can help physicians to come away from even high-risk encounters with the conviction that they have exercised power ethically in the service of the patient and the community.

Third, making every effort to work with the patient therapeutically is essential. Recommendations for such work are listed in Table 5–2. Important strategies in this process include treating individuals with respect, compassion, and dignity; helping them to recognize their need for care; working together to find acceptable and safe options; and integrating duties to report and to warn into treatment interactions. Many clinicians and ethicists have been concerned that they must assume a policelike or judicial role that is contrary to their mission as patient advocates and healers. Psychotherapists in particular may feel that the trust and confidentiality crucial to effect personal change may not be possible under current legal mandates and political pressure. For these reasons, individual clinicians must search their hearts and know their societally mandated and professionally affirmed duties to arrive at acceptable approaches to dealing with these complicated, multifaceted issues with their patients.

CASE SCENARIOS

■ An unemployed man with a severe depressive episode voices the intent to kill his wife, children, and himself because he feels that they would all be "better off." He has a loaded gun in his closet.

■ An agitated patient verbally threatens and physically strikes a nurse who attempts to accompany him to a secure evaluation room in the emergency department.

■ An elderly woman with delirium postoperatively is placed in soft restraints in her hospital room.

■ A patient with posttraumatic stress disorder and alcohol dependence who made a serious suicide attempt 4 weeks earlier is experiencing suicidal ideation and insomnia but denies intent or plan to harm herself.

■ A university student behaves secretively and engages in hoarding, entirely unlike his past behaviors. He breaks up with his girlfriend and fills a notebook with racially charged hate statements. He begins watching violent television shows and posting violent messages on social media accounts.

6

Confidentiality and Truth Telling

Laura Weiss Roberts, M.D., M.A.

Psychiatrists acquire special knowledge about their patients and colleagues. In the course of gathering personal histories, reviewing medical records, and performing physical evaluations, mental status examinations, and other assessments (e.g., HIV or genetic tests, psychological tests, imaging studies), psychiatrists are invited into the intimate lives of their patients. Similarly, as clinicians, they are uniquely positioned to observe and evaluate the everyday professional practices of their colleagues as they respond to patient care situations that range from subtle to dramatic. With this special knowledge come two important professional ethics responsibilities: safeguarding confidentiality and truth telling.

Safeguarding patient confidentiality has been an enduring duty of physicians since the time of Hippocrates, who wrote in The Oath: "What I may see or hear in the course of treatment...in regard to the life of men...I will keep to myself, holding such things shameful to be spoken about." This duty derives from the broader philosophical concept of privacy—a notion that is highly valued in many cultures and encompasses nonintrusion, freedom to act without interference, and keeping personal information safe. *Protecting confidentiality* is simply defined as the duty not to disclose patient information without clear permission or in the absence of overriding legal imperatives.

Truth telling—the act of sharing one's knowledge and the limitations of one's knowledge with accuracy and sensitivity to the clinical impact of the disclosure—is also an ethical imperative in medicine as practiced in the United States. The truth-telling duty derives from the philosophical principle of respect for the truth (i.e., veracity). Truth telling entails that information be trustworthy and conveyed in a manner that the patient can understand and meaningfully apply. Beyond these responsibilities of individual clinicians, truth telling is an important principle in the structuring of health care systems to act honestly and foster accurate disclosure of information (e.g., when medical mistakes occur or decisions about covered services are made). *Deception*, in contrast, is the purposeful act of leading another individual to adopt a belief that is known to be untrue, through either direct misinformation or incomplete information. Truth telling is especially important in speaking with patients about the unfortunate realities of their illnesses, uncertainties and risks associated with treatment or research protocols, and medical mistakes. Truth telling is thus at the heart of informed consent (see Chapter 4, "Informed Consent and Decisional Capacity"). Truth telling is also crucial for preserving trust and integrity in the profession of medicine, resulting at times in therapeutic interventions with impaired colleagues and formal whistle-blowing efforts to prevent potential harm to patients or protocol participants. These aspects of the clinician's duty to tell the truth are reflected in the American Medical Association's (2001) *Principles of Medical Ethics:* "A physician shall uphold the standards of professionalism, be honest in all professional interactions, and strive to report physicians deficient in character or competence, or engaging in fraud or deception, to appropriate entities."

The tensions between clinicians' duties of confidentiality and truth telling often give rise to ethical dilemmas. Clinicians who respect local law and comply with mandatory reporting guidelines—for example, in situations of suspected child abuse—may fulfill their responsibility to tell the truth in their professional role but may also act against patients' confidentiality wishes in the process. As another example, not disclosing a patient's diagnosis of HIV-related mania, encompassing sexual impulsivity and compromised judgment, to the patient's spouse may be respectful of the patient's confidentiality preferences—and, in many states, the law—but may also undermine the clinician's sense of dealing honestly within the patient care situation.

Documentation in the medical record may be similarly riddled with ethical problems. Clinicians may be tempted to omit or "tailor" patient information to achieve certain aims—for example, obscuring data that are embarrassing to the patient or framing patient information in a manner that facilitates insurance reimbursement. More worrisome perhaps would be the inclination to minimize information related to mistakes that may have occurred in the course of a patient's care to protect against legal liability. Such practices violate ethical expectations within the medical professions but nevertheless occur. For these reasons, confidentiality and truth telling are linked, and clinical decision making often entails finding an ethically sound balance between these professional duties within the legal context of medical practice.

EXAMPLES OF EMPIRICAL STUDIES

Confidentiality

Long before the electronic medical record, physician-ethicist Mark Siegler (1982) conducted a study in an attempt to allay the concerns of a fellow faculty member who wanted privacy while admitted to an academic hospital. His colleague's fears were heightened rather than allayed when Siegler found that roughly 75 health care personnel, including 6 attending physicians, 20 nurses, 15 students, 12 residents, 4 financial officers, and 4 hospital reviewers, among others, legitimately had access to the chart of one patient during the course of a single, brief hospital stay. The exasperated colleague remarked, "Perhaps you should tell me just what you people mean by 'confidentiality'!" In this day of managed systems of clinical care, with computerized medical charts, laboratory reports, complex billing procedures, and broad-scale sharing of data for research, it would be nearly impossible to develop an accurate estimate of the vast number of individuals with potential access to an individual patient's clinical records.

Empirical work on confidentiality in the era before the electronic medical record is limited, but early studies suggest that efforts to protect patient confidentiality were variable and success was difficult to attain. In a self-report, structured interview study with 747 adolescents, for example, 76% indicated that their confidentiality had been violated by a clinician in the past (Cogswell 1985). Female participants in this study identified confidentiality breaches far more often than did their male peers, especially for reproductive health issues (72%) as opposed to general health issues (28%). In a novel study examining the actual behaviors of health professionals, Ubel et al. (1995) observed inappropriate disclosures of patient information on 14% of 259 observed hospital elevator rides at one institution. A questionnaire study with 177 patients, 109 house staff, and 53 medical students further revealed that patients expect greater levels of respect for patient confidentiality than actually are present in the training hospital setting (Weiss 1982). For example, whereas only 17% of patients thought that medical personnel commonly talked with their spouses or partners about patient cases, 51% of house officers and 70% of students reported this perception. Only 9% of patients thought that clinicians would talk about patients as interesting stories at parties; 45% of students and 36% of house officers, however, responded that such talk was common.

Data breaches have occurred in numerous private and public health systems, the federal government, and the Veterans Affairs system over the past few years. Since 2009, for example, private medical information of more than 154 million people was reported to have been disclosed due to employee carelessness, people acting with criminal intent, and hackers (U.S. Department of Health and Human Services 2016); and in 2015, the U.S. Office of Personnel Management disclosed that the personnel data of a total of 25.7 million people had been stolen, including potential, current, and former federal government employees (Davis 2015). The U.S. Department of Veterans Affairs experienced 14,215 privacy breaches affecting more than 100,000 veterans cared for in more than 100 facilities between 2010 and early 2013 (Prine 2013). Efforts to ensure cybersecurity across most health systems in the United States have failed, and many health systems have received penalties amounting to multimillion dollars for insufficient safeguards to protect patient data. Each year, new and stricter policies, procedures, and regulations are introduced to protect against system vulnerabilities, as reflected in ever-growing notices on governmental Web sites.

Early studies of patients with mental illness have shown that about half experience significant concern about confidentiality but only a small proportion are aware of confidentiality measures that exist for their protection, such as those surrounding documentation of sexual health issues or substance abuse treatment (Lindenthal and Thomas 1982; Wettstein 1994). Such findings are especially ominous in view of the fact that fears of confidentiality breaches may contribute to other worries patients may have that interfere with their seeking or engaging fully in necessary mental health care.

In general medical care, the clinical value of protecting sensitive patient information has also been demonstrated empirically. In a study of 56 adult women patients, 91% indicated security, trust, and confidentiality as among the top five qualities desired in a physician being consulted for advice on sexual health matters (Metz and Seifert 1988). Participants in a survey of 102 self-identified gay, lesbian, and bisexual youth ages 18–23 years reported far greater willingness to discuss their sexual orientation, sexual health concerns, and sexually risky behaviors after receiving accurate information and reassurance about confidentiality safeguards related to their care (Allen et al. 1998). An anonymous survey of 1,295 high school students revealed that 25% would forgo necessary treatment if their parents might find out (Cheng et al. 1993). Such findings underscore the importance of confidentiality protections to the use of health services and the effectiveness of clinical assessment and treatment planning.

Truth Telling

A number of empirical studies have examined truth telling in clinical care. Case reports and empirical studies entered the literature before the turn of the century (e.g., Baylis 1973; Finkelstein 1974). Mazor et al. (2004) reviewed the early literature and found that patients and the public support disclosure of medical mistakes and that although physicians also support disclosure, they often do not disclose. A systematic review (Kaldjian et al. 2006) examining the motivational context surrounding the decision to disclose an error identified four factors that facilitate truthful disclosure of a mistake by a physician: responsibility to 1) the patient, 2) the profession, 3) oneself as a physician, and 4) the community. Factors that impeded physician disclosure practices, however, were numerous, diverse, and potent, such as attitudinal barriers, feelings of helplessness and uncertainty, and fears regarding negative consequences.

In an early study, Sweet and Bernat (1997) randomly selected 150 medical students, house officers, and attending physicians to consider two vignettes in which an error of commission occurred (i.e., a physician's medication error resulting in coma, seizures, and enduring pain and a physician's medication error resulting in patient death) and one vignette in which an error of omission occurred (i.e., a referral physician's failure to diagnose a patient's cancer, leading to unnecessary paralysis). A majority of participants indicated that they would tell the patient or the family truthfully about the mistake in the first two scenarios (95% and 79%), but only 19% indicated that they would report the error of the colleague in the third scenario.

Since the publication by the Institute of Medicine in 2000 of a highly influential report on the topic of medical mistakes, accurate disclosure of medical mistakes has received tremendous attention as one element of patient safety. Empirical studies subsequent to this report have shown that physicians believe in the importance of quality and safety in the health care environment and strongly affirm the need for hospitals, for example, to provide accurate data on the health outcomes of patients. Professionals in medicine and other health fields such as nursing indicate less certainty, however, about the best way to approach disclosure of specific errors in the care of individual patients. Barriers to disclosure identified in the literature have been conceptualized in four areas: intrapersonal, interpersonal, institutional, and societal (Perez et al. 2014). Substantive efforts to prevent medical mistakes have been accompanied by valuable efforts to overcome barriers to disclosing when errors have taken place (Wittich et al. 2014). Taken together, this work has contributed greatly to the momentum around the current health safety and quality movement (Brennan et al. 2004; Kitson et al. 2013; Kitto et al. 2013; Mathews and Pronovost 2012; McDonald et al. 2013; Myers and Nash 2014; Rubin and Zoloth 2000).

A number of studies reflect a range of views held by clinicians and patients about the manner and completeness in which difficult diagnoses are revealed. An early structured interview study of 32 U.S. physicians related to care of the terminally ill revealed that in truthfully delivering "bad news," such as a poor-prognosis diagnosis to patients, only 47% would tell the patient the diagnosis explicitly, whereas 22% would speak euphemistically and 31% would not tell the patient at all (Miyaji 1993). In a cross-cultural study, Blackhall et al. (2001) surveyed 200 elderly residents of Los Angeles regarding truth-telling issues in diagnosing and treating terminal illness. The study found that lower percentages of Korean American (47%) and Mexican American (65%) participants were likely to believe that a patient should be told the diagnosis of metastatic cancer as compared with Anglo (87%) and African American (88%) participants, and strong cultural differences were also found in opinions regarding the role of families and the relative influence of clinicians in making end-of-life decisions. (See Chapter 10, "People From Culturally Distinct Populations," for a more in-depth discussion of cultural issues in psychiatric ethics.) A study of 677 medical geneticists in 18 nations similarly revealed considerable variability in their responses regarding whether they would 1) disclose the diagnosis of XY genotype in a female patient, 2) indicate which parent carries a translocation causing Down syndrome, or 3) reveal a diagnosis of Huntington's disease or hemophilia A against the wishes of the patient who was tested (Wertz et al. 1990). Interestingly, the ethics of withholding information from patients was the top-ranked topic (75% of respondents) reported as deserving more curricular attention in a study of 181 psychiatry residents at 10 training programs (Roberts et al. 1996).

Significant disagreement exists regarding standards for ethical disclosure of patient information even in situations in which reporting is mandatory. Indeed, one study showed that up to 75% of clinicians would elect not to report a case of suspected child abuse, despite the fact that this omission would violate the law (Wettstein 1994). A U.S. survey with 211 physician participants revealed that a majority were willing to misrepresent a screening test as a diagnostic test to obtain insurance reimbursement. One-third said that they would offer incomplete or misleading information to family members regarding a medical mistake resulting in the death of a patient. Only 25% indicated that they never employed deception of any kind in patient care, and 27% agreed with the statement that patients "expected" them to "utilize deception" for patient benefit (Novack et al. 1989). A survey of 510 Kansas family and general practitioners revealed that small community size was a critical problem affecting patient privacy and physicians' behaviors related to confidentiality and truth telling. These physicians' techniques to protect patient confidentiality included speaking with office staff about confidentiality (88%), omitting details from the medical record (69%), charting the importance of confidentiality (46%), omitting details from insurance forms (37%), failing to notify public health officials (21%), and misrepresenting facts in the medical record (6%) or on insurance forms (5%) (Ullom-Minnich and Kallail 1993).

Only limited data have been reported on the ethical imperative to tell the truth as it relates to whistle-blowing (Jackson et al. 2014). For instance, case data published by the Office of Research Integrity within the U.S. Public Health Service revealed 986 allegations of research misconduct in the 5-year period 1993–1997 inclusively (Price 1998). In 1996, a total of 3,653 disciplinary actions against physicians occurred due to alleged violations of law, ethics, or practice standards in the United States. From 1992 to 2001, a total of 529 (of 3,662) institutions or organizations reported research misconduct (Rhoades 2004). No data currently exist on failure to report unethical colleague behavior in either the research or the clinical domain.

CONFIDENTIALITY AND TRUTH-TELLING DILEMMAS

There are circumstances in which the risks associated with nondisclosure of patient information in mental health care are very great and outweigh the individual's privilege of confidentiality. Reporting clinical findings becomes ethically and legally justified when there is a serious and imminent threat of physical harm to an identifiable and specific person, when breaking the confidence is likely to do good and to prevent harm (e.g., protection of the intended victim), and when other efforts to address the situation have failed or are insufficient clinically or legally. The good-outweighing-the-bad logic is the basis for mandatory reporting in the diagnosis of communicable diseases, the discovery of gunshot or other crime-related wounds, the suspicion of child or dependent-elder abuse, and drivers who are dangerous due to serious mental illness, epilepsy, or other conditions. Such disclosures are viewed as imperative in light of the need to protect vulnerable individuals and/or society.

The landmark legal case of *Tarasoff v. Regents of the University of California*, 1974 and 1976, serves as a dramatic illustration. In this tragic case, a young woman named Tatiana Tarasoff was murdered by a graduate student, Prosenjit Poddar, who stabbed and shot her. Mr. Poddar had previously disclosed his intention to kill Ms. Tarasoff during the course of psychiatric care. Although the clinicians involved in Mr. Poddar's treatment took his threats seriously, their efforts to commit him involuntarily for inpatient psychiatric care and to retain him in outpatient treatment by the University of California failed. Although his attorneys argued that he had diminished capacity due to mental illness, the Superior Court of Alameda County, California, found Mr. Poddar guilty of second-degree murder in 1974. This verdict was overturned as the result of errors made by the judge in instructing the jury. Mr. Poddar was subsequently allowed to return to India. Because of the immense controversy the case caused, it was re-reviewed by the California court system in 1976, leading indelibly to the clinician's legal duty to protect potential victims of threatened violence.

From an ethical perspective, the tension between the professional principles of autonomy (i.e., furthering the rights and beliefs of patients) and nonmaleficence and beneficence (i.e., ultimately protecting the well-being of individuals) was central to the *Tarasoff* case. With the *Tarasoff* legal decision, fulfilling the responsibility to protect innocent others and society at large in circumstances in which patients may endanger the lives of others became the predominant and enduring ethical imperative. Indeed, forensic issues often are predominant in making confidentiality decisions in clinical care. Specifically, in five situations significant legal precedents suggest that it is justifiable to disclose a patient's personal information without explicit permission:

1. In a clinical emergency
2. In the context of involuntary commitment
3. When necessary to protect third parties
4. In compliance with statutory reporting requirements
5. When speaking with colleagues to develop multidisciplinary clinical care plans

Within these legal parameters, however, a number of ethical judgments must be made. Consider, for instance, a hospitalized, delusional patient who expresses homicidal intent but without reference to a specific individual. The patient is under close supervision, has no history of violence, and is accepting medication. Is there any immediate need to take action to curtail the liberties of the patient or report the patient to local officials? How about if the psychiatrist knows that the patient has a long-standing paranoid belief about a next-door neighbor and has made threats toward the neighbor in the past—is this sufficient to warrant action? What if the patient then leaves the ward without the knowledge or permission of the staff? Consider a second example related to the timing of a mandated report of suspected child abuse. How much data gathering should the clinician engage in before complying with legal imperatives to disclose information to state or county agencies? Which member of the multidisciplinary treatment team should make the report? How should the process around reporting the situation be documented in the parent's and the child's medical charts?

Confidentiality issues arising in more mundane, everyday situations are also complex. Consider the situation of treatment planning among multidisciplinary team members: Patient information disclosed or discovered in the context of a therapeutic relationship may be discussed openly by members of a large clinical care team. Patient information is also commonly entered into a written medical record or computer database. Similarly, in teaching settings, it is essential that trainees obtain guidance from their supervisors regarding all significant patient care matters. What confidentiality protections exist in these discussions? Is every aspect of the patient's life history included? How should sensitive material (e.g., related to drug use, sexual behavior, violence history, or HIV status) be documented? What limitations are placed on access to the patient's chart or to the computer database? What if a patient is also a part-time employee at the clinic where he or she is receiving care, because the group insurance policy requires this? Other routine situations in which confidentiality decisions arise include elective patient consultations; disclosures of patient data to insurance reviewers, managed care companies, or legal agencies; and appropriate disguise of protected patient information in clinical presentations and scientific papers. These widely ranging situations are often very difficult and may create significant ethical binds for clinicians.

The Health Insurance Portability and Accountability Act of 1996 (HIPAA) offers additional protections for patients' medical records. According to the U.S. Department of Health and Human Services, the aim of this set of regulations was to increase confidentiality protections and to balance the privacy needs of individuals with societal needs—such as public health, medical research, and quality assurance efforts and greater accountability around health care fraud and abuse. HIPAA affects many different organizations and entities, including health insurers, health care providers, health care clearinghouses such as billing companies, and other businesses that handle identifiable health information. Key features of HIPAA include limitations on the use of personal health information by agencies and institutions for reasons other than direct clinical care (e.g., restrictions on use of data for research purposes), increased access by patients to their health records, increased access to patient data by governmental entities under some circumstances, and strengthened rights of patients regarding explicit advance consent procedures for the release of identifiable data.

RESPONDING TO CONFIDENTIALITY AND TRUTH-TELLING DILEMMAS

Three general principles guide the resolution of confidentiality and truth-telling dilemmas in clinical ethics:

1. Respect for individuals and their privacy
2. Respect for the truth
3. Respect for the law

Although the three principles may be in tension, as noted in the previous illustrations, they often are congruent or can be combined harmoniously within the context of the therapeutic relationship of the psychiatrist and patient. For example, when assessment of a family reveals evidence of emotional, physical, or sexual abuse of a child, mandatory reporting can be integrated constructively into the therapy by 1) informing the parents of the clinician's responsibility to protect the child, including the legal duty to notify authorities about the situation; 2) clarifying what the possible consequences of reporting may be and addressing the parents' fears; 3) inviting the parents to take responsibility for immediately reporting the situation in the presence of, and with support from, the clinician; 4) mobilizing additional clinical services to help the family cope in the crisis situation; and 5) offering reassurance that the family will not be abandoned by the clinician. Through such efforts, it is possible to act therapeutically and to embody respect for individuals, the truth, and the law.

In general, strategies for resolving dilemmas related to confidentiality and truth telling involve several components. These components are summarized in Table 6–1 and discussed further below.

First, it is critical to inform patients of confidentiality issues very early in the therapeutic relationship (i.e., usually in the first encounter) and to explain how the professional and legal obligations of the clinician fit within

---

TABLE 6–1.   Summary of strategies for resolving dilemmas related to confidentiality and truth telling

1. Inform patients of confidentiality issues very early in the therapeutic relationship.

2. Gather additional information and guidance from supervisors and colleagues, especially for novel or difficult ethical dilemmas.

3. Think carefully about who has access to patient data and how much such information is shared.

4. Adopt the practice of revealing only what is absolutely necessary in all interactions outside the clinician–patient relationship.

5. Look for ways to improve how patient information is dealt with in the clinical care setting and clinical system.

6. When dealing with threatening, abusive, or neglectful patient behavior that falls under mandatory reporting laws or with colleague incompetence or impairment, set up a safe and supportive situation in which patients or colleagues may report their own behavior directly.

---

this relationship. It is important to offer accurate explanations of confidentiality protections and their realistic limitations, given the clinical care context. It is helpful to foreshadow for the patient how specific consent will be sought for voluntary disclosures of personal information—for example, in family meetings or to insurance company reviewers. This early foreshadowing is especially crucial in discussing potentially stigmatizing health issues, such as symptoms of mental illness, sexual behaviors, genetic information, HIV risks, and patterns of substance use. In this same conversation, it is possible to introduce the topic of disclosure practices that arise due to legal imperatives, such as when threatening, neglectful, or harmful behaviors fall under mandatory reporting laws. When dealing with health data that might affect insurance or employment status, it is also valuable to clarify the patient's understanding of the impact of disclosure and the clinician's responsibilities for documenting and reporting data revealed in the course of clinical care. With some very difficult patients who may purposely seek to pressure or even intimidate patients and staff—for instance, in some drug treatment programs or inpatient units—this material may be introduced very naturally into larger discussions of behavioral expectations and consequences within the treatment setting.

Second, gathering additional information and guidance from supervisors and colleagues is important for novel or especially difficult ethical dilemmas related to confidentiality and truth telling. For example, a clinician caring for a patient with newly emerging substance abuse problems and a high-stress job involving the safety of others (e.g., air traffic control, military duty) may wish to speak with a specialist in chemical dependence to discuss indicators of more serious symptoms, appropriate treatment-adherence strategies, and professional obligations in the specific clinical context. In addition, to fulfill basic standards of care, all clinicians need to provide patients with complete and timely information about their diagnoses, prognoses, and potential therapeutic options, including the option of no treatment at all. Any deviation from this expectation for truth telling in ethics practice requires careful justification, reflection, and documentation and should be undertaken only after consultation with knowledgeable colleagues.

Third, it is important for clinicians to think carefully about who has access to patient data and how such information is shared. Legally, patients own their personal information, whereas the psychiatrist's health care system or institution owns the actual clinical chart or computerized record. Although this position has been maintained historically, safeguards are being eroded by the existence of large databases (some of which contain genetic data in addition to general health data), insufficient cybersecurity efforts, and robust activities aimed at breaching data systems. Moreover, many individuals legitimately have access to the chart or computerized record in the clinical institutional setting (e.g., for direct patient care or quality assurance reasons), and when insurance releases have been obtained, the numbers of individuals with access to detailed information about individual patients can be very high. In answering the question of who should see or receive information from a patient's medical record, HIPAA regulations offer additional protections to patients when information is sought for reasons other than direct patient care. Clearly, however, personal health information is no longer truly secure in the current technologically rich and fast-paced society.

Other ethically important issues arise when information is given to patients or legal guardians. In accordance with HIPAA regulations, the majority of U.S. states have laws explicitly allowing patients and guardians to have direct access to the medical chart. Sharing of information with patients and families must be understood within a therapeutic framework, however. Wilson et al. (2014) queried 179 family members or caregivers who provide care and support to individuals with serious mental illness—on average for more than 14 years overall and more than 20 hours each week—and found that these caregivers commonly encountered difficulty obtaining necessary health information regarding the ill individuals for whom they cared. The reasons for withheld information included lack of patient consent (46%) and unavailability of a health team member (46%), and caregivers expressed concern that they did not have the information they needed to serve the well-being and interests of the patients. Under ideal circumstances, patients and family members or other caregivers should be given the opportunity to discuss relevant health information. They should be observed and supported during the process of reviewing the record itself, if it is shared. Alternatively, many clinicians will choose to sit with the patient and orally summarize and interpret the often confusing, potentially disturbing entries in the chart. Because the clinic, hospital, or medical facility actually possesses the chart and is legally responsible for it, patients should not be allowed to remove the record from the immediate care site. For these reasons, whenever possible, a secure, supervised area should be provided for chart review in health care settings.

A fourth strategy that is highly important, from an ethical perspective, in dealing with confidentiality dilemmas is adopting the practice of revealing only what is absolutely necessary in all interactions outside the clinician–patient relationship. This practice is important in both voluntary and involuntary disclosures in which personal information is released to anyone other than the patient (e.g., family members, insurers). The approach is also important in gathering advice from clinical colleagues. In general, personal information, including health data, should not be shared with an employer, unless this disclosure is clearly arranged and the patient formally consents to it at the time of the evaluation or is subject to mandatory reporting laws (e.g., uncontrolled seizure disorder in a school bus driver, suicidality in an airplane pilot with major depression). With very few exceptions, the chart and the data contained in it should never be given over as a whole to anyone outside the clinical care team or appropriate medical facility personnel. The practice of tailoring the disclosure to the specific request is important even in cases in which there are legal imperatives (e.g., caring for victims of criminal assault such as rape), because the chart often contains a wide range of personal material that is not germane to the situation and may be damaging to the patient if released. For these reasons, to comply with the law while also affording maximal protection to the patient, the clinician may find it necessary to provide only portions of the charted data or to review the relevant material verbally with the outside reviewer. Even though it may be very burdensome, the clinician's ethical duty to protect patient information is not abdicated in such circumstances.

Furthermore, clinicians, policy makers, and ethicists have reflected carefully on the professional responsibility to ensure health care quality and how best to prevent and handle medical mistakes. The landmark Institute of Medicine (2000) report focused specifically on the issue of medical mistakes and their importance to health care systems as well as to individual patients. Mistakes may take many forms and in clinical settings may have effects that range from essentially unnoticeable to truly life threatening. For the clinician, recognition of a mistake can trigger a number of reactions; certainly concern for the well-being of the patient is foremost in the minds of most clinicians, but embarrassment and fear (e.g., of being blamed or of a malpractice issue) are feelings that also may arise. To ensure patient safety, to continue to learn and improve care practices, to prevent future mistakes of a similar nature, and to minimize the risk of litigation, it is important to address specific mistakes as well as to assess the overall quality of care in health care settings. Best-practice recommendations regarding disclosure of a medical error entail several elements:

- Upon discovering that an error has occurred, the clinician should first take steps to ensure the patient's safety and well-being to the extent possible.
- The clinician should confer with the hospital's attorney and clarify whether there is an institutional policy or approach to disclosing mistakes to patients and their families.
- When speaking with a patient about a mistake, it is important to express regret, to explain the nature of the error, to talk about the known or anticipated consequences of the error, and to provide a plan to follow up on issues related to the patient's needs or concerns.
- It is important to discuss the measures being undertaken to review the situation and prevent similar errors in the future.

Fifth, it is important to look for ways to improve how patient information is dealt with in the clinical care setting and clinical system. Sensitizing health care staff to the complex issues surrounding patient privacy and offering constructive guidelines for the workplace are critically important interventions for ensuring patient confidentiality. Maintaining secure and appropriately detailed personal notes, or perhaps "shadow" charts—with clear notations in the "main" clinical record, including reference to the existence of the parallel, protected chart—is a reasonable solution that many clinicians may employ when caring for patients with stigmatizing illnesses. This practice may be prohibited in many settings. In all circumstances, the main clinical record must document all key information needed to care for the patient. The development and implementation of appropriate procedures to protect patient information contained on computerized databases serves as a second example. Simple measures that health care facilities may adopt include use of passwords and encrypted codes that are periodically revised. Limiting access to those portions of the database that contain potentially stigmatizing information is also crucial. Encouraging employees to position their monitors so that data presented on their computer screens are not visible to passersby may also be helpful on an individual user basis. Similarly, efforts to minimize clinical interactions in public areas, such as hallways and elevators, will help prevent inadvertent breaches of patient confidentiality.

Finally, when dealing with threatening, abusive, or neglectful patient behavior that falls under mandatory reporting laws (e.g., harm to a child or a dependent adult) or when dealing with colleague incompetence or impairment, it is ideal to set up a safe and supportive situation in which patients or colleagues may report their own behavior directly. Individuals who are ill, who have compromised judgment, and whose behavior is actually or potentially dangerous will benefit from a process in which they assume responsibility and take the initiative to help themselves.

A wide range of approaches are available to clinicians in resolving subtler everyday patient care dilemmas related to confidentiality and truth telling (Roberts et al. 2002). Table 6–2 lists guidelines for protecting confidentiality. From the perspectives of the law and ethical practice standards, some of these approaches are good, and some are not so good. Purposefully inaccurate documentation of patient information on an insurance form, for example, is not an acceptable ethical solution to the problem of safeguarding patient privacy. Nevertheless, clinicians may choose, ethically, not to document their *speculations* about a specific patient care situation if they are in the process of gathering information and expertise that may help clarify the issues involved. In some cases, however, even this may be ethically problematic—for example, when legal imperatives relate to clinicians' best judgments in the absence of complete information, such as mandatory reporting of suspicion of abuse. The duty to be law abiding and the duty to be truthful, even about clinical impressions based partly on evidence and partly on intuition, compel the clinician to explore the situation in order to substantiate or discard the hypothesis about the patient and then to act accordingly.

There is one interesting exception in which "deception" has been viewed by the profession of medicine as ethically acceptable: the publication of case studies in which identification of the patient would be possible unless certain historical details are obscured in the presentation. Although it is optimal to obtain prospective consent for writing up a case, explicit consent may not always be possible. In such situations, it is within the traditions of clinical medicine to present cases in a manner that disguises the patient appropriately. This allowance does not give permission for all types of inaccuracies, however. In composing these case studies, it is incumbent upon clinicians to use a minimum of false information in protecting the patient's identity and to alter no fundamental features of the case such that the

TABLE 6–2.   Guidelines for protecting confidentiality

Confidentiality issue	Don't	Do
Patient information	Don't assure patients that whatever they say is confidential.	Do provide accurate information to patients about the limits of confidentiality in their clinical care.
Medical records	Don't assure patients that the medical record—whether printed or electronic—is confidential.	Do explain that the purpose of the medical record is to be read so that optimal care may be given.
Stigmatizing conditions	Don't avoid discussing the difficult issues that surround stigmatizing disorders.	Do strategize explicitly with patients about potential confidentiality problems.
"Tailoring" the chart	Don't use practices that violate legal and ethical standards.	Do consider how to reconcile accuracy and privacy in all forms of documentation.
Significant others	Don't talk to patients' significant others without their permission.	Do remember to inquire about patients' important relationships.
Law and professional standards	Don't break the law or violate professional standards in the process of respecting confidentiality.	Do actively work to change confidentiality-related laws and policies that you think are unethical.
Lifelong learning	Don't neglect your commitment to lifelong learning—including ethical and legal considerations in confidentiality.	Do continue to learn about professional aspects of medicine and share this knowledge with colleagues.
Consultation	Don't feel that you must be on your own when confronting difficult confidentiality questions.	Do seek consultation and direction from other sources: books, articles, continuing medical education, Internet sites, ethics consultants, and ethics committees.

Source.   Adapted from Roberts LW, Geppert CM, Bailey R: "Ethics in Psychiatric Practice: Essential Ethics Skills, Informed Consent, the Therapeutic Relationship, and Confidentiality." *Journal of Psychiatric Practice* 8(5):290–305, 2002. Used with permission.

clinical teaching point is itself based on an inaccuracy. For example, the clinician should not claim that an adult patient is a child in a published report in order to characterize a childhood syndrome. Similarly, the clinician should not present imagined therapeutic processes and outcomes as factual when describing a novel patient care situation in a case report. However, stating that the patient grew up in "a small family in the Midwest" when the patient actually grew up in a large family in the Pacific Northwest, if these factors are not relevant to the clinical situation but can help protect the patient, is, in this special circumstance, viewed as ethically acceptable. When developing a publication of this type, authors ideally will seek advice and collaboration from others in making judgments about how much of the truth to reveal, how much to omit, and what kinds of purposefully inaccurate information to include so as to adequately disguise and protect the patient. In many circumstances, it may also be appropriate for the authors to acknowledge explicitly their efforts to guard the identity of the patient through such strategies in the published report. The fact that some information in the case study is altered must be noted for the editors at the time of submission as well.

CONCLUSION

Psychiatrists have the positive duty to protect the personal information of their patients, as well as observations and findings that arise in the care of patients, except where legal obligations supersede this duty. Psychiatrists also have the duty to tell the truth—that is, to be honest and avoid deception. These ethical duties may seem straightforward, yet situations do arise that present questions for clinicians: How much does the clinician tell parents about the distress of their child? Does the clinician have a responsibility to talk about the likelihood of a health condition with a discouraging prognosis when the evidence is not yet clear? How much information is too much? How much information is too little? As in other ethically challenging aspects of clinical care, it is helpful to gather additional information and guidance and to implement safeguards in the clinical care situation. Through such practices, the clinician can ensure that the well-being and rights of the patient are protected and that the activities of the clinician adhere to expected legal and ethical standards of the profession.

CASE SCENARIOS

- A 17-year-old has been in psychotherapy for 2 years. He has generally been doing well in school and at home but continues to have irritable periods and occasional outbursts of anger that are frightening to him and to his family. His mother calls the therapist and asks, "What is going on with my son?"

- At a party, a stranger physically assaulted a 22-year-old woman. She is evaluated in an emergency room, and the physician becomes concerned about alcohol use and depressed mood that the patient reports occurring over the previous year. Her father, who holds a very high-ranking position within the community hospital, asks that the physician not document these concerns or the circumstances of the assault in the patient's chart.

- An employer calls a community psychiatrist to request information about a worker's mental health and addiction history. The employer tells the clinician that the company is entitled to this information because the company pays for the patient's insurance, and the patient must be in good health to do the job.

- The chief administrative officer of a large health system calls the chairman of the department of psychiatry to request treatment for his 15-year-old-son but asks that the care occur "off the books" to prevent any form of documentation.

- A 34-year-old mother of three small children sees a psychiatrist for panic attacks that began after she was in a car accident at age 17 years. She has been psychiatrically stable for years and requires only semiannual "checkups." At her most recent visit, she tearfully confides in her psychiatrist, "I'm worried about my temper with my kids. I feel like a terrible mother, and I can't keep myself from spanking them."

II

Caring for Special Populations

7

Children and Transitional Age Youth

Jerald Belitz, Ph.D.
Laura Weiss Roberts, M.D., M.A.

Clinical work with children and adolescents—particularly those with psychiatric disease, neurodevelopmental conditions, or behavioral disorders—is demanding and complex. Mental health issues, moreover, are common among young people. Current estimates for the United States suggest that roughly 20% of young people are struggling with a psychiatric disorder, and the 12-month prevalence for children ages 8–15 years for any disorder is 13% (National Institute of Mental Health 2016a). Many neurodevelopmental disorders manifest in the first few months of life, and severe and persistent mental illnesses may first emerge in older youth, bringing overwhelming health needs to families that are unprepared for the resulting challenges they will face.

Inimitable challenges exist for chronically mentally ill adolescents transitioning to adult services. These young adults have required the most comprehensive and coordinated care, customarily including the adolescent, guardians, psychiatrists, psychotherapists, case managers, and other health care providers. The youth is leaving a treatment culture that is often family centered, interdisciplinary, psychosocially developmental, and psychosocially contextual to a culture that is more focused on individually based care and disease management (van Staa et al. 2011).

In contrast to mature minors, these young adults may need ongoing involvement and support from their family. Providers have an obligation to assess the developmental level of the youth to determine the appropriate degree of guardian involvement. Both the adolescents and guardians must be apprised of the confidentiality, privacy and informed consent rules that govern adult care. The Society for Adolescent Medicine (Rosen et al. 2003) has developed guidelines to assist in the transition process. These guidelines call for a specific provider to coordinate the transition, a portable and accessible summary of care, a detailed transition plan that has involved the youth, and identification of the skills required by the adult provider to ensure the ongoing provision of developmentally appropriate care. Optimal care may be secured if the adult program has a self-selected corps of providers that specializes in the care of young adults (McManus et al. 2015). Essentially, the transition process should start before the youth reaches the age of majority and be a collaborative effort among the youth, the family, and the child and adult providers.

When ethical and legal regulations are added to the therapeutic mosaic, clinical work becomes even more challenging. Every state has statutes delineating the legal rights of children and adolescents; however, few professional codes focus on the delivery of services to children, transitional age youth (i.e., those ages 12–24 years), or their families. Psychiatrists and other mental health professionals need to familiarize themselves with all relevant laws and practice-of-care standards, examine their values, and collaborate with colleagues to ensure that ethical and quality care is provided to children and transitional age youth.

PROFESSIONAL COMPETENCE

Each professional code of ethics emphasizes the necessity of practicing within the scope of professional competency (American Academy of Child and Adolescent Psychiatry 2014). Proficiency as a child clinician or researcher is attained through formal education, training, and supervision. Clinical competency requires a thorough understanding of developmental processes in the domains of cognitive, emotional, social, and moral development; impulse and behavior regulation; identity formation; and family systems. It further demands an understanding of childhood psychopathology, developmental disorders, and learning disorders.

Children and adolescents are legally defined as minors and consequently are not sanctioned as independent and autonomous members of the community. Instead, children have parents or guardians who are legally entrusted with the authority to make decisions for them. Both case law and state statutes have confirmed the primacy of parents in the lives of their children. Additionally, adults other than parents are important in the socialization and care of children. These other adults can include relatives, teachers, clergy, coaches, health care providers, neighbors, and social service workers. Also, families are now defined in a multitude of ways.

Because children function in multiple environments, clinicians are advised to adopt an ecological approach in their work with children and families. An *ecological or contextual view* incorporates an understanding of the many systems that influence children, including the nuclear and extended family, educational systems, churches and religious beliefs, community standards, and sociocultural variables such as culture, ethnicity, and socioeconomic status. Correspondingly, clinicians need to learn to be comfortable with and diligent about the task of communicating with the important adults in a child's life and to coordinate the child's care with other professionals and agencies. Clinicians usually deliver care to children as part of a multidisciplinary treatment team. This collaborative approach requires all providers not only to understand the scope of their professional practices but also to recognize and respect the important contributions of the other team members.

Professional competence demands that child specialists examine their attitudes about children and adolescents, young adults, marriage, families, and child-rearing practices. Such examination may precipitate an exploration of the professional's childhood. Professional competence further demands clinicians' self-awareness about their motivations for working with children. Unless clinicians become conscious of these underlying processes, they are at risk of abusing their power with children and families. Therapists may act out wishes of being the child's protector or ideal parent rather than focusing on the child's and family's needs and strengths. This phenomenon serves as a cardinal example of self-gratification, rather than fulfilling the primary obligation of serving the interests of the patient and, when necessary, setting aside the clinician's personal interests (i.e., the principle of beneficence and the virtues of self-effacement and self-sacrifice). Psychiatrists and other mental health professionals who have unresolved parent–child conflicts may unknowingly precipitate clashes between the child and family or develop a nontherapeutic alliance with either the child or the adult. Any behavior that undermines or devalues the child, parent, or family is a misuse of power. Child specialists are obligated to use their assigned authority and power only in the service of advancing the well-being of their patients.

CLINICAL TREATMENT ISSUES

Psychiatric treatment with children and transitional age youth presents unique challenges to the clinician. These special issues involve consent, confidentiality, boundaries and practice dilemmas, and protecting children and reporting child abuse.

In addition to considering questions about consent, the clinician must sort out ambiguities associated with confidential information, parental access to the medical record, documentation about other family members, and defining treatment goals.

Consent

Parental consent or permission is generally required before children can receive medical or mental health interventions; however, existing state laws allow children and adolescents a degree of autonomy in consenting to psychotherapy and other types of treatments. In addition to recognizing emancipated minors, such as those who are married, in the armed services, or emancipated by the courts, many states recognize the rights of mature minors. A mature minor possesses the requisite cognitive ability and maturity to understand the meaning and consequences of the proposed treatment and is capable of providing informed consent. Most states at this time explicitly authorize minors to consent to health care associated with substance abuse, mental health, and sexual activity without the mandate of parental notification. The decision to notify parents is made only when the health care provider determines that such notification is in the best interest of the minor. In a review of state laws, Boonstra and Nash (2000) reported that all 50 states and the District of Columbia allowed minors to consent to testing for and treatment of sexually transmitted diseases, 44 states and the District of Columbia allowed minors who abuse alcohol or drugs to receive confidential treatment, and 20 states and the District of Columbia permitted minors to consent to outpatient mental health services.

Knowledge of state regulations does not eliminate ethical questions in the outpatient care of minors. Providers must use clinical judgment, knowledge of state laws, and professional guidelines to inform their decisions. Parental notification may be circumvented if the minor is approaching emancipation or if parental involvement is likely to be deleterious to the minor. Failure to notify or involve parents may alienate the guardian system and may make successful treatment more difficult. In most instances, parental or guardian contribution will facilitate more effective treatment. Parental awareness and support of treatment is preferable because minors live with their parents and families, or foster parents, and depend on these adults for their well-being. Amelioration of the child's symptoms often requires modifications in the parents' behaviors, and such modifications cannot be achieved without their participation. Also, access to the other systems in which the child functions may not be possible without parental permission. Moreover, issues around consent for treatment become particularly complex when the child or adolescent receives services from a clinician within a health care setting or system and the parent is asked to be financially responsible for the care.

Confidentiality

Only the individual who consents to treatment can authorize the release of confidential information to a third party. With children, the adult guardian who provided informed consent for the treatment has the privilege of approving a release of information. Even when a state statute allows minors to consent to confidential alcohol, drug, or outpatient mental health treatment, minors may not possess the right to authorize the release of information to third parties other than their guardians. In many states, the laws require the guardian of a minor younger than 14 years to permit information to be shared with third parties. Typically, minors can release their confidential information if they have legally consented to their treatment. Virtually every state allows health care providers to share information with other providers without explicit parental permission when that information is considered necessary for the continuity of the minor's treatment or is necessary to protect the minor or others against imminent harm or death. The 1976 decision in the *Tarasoff v. Regents of the University of California* case, which detailed the duty of clinicians to protect identifiable third parties from harm, applies for clinical work with patients of all ages.

Questions regarding the protection of confidential material from parents are more complicated. Many states allow minors to receive confidential treatment for problems related to substance abuse and sexuality. Although many states allow mature minors to consent to outpatient mental health treatment, providers retain the right to notify the guardians when it is in the best interest of the minor. Furthermore, a guardian has the right to access his or her child's medical record, even when the minor legally consented to the treatment. The Health Insurance Portability and Accountability Act of 1996 (HIPAA) allows a licensed health care professional to deny a parent access to a minor's protected health information if, in the professional's judgment, access would likely cause substantial harm to the minor.

Regulations can help inform practice guidelines. They do not, however, resolve the most difficult ethical quandary: When is it appropriate to share confidential information with a parent? The distilled answer: when such disclosure is in the best interest of the child. Of course, determining what is in the child's best interest is a complex process. Successful resolution of this question begins at the initiation of treatment, when the clinician communicates the standards pertaining to confidentiality. This discussion, conducted in a manner congruent with the child's age and developmental level, identifies the particulars of sharing information with parents. At this point, the clinician clarifies whether the patient is the child, the parents, or the family and specifies the professional's relationship with each. As treatment progresses and the child matures, the guidelines concerning confidentiality may be modified.

Younger and more dependent children require a greater measure of parental involvement. Dilemmas usually occur with adolescents, who are struggling with autonomy and identity issues and may engage in high-risk behaviors. It is respectful to explore with adolescents the process of sharing information with parents at the beginning of treatment and again when the need arises. More specifically, this decision to potentially share information with parents entails deciding whether the adolescent, the therapist, or both will communicate with the parent and the context in which information is shared.

When adolescents are apprised of the limits of confidentiality, they can make informed decisions about disclosing information to the therapist. Clinicians are advised to clearly convey their definition of high-risk behavior, dangerous situations, personal neglect, self-injury, and other circumstances that may warrant parental notification. Potential high-risk situations might include substance use, sexual activity, truancy, gang involvement, irresponsible driving behavior, extreme religious practices, unorthodox dieting practices, fascination with guns and other weapons, and illegal behaviors. Undoubtedly, every clinician has a list of dangerous scenarios that can trigger the process of communication with guardians. Central to the decision-making process is the clinician's understanding of the meaning of the specific behavior to the adolescent, the adolescent's view of the parent's capacity to emotionally support the child, and the family's cultural and religious beliefs. Also, mental health professionals need to understand their feelings about their adolescent patients and their own moral principles about the behaviors in question. This ethics skill and other ethics skills of the astute practitioner are highlighted in Chapter 2, "Clinical Decision-Making and Ethics Skills." See Table 7–1 for a summary of essential clinical and ethical skills in caring for children and transitional age youth.

For transitional age youth on college campuses (Balon et al. 2015), the availability of student insurance can provide an opportunity to obtain care

TABLE 7–1.   Essential clinical and ethical skills of clinicians caring for children and transitional age youth

Remain attentive to the vulnerability of children and adolescents.

Hone a broad repertoire of abilities to assess, treat, protect, and advocate for children.

Develop skills to work with families, agencies, and systems.

Strive for self-awareness and courage.

Master information-gathering strategies to help resolve dilemmas.

Seek consultation and advice.

Monitor one's own actions and motivations.

Maintain an absolute commitment to the safety and well-being of the patient.

Source.   Adapted from Roberts LW, Dyer AR: *Concise Guide to Ethics in Mental Health Care.* Washington, DC, American Psychiatric Publishing, 2004, p. 133. Copyright © 2004 American Psychiatric Publishing. Used with permission.

without their parents' direct knowledge of the fact of treatment or the nature of the condition being treated. When students decline the school's insurance offerings and use their parents' insurance, now possible until age 26 because of the Affordable Care Act, parents may learn of the fact of care and even the nature of the condition being treated. This problem with protecting the confidentiality of young people on college campuses has proven to be a barrier to students' seeking necessary health care. In light of the serious issues around suicide among students in higher education in the United States, stigma and lack of confidentiality represent important issues in psychiatry.

Problems related to documentation about family members are also common. Many parents release confidential information about their children without realizing that the medical record contains data about themselves or other family members. Clinicians are encouraged to educate parents about this potential release of private information. Possible options for preventing such unwanted disclosures include maintaining a separate record on each family member, obtaining a separate release of information for each member, or deleting nonpatient material from the record before disclosing it to a third party. Many mental health providers are conscious of this possible exposure of private family information and are careful to document personal information only about the client.

Boundaries and Practice Dilemmas

Clinical work with children presents unique practice predicaments (Table 7–2). An early survey of Minnesota psychologists noted several ethical problems associated with clinical boundaries: accepting hugs from clients, restraining out-of-control clients, giving food as a reward, accepting invitations to significant events in clients' lives, buying fund-raising items, giving gifts to clients, escorting clients to the restroom, and assisting preschoolers with toileting (Mannheim et al. 2002). The child's age and the situational context were the key variables that influenced the respondents' ethical assessments of these behaviors. Generally, these clinician behaviors were viewed as more acceptable with younger children.

Boundary dilemmas about self-disclosures also exist. It is common for children to ask personal questions of the clinician, ranging from "Do you have children?" to "Did you use drugs when you were a teenager?" Clinicians are advised to maintain their focus always on the needs of their patients. It is important for psychiatrists and other mental health professionals to understand the questions within the context of the patients' psychic world and the manner in which the clinician is affected by certain questions and patients.

Competing worldviews held by the child and the parent represent another dilemma. This predicament is manifested early in treatment when the child disagrees with the parent's conception of the problem and treatment objectives. A therapeutic alliance is difficult to achieve if the young person perceives the clinician as an extension of the parents. Effective and ethical treatment is contingent on actively engaging the child or adolescent in the process of identifying the problems, developing a treatment plan, and establishing discharge criteria. Clinicians are responsible for facilitating communication between the child and parent and for mediating differing values and goals. When parents maintain unusual beliefs that do not fit within larger societal norms, psychiatrists and other members of the multidisciplinary team may face very difficult dilemmas. For example, when parents do not believe in the use of medications, the child may be placed at unnecessary risk for serious, persistent, or life-threatening illness. In such situations, the psychiatrist should attempt to find common ground but ensure the safety of the child or adolescent and seek to implement appropriate standards of clinical treatment. This duty to preserve the child's safety may at times entail the use of legal systems to protect the child's best interests and well-being.

Another critical question pertains to the scarcity of resources for mental health care for children. Barriers to care may be concrete, such as the ab-

TABLE 7–2.   Examples of dilemmas in caring for children and transitional age youth

Clinical boundaries: giving and accepting gifts, restraining patients, using rewards, and accepting invitations to significant events in patients' lives

Self-disclosure about own childhood and children

Competing worldviews of child and parent regarding the clinical problem and treatment objectives

Reporting child abuse while trying to preserve the therapeutic alliance

Scarcity of mental health resources and their allocation and use

Source.   Adapted from Roberts LW, Dyer AR: *Concise Guide to Ethics in Mental Health Care.* Washington, DC, American Psychiatric Publishing, 2004, p. 126. Copyright © 2004 American Psychiatric Publishing. Used with permission.

sence of mental health care services in certain rural and frontier regions of the United States, or invisible and poorly identified, such as the obstacles to care for children who are poor, homeless, or recent immigrants or who have multiple problems and are difficult to treat. This pattern is long-standing. As an example, nearly 25% of low-income children in the United States did not have any health insurance in 1996 (Annie E. Casey Foundation 2000), and in 2013, the uninsured rate for children under age 19 in poverty was 9.8% (United States Census Bureau 2014), even with significant health care reform in the United States.

This insufficiency of mental health resources has been identified as a current health care crisis throughout the world. In the United States, only half of young people with mental disorders receive mental health services, according to the Centers for Disease Control and Prevention (National Institute of Mental Health 2016b). Adolescents receive more services than do younger children, girls are far less likely to receive needed services, and interestingly, young people with anxiety disorders were the least likely to receive services (Merikangas et al. 2011). Since the 1990s, the Surgeon General reported that an unnecessarily large number of children fail to have their emotional, behavioral, and developmental needs met because of the inadequacy of early intervention and treatment programs and the lack of an infrastructure dedicated to children's mental health services.

Protecting Children and Reporting Child Abuse

Physicians and multidisciplinary mental health providers who care for children have special obligations to help protect children from harm. This obligation translates to ensuring the safety of children who are self-harming or suicidal or who may be neglected or abused at home. These duties guide treatment practices as well, in that they preclude the use of highly restrictive treatment procedures and severe discipline (e.g., inappropriate use of seclusion and restraint, purposely creating pain or discomfort with the goal of altering the behavior of a child). Since the 1970s, every state has had a statute requiring mental health professionals to report suspected child abuse to an identified state agency. States impose penalties for failure to report and provide immunity from liability against good-faith reports.

As a point of reference, in 2011, there were approximately 742,000 instances of confirmed child maltreatment. The overall national rate of abuse and neglect was 9.9 child victims per 1,000 children. The rates of child victims by state ranged from 1.2 per 1,000 to 24.0 per 1,000, according to a report of the U.S. Department of Health and Human Services (2013). Children in the foster care system typically have experienced abuse and neglect. On the last day of 2011, there were 407,000 children in foster care in the United States. This number represents a significant decrease from the prior decade. Most children in foster care are members of underrepresented minority groups. Finding permanent homes for children in foster care is very difficult, an observation that further raises health and racial disparity concerns for the United States.

Ethical conflicts are most frequently connected to reports of child abuse. These reports challenge the principles of confidentiality and threaten the therapeutic relationship. Often, children and parents feel betrayed when a report is made, especially if the limits of confidentiality were not discussed at the beginning of treatment. Typically, the conflicts revolve around the questions of when and how to report. Determining what constitutes abuse is also difficult. Most states do not specifically define abuse or establish a threshold for suspicion. Local state agencies can provide examples of reportable abuse. Clinicians are counseled to explore their values and beliefs about corporal punishment, shouting, and other discipline styles before concluding whether a child is or is not being abused. The decision to report needs to be independent of the clinician's attitude about child protective service agencies and past experiences with reporting. However, the process of reporting may be affected by these variables.

There are a number of possible options for how to report; for example, the child or the parent may report, the clinician may report in the presence of the child or parent, the clinician may inform the child or parent either before or after the report, and the clinician may not inform the parent about the report. The decision of how to report depends on the provider's assessment of the psychological status of the child and parent and the parent's likely response to the report. It is ideal to integrate the call to protective services with the therapeutic alliance by supporting the parent in his or her effort to care for and protect the child. The guiding principles are to act in the best interests of the child while complying with the law and using every clinical effort to maintain the therapeutic relationship with the child and the family.

Although psychiatrists who do report child abuse and neglect are abiding by the law, they may experience difficult feelings, particularly if a child is then placed outside of the home with other family members or in the foster care system. In addition, new issues surrounding sexual exploitation of children, including young people who have come from other countries and/or are separated from their parents, are increasingly recognized. Many young people who have been sexually abused and exploited, at home and outside of the home, are entering the foster care system, escalating the need for intensive mental health services. These issues are also difficult to confront and may challenge the worldviews of psychiatrists and other mental health professionals. Ongoing supervision and consultation can help the practitioner manage such feelings while developing constructive approaches to care of the child.

CONCLUSION

Caring for children and adolescents with mental illness and seeking to improve their well-being until they reach young adulthood involve clinical and ethical complexities that do not exist in work with older adults. Mental health practitioners who work with young people must remain attentive to the vulnerability of their young patients. Moreover, these professionals must have a broad repertoire of skills and abilities that allows them to assess, treat, and protect children; to advocate for them; and to work with families, agencies, and systems (see Table 7–1). They must also have the requisite courage and self-honesty for this ethically unique work. When ethical dilemmas arise in the care of children, it is valuable to remember the basic steps used in resolving clinical dilemmas: gathering more information, seeking consultation and advice, monitoring one's motivations and actions, and maintaining an absolute commitment to preserving the physical and emotional safety of the child.

CASE SCENARIOS

- Psychotropic medication for a child with depression and attention-deficit/hyperactivity disorder has a known risk of sudden cardiac death.

- A psychiatrist begins to develop feelings of dread before seeing a particular child and her parents for a family evaluation. They were referred by a local school where a teacher has been accused of sexually abusing children.

- In play therapy, a 7-year-old child who has been irritable and withdrawn begins to act out sexual behaviors. She becomes very distressed and tearful, and she appears frightened when it is time for her to return home with her mother and her mother's new boyfriend.

- A 4-year-old boy with autism spectrum disorder would benefit from more intensive health care services, but the parents' health insurance does not cover these services and the psychiatrist works in a small multidisciplinary practice with few resources.

- A 17-year-old is brought to a psychiatric emergency room by campus police, apparently intoxicated and the victim of a sexual assault.

8

People in Small Communities

Laura Weiss Roberts, M.D., M.A.

Special ethical problems arise in small communities, including, for example, family villages in the Alaskan bush, college campuses in Iowa, communities in rural Kentucky, and ethnic enclaves in New York City. Patients in small communities are often isolated, have limited access to health care services, hold distinct cultural beliefs related to health and illness, and seek care from clinicians who are also neighbors, friends, family, or professional colleagues. Clinicians in these communities struggle with problems inherent to the context: helping to overcome geographic, resource, and/or attitudinal barriers to care; choosing which patients receive which health services; deciding how much to say or not say in social situations; providing care for their own child or other family members in an emergency situation; functioning without multidisciplinary specialist support; and coping with exhaustion and stresses.

Ethical dilemmas faced by clinicians in small communities have been poorly recognized and are heightened when stigmatizing disorders (e.g., substance dependence, mental illness) are involved. Furthermore, these dilemmas are not easily remedied by ethics guidelines that derive from larger, richer, and more flexible contexts. Nevertheless, rural clinicians comment on the positive aspects of their work and the important roles they play in caring for patients and families and in serving their communities. Insight into the distinct ethical attributes of small communities and several clinical ethics problem-solving strategies may assist clinicians and trainees working in these special circumstances.

Small-community ethics dilemmas primarily relate to five issues (Table 8–1): 1) overlapping relationships, conflicting roles, and altered therapeutic boundaries; 2) confidentiality; 3) cultural dimensions of care; 4) limited access to clinical care, mental health, and ethics resources; and 5) special stresses of small-community clinicians.

OVERLAPPING RELATIONSHIPS

Overlapping relationships are the rule rather than the exception in small towns—for example, the doctor and the patient grew up on neighboring farms; the clinic nurse attended high school with the patient's daughter; the office manager and the patient are members of the same church; and the patients all talk to one another in the coffee shop while waiting for their appointments. Medical schools and college campuses resemble small towns in that the student may need to seek care from a faculty supervisor or through an undergraduate advisor—that is, someone who plays an important educational role in the student's life and may greatly influence future professional opportunities. Especially in more remote, tightly knit, or restricted communities, health providers routinely interact with patients in nonmedical, overlapping roles.

In one poignant example, a patient drove several hours to a university hospital emergency room for help with a substance abuse problem. He said that he could not seek care at home because his aunt worked at the mental health clinic. The distance this man traveled to obtain care ultimately became burdensome to him and was identified as a reason for the patient's nonadherence with subsequent treatment. The overlapping role with a clinical staff member in this case led to a series of significant barriers for necessary care.

Overlapping relationships are ethically complex because they bring differing roles, duties, and motivations to clinician–patient interactions. Instead of focusing exclusively on the well-being of the patient, for instance, small-community clinicians may feel caught between serving the needs of the patient and responding to the needs of their shared community. This issue of overlapping relationships is apparent in the example of a physician, living adjacent to a rural Native American reservation, who discovered that his patient, a very powerful tribal council member, had sexually abused a number of children nearby. The physician complied with the mandatory reporting law in that state, even though he knew that the tribal council, his

TABLE 8–1. Small-community ethical problems and solutions

Issue	Problem areas	Solutions
Overlapping relationships: complex and differing roles, duties and motivations brought to clinician–patient relationship	Personal and professional roles routinely overlap in community life. Clinicians may be caught in binds between serving needs of patient and community. Clinicians may have difficulty maintaining therapeutic boundaries.	Educate office staff and colleagues about problems with personal and professional relationships in small communities. Establish backup arrangements so that team members may be excused from sensitive situations. Build a reciprocal referral network in neighboring communities. Discuss overlapping relationships with patients to minimize impact on care, and separate conflicting roles where possible.
Confidentiality: respect for patient privacy	Patients may be uncomfortable seeking treatment for stigmatizing conditions as a result of overlapping relationships. Office breaches of confidentiality cause harm to patient, such as loss of respect or employment. Patients may not seek care or may leave care prematurely, and the duty to continually keep secrets may cause physicians to feel isolated.	Implement confidentiality routines (e.g., keep charts and computer screens out of sight, discuss patient care only behind closed doors, use shadow charts and encoding). Follow up on leaks of information to reinforce policies for protecting patient privacy. Provide medical and mental health services through a single clinic to avoid stigma.

TABLE 8–1.   Small-community ethical problems and solutions (*continued*)

Issue	Problem areas	Solutions
Cultural issues: values and beliefs affecting recognition of illness, pursuit of care, perception of consent, medical preferences, and views of clinicians and treatment	Mental illnesses may not be culturally sanctioned or may be defined alternatively, and degree of truth telling and decision making may differ among cultural groups. Ethical mistakes may arise through ignorance or disregard of cultural values. An overemphasis on cultural values may lead to ethical mistakes and the erosion of professional values.	Enlist the help of community leaders to design culturally effective approaches. Be aware of influence of personal cultural beliefs for the clinical role without losing one's cultural identity. Address clinical mistakes in a culturally congruent manner. Communicate decisions, especially when they are at odds with community standards and when the values underlying them are a manifestation of medical necessity and professional integrity.
Limited access to clinical care: resource limitations in continuity of care, effectiveness of service, and ability and willingness of patients to use services	Rural areas may lack emergency, urgent care, or specialty care facilities or clinicians. Nonphysician providers have increased responsibility without additional training. Few hospital-based supports—such as ethics committees and consultants and multidisciplinary teams—are available. Distance, ethnic and language differences, time of year, and physician openness to alternative treatments all affect actual use of services.	Develop collegial relationships for support and guidance. Use the Internet and video conferencing to build a consultation network. Advocate for and educate others about rural health needs.

TABLE 8–1. Small-community ethical problems and solutions *(continued)*

Issue	Problem areas	Solutions
Small-community clinician stress: unique stresses as a result of overlapping roles, long hours, little support, and isolation	Clinicians who follow their own ethical guidelines may risk ethical and/or legal problems. Because specialists often are not available, physicians may practice outside of their expertise. Clinician and resource shortages may lead to burnout and cynicism. Overlapping roles and distance may result in personal and professional isolation.	Identify and minimize career-related stresses and role conflicts. Balance practice patterns and caseloads. Advocate for and educate others about rural health needs. Develop adequate backup coverage to allow vacations. Attend to self-care, including physical, emotional, and social health.

Source. Adapted from Roberts LW, Dyer AR: *Concise Guide to Ethics in Mental Health Care.* Washington, DC, American Psychiatric Publishing, 2004, pp. 169–171. Copyright © 2004 American Psychiatric Publishing. Used with permission.

employer, and his neighbors and friends in the broader community would be divided about the decision. This problem of overlapping relationships is also apparent in the example of a medical school clerkship director who works in a student health clinic and determines that a student-patient has a serious substance dependence problem. Intervening therapeutically, fulfilling mandatory reporting requirements for the state and for the institution, and evaluating the student academically in a fair manner, taken together, are very challenging. In both of these situations, the clinician may make a number of ethical errors of omission (e.g., overlooking the problems identified or failing to report them in compliance with the law) or commission (e.g., using or talking about sensitive personal information derived from the patient encounter in other contexts).

Overlapping relationships also generate ethical problems because of conflicting roles and their adverse effects on treatment boundaries. As described in Chapter 3, "The Tradition of the Psychotherapeutic Relationship," *treatment boundaries* are defined as the rules and conduct that establish the professional relationship as distinct from other relationships and as fundamentally respectful and protective of patients. In some small villages, clinicians must seek goods and services from patients; indeed, bartering or bickering over prices is often part of the community culture. Typically, the nature of the relationship between buyer and seller influences the terms and process of negotiation. In such circumstances, it is difficult to address the inequalities of the clinician–patient relationship squarely and in a manner that is not exploitative. In one situation, an Alaskan psychiatrist was asked to perform forensic evaluations of his patients for the state court system because no other doctoral-level mental health professional was available in the region. He felt conflicted about acting as a dual agent in this way, because his opinions offered in the service of the court would directly affect the sentencing process. Because of such pressures associated with overlapping roles in small communities, physicians may ultimately—if unknowingly—serve interests and concerns other than those of their patients. In addition, because guidelines followed by centralized licensing boards and nationally based professional organizations may not reflect attunement to the small-community context, clinicians in small communities may be judged by incorrect standards when claims of ethical misconduct arise.

CONFIDENTIALITY

Respect for patient privacy—a crucial element of trust in the clinical relationship (see Chapter 6, "Confidentiality and Truth Telling")—is often tested in small communities. As one rural inhabitant remarked, "We may not have a lot of people, but we sure do have a lot of talk!" Another person who grew up in a small town commented, "Everybody watches who goes into the clinic on Wednesdays when the mental health counselor visits.... Heaven forbid that you get a sore throat on Tuesday night!" Particularly when stigmatizing health issues emerge, such as those associated with mental illness, sexuality, relationship stresses, or substance use, small-community residents may become acutely uncomfortable with the prospect of disclosing intimate information to their clinicians. Even when patients overcome this barrier, they may reasonably fear that office staff will learn of their personal health concerns. This is true for rural patients in the doctor's office and college professors at the university health clinic alike. Moreover, it may be a realistic worry, because losses—ranging from respect to employment—may result from confidentiality breaches in the context of a small, closed community. Because of these concerns, patients may not seek necessary care or they may later be lost from the therapeutic alliance. This may be the case even for patients with very serious disorders. This poorly recognized barrier to care was shown in a survey study of 160 multidisciplinary clinicians in Alaska and New Mexico, in which clinicians in communities of less than 2,500 people expressed greater agreement with the statement that confidentiality concerns interfere with patients' willingness to talk openly about sensitive issues (Roberts et al. 2003b).

CULTURAL DIMENSIONS OF CARE

Cultural issues influence health care in small-community contexts (see Chapter 10, "People From Culturally Distinct Populations"). Cultural values and beliefs affect recognition of illness, pursuit of care, perceptions of informed consent, expression of medical preferences, and attitudes toward clinicians and health care interventions. Certain forms of mental illness are not recognized or even given a name in some cultures. Alternative explanations or attributions are proffered instead; for example, a depressed person might be said to lack "moral fiber," or a psychotic person might be said to have "witch sickness" because of a spiritual imbalance or problem within the larger community or because the person failed to undergo ritual cleansing after having come into contact with a corpse.

Similarly, how clinical information and guidance are disclosed varies among rural populations. For instance, definitions of physical and psychological health were explored among 62 men and women from 13 rural counties in Montana (Weinert and Long 1987). The investigators noted that individuals in this group defined health as "the ability to work or to be productive in one's role. Ranchers and farmers stated that pain would be

tolerated for extended periods so long as it did not interfere [with work]....
Mental health problems were rarely mentioned" (p. 452). Indeed, individuals from different cultural backgrounds differ in their views of pain, stoicism, concepts of disease, etiological explanations for sicknesses, patterns of use of folk healers and alternative medicines, tolerance of illness, and acceptance of technological interventions.

The ethical principles of respect for persons and justice necessitate that care provided in small communities reflect attunement to the cultural beliefs and expectations of both the patient and the community. Cultural ethical mistakes may arise when clinicians manifest unawareness of or disregard for indigenous values and behaviors by, for example, interfering with a healing ceremony, failing to work with the natural supports within families and communities, inappropriately interpreting interpersonal cues on the mental status examination, or disregarding a patient's choices and personal beliefs.

A second kind of ethical mistake may occur when the clinician overemphasizes indigenous values to the point of diminishing the clinician's professional values and ethics—values and ethics that admittedly have derived from the larger culture but are the basic guideposts for decision making in most clinical situations. This emphasis, which some authors have referred to as romanticizing different cultures, may lead to underdiagnosis and poor treatment of patients, as described in Chapter 10. It also may give rise to inadvertent collusion with the maladaptive behaviors and coping problems of the patient. Examples include not confronting the therapy patient who often arrives late for or misses appointments because the behavior is ascribed to cultural factors, or missing observable cues of depression (e.g., restricted affect, poor eye contact) because they are culturally congruent. These cultural considerations are clinical hypotheses to be tested. Moreover, they fall within the purview of psychiatric clinical ethics because of the heightened responsibility of mental health providers to be attuned to the concerns and experiences of patients in the context of serving their health and well-being. Beyond this, mental health providers have a special responsibility to observe themselves in the therapeutic interaction and therefore to monitor their assumptions about cultural influences on patient care.

LIMITED ACCESS TO CLINICAL CARE, MENTAL HEALTH, AND ETHICS RESOURCES

Resource limitations generate numerous ethical problems for psychiatrists and other clinicians in small communities. Obstacles to health care access include limitations in the continuum of services, relative effectiveness of services, actual use of services, willingness to use services, and ability to use services. Many rural areas, for example, do not have emergency, urgent care, or specialty care facilities. Rural areas have physician shortages; as noted by Khazan (2014), "About a fifth of Americans live in rural areas, but barely a tenth of physicians practice there." As a result, rural nurses often have expanded roles and responsibilities, with greater autonomy and the need for extensive knowledge but with less training and fewer resources than urban nurses. Nurses and nursing assistants, physician assistants, social workers and aides, and "deputized" local citizens often serve as care providers in small communities. In frontier villages in the United States, a patient's entire treatment team may consist of family members who have no training and little support from care providers. Problems related both to professional responsibility and personal exhaustion commonly arise for individuals when keeping watch over suicidal, manic, or psychotic patients under such circumstances.

Many small communities also do not have hospitals or hospital-based supports, including specialty consultants who can help improve clinical standards of care. Relative effectiveness of care may be limited by poor multidisciplinary care services, which can lead, for example, to insufficient physical and psychological therapies and/or late detection of illness. Willingness to pursue and accept care and the actual use of services may be affected by a wide variety of factors, such as the ethnicity and cultural background of the care providers, perceived quality of past treatment, time of year (e.g., harvest season), language(s) spoken in the clinic, and attitudinal factors such as the clinician's acceptance of alternative healing practices (Chipp et al. 2011; Henderson et al. 1997; Roberts et al. 2005c, 2007). Rural patients have been found to be twice as likely as urban patients to have to travel for over 30 minutes to reach their usual source of health care. Rural clinics may also be less well equipped than urban centers to handle the special requirements of disabled patients. Rural clinicians may hesitate to send patients far from home for serious medical conditions because of the absence of supports in these distant cities; their patients may not have transportation or money for such outside care. These rural health care attributes affect patients' ability to use services. Overall, access considerations have become more severe as managed care companies and capitated care systems have entered rural areas. Many similar problems are mirrored in urban areas with distinct subpopulations, such as immigrants or religious groups. In response to such resource limitations, clinicians may be forced to provide care outside of their usual areas of expertise, a practice that poses risk for both clinical and ethical errors. Greater attention to care issues in small communities or subcommunities in large urban areas is thus critical in terms of the fair distribution of medical resources, a key social justice issue in the United States.

Ethically sound care in complex cases often entails a consultative process with a bioethics committee, an ethics or legal expert, or a knowledgeable colleague. Ethics review processes, both formal and informal, are not readily available in many small-community situations, however. Ethics committees do not exist in most small-town hospitals and clinics, and when they do, these groups grapple with the same overlapping-role and role-conflict issues, confidentiality problems, and other dilemmas of rural providers. Ethics experts and specialist colleagues, peers, and supervisors may not always be available in isolated areas. Even in urban small communities, outside consultants may not appreciate the subtleties of the patient's immediately surrounding culture and expectations or the small-community clinician's special conflicts.

Psychiatrists and other clinicians in these areas often feel that sources of information on identifying and resolving clinical ethical dilemmas (e.g., bioethics literature, forensic textbooks, professional ethics codes) are so "out of touch" or incongruent with the realities of the small-community context that they are unhelpful. Because of these problems, small-community clinicians sometimes develop guidelines for resolving ethical problems. Because these innovative "solutions" may deviate from national standards, these factors place the small-community practitioner at risk for true ethical misjudgments as well as complaints of perceived misconduct. Consequently, greater availability of ethics resources and special efforts to address the dilemmas encountered by small-community clinicians may help bring about problem-solving strategies that may differ with approaches in other communities but do not violate basic ethics principles and professional values held more widely throughout medicine.

STRESSES OF SMALL-COMMUNITY CLINICIANS

Although small-community psychiatrists and other clinicians are highly valued individuals, they experience unique stresses from their overlapping roles, rigorous daily work responsibilities in the absence of adequate support and expertise, and personal and professional isolation (Bonham et al. 2014; Roberts et al. 1999a). Relentless visibility and limited time and health care access may be poorly appreciated obstacles to self-care for rural clinicians. Exhaustion, burnout, cynicism, and impairment are predictable outcomes of such stresses. These factors, in turn, may contribute to the short tenure and frequent relocation of rural practitioners. Positive protective forces such as community support, hardiness, and affirmation of the clinician's professional role may help mitigate these pressures. Nevertheless, from an ethics perspective, these context-driven stresses may narrow the repertoire of problem-solving approaches that a clinician may draw upon in comparison with other situations that have more opportunities for reflection, management of stress, and expert supervision and consultation.

CONSTRUCTIVE APPROACHES

Small-community clinicians are highly dedicated individuals—people who undertake the special challenges of their situation, often in fulfillment of deeply held personal and professional values. Small-community practitioners often feel a special commitment to promoting the processes of health and recovery seen throughout their communities. These thoughtful clinicians continually create constructive approaches to the therapeutic relationship dilemmas, problems of limited resources, stresses, and moral binds they experience.

Positive strategies for dealing with ethical dilemmas in small-community settings are several. Many of the solutions discussed further below are listed in Table 8–1, which appeared earlier in this chapter.

First, maintaining relationships with colleagues in other geographic and specialty areas will help lessen the sense of isolation and disconnection from the profession. Connection is very important, because colleagues with clinical, legal, or ethics expertise (e.g., on hospital-based ethics committees) are often not available in small communities to provide information, guidance, or support for small-community care providers. Participating in telehealth projects and postgraduate and continuing education activities are also valuable for learning about evolving clinical and ethical standards of care. Building a network of multidisciplinary experts through innovative technology such as the Internet and telemedicine will allow for consultation or referral on difficult cases. In this process, seeking to educate colleagues regionally and nationally about the challenges of small-community care is critically important. Active involvement with consumer groups, professional organizations, local leaders, and agency representatives may help bring attention and resources to underserved communities. Moreover, advocating for health service resources and suggesting adaptive and appropriate revisions of extant ethics guidelines can help future clinicians who serve in small-community settings. Increasing awareness of the issues will help these practitioners deal with the distress and aloneness they may experience as a result of ethical complexities inherent to their situation.

Second, when it is necessary to take actions that would appear to differ from national ethics standards, it is important to think through the reasons and implications of this choice from an ethical perspective. Furthermore, it is optimal to take several steps to ensure that patients are sufficiently safeguarded. For instance, in an interdependent frontier community, accepting gifts or bartering for services may be fundamental to the shared life and practices of the community. Even so, there may be gifts that are too large to accept ethically or individuals from whom services and resources should not be traded because of the specific unequal nature of the professional–patient relationship. In such situations where urban ethics rules and guidelines are not readily applied, the processes by which the rural clinician seeks to act ethically gain immense importance. Important process steps for ethical clinicians include comparing their practices with those of other rural and frontier clinicians, seeking consultation from trusted colleagues, developing written clinic policies, documenting decisions, and accurately disclosing what they have chosen to do.

Third, proactively addressing the interconnected issues of overlapping roles and confidentiality is very important for small-community clinicians. Talking with office staff and multidisciplinary team members about the ethical problems associated with personal and professional relationships in small communities, for instance, is a crucial measure employed by many wise rural clinicians. In this process, it is important to follow up on any leaks or slips of patient information that may occur so that the message of protecting patients is unambiguous. Creating backup arrangements so that members of the clinical care team may excuse themselves from sensitive situations such as caring for family members, without leaving their colleagues in the lurch, is important for patients and colleagues. At times, it may be necessary to refer patients to receive care in neighboring communities. Over time, it may be possible to build collaborative networks of reciprocal care across communities to help in such situations. Conscientious clinicians will also remain attentive to the impact of overlapping roles on the patient perspective—how patients may feel apprehensive about the conflicts associated with these roles and how these conflicts may create barriers to pursuing or accepting care. Talking through the challenges of overlapping relationships with patients is also constructive. Efforts to separate personal and professional roles to whatever extent is possible will help with these conflicts. Psychiatrists may wish to address their patients on a first-name basis at the post office or the ballpark, for instance, but choose to talk with their patients on a more formal basis at the clinic (e.g., calling them Mrs. Jones or Mr. McDonald).

Efforts to address confidentiality in small communities ranging from the medical school student health clinic to a Native American pueblo include careful confidentiality routines, such as keeping computer screens and private records out of sight; conducting telephone conversations (e.g., to the pharmacy or a consulting clinician) behind closed doors; maintaining separate, shadow charts when necessary; and encoding patient material in both written charts and computer databases. It is helpful when medical and psychiatric or psychological services are both available through a single clinic so that the stigma associated with the need for mental health care is minimized.

Fourth, the psychiatrist or other mental health professional should enlist the help of leaders in the community in building effective strategies for dealing with the specific cultural and mental health issues that are faced. Clinicians who are new to a community should expect a period of intensive learning and testing initially. Psychiatrists who seek to understand their community's history and their patients' authentic concerns will often be well accepted, if only from necessity, even if the clinicians come from personal backgrounds that are very different from those of their patients. Indeed, it is not necessary for clinicians to blend in or to lose their identity in order to be an effective doctor or healer. It is nevertheless essential to have a sense of their own cultural beliefs and to reflect on the influence of those beliefs in the clinician–patient relationship. Fidelity to the well-being of the patient in the context of the patient's background and value system is often the key to this process. Consequently, small-community clinicians need to remain flexible—but to a limit. For instance, if the psychiatrist is asked, implicitly or explicitly, to make choices that vary greatly from other communities' standards, it will be important to obtain supervision and support from colleagues. When making decisions that are at odds with the preferences of the community, it will be important to communicate the values and restrictions that underlie these decisions. Framing the decisions as reflections of clinical necessity or as manifestations of professional integrity will at least help the community to understand what is happening. Moreover, addressing clinical mistakes in a culturally congruent manner will do much to establish the credibility of the small-community practitioner. Finally, for psychiatrists or other mental health professionals who have grown up or practiced for a long time in a particular community, it will be necessary to think through and periodically reconsider their assumptions about cultural expectations, which may be rapidly evolving given the growing influence of urban values through media and other avenues of communication. In this context, small-community practitioners will also need to be mindful of the cultural significance of their clinical role for their patients by virtue of their ethnicity, gender, age, urban training and education, community status, and other personal attributes.

Finally, personal self-care is an important professional task for small-community clinicians. Identifying and minimizing career-related stresses, pursuing ways of reducing role conflicts, balancing caseload and pacing practice patterns, taking vacations, developing adequate backup coverage approaches, obtaining personal health care such as annual physical examinations, and other activities are crucial. These efforts will help the practitioner to be emotionally and physically healthy and to remain able to do the hard work of small-community care.

CONCLUSION

Small communities present special ethical dilemmas. Wise practitioners identify distinct and constructive strategies for fulfilling ethical standards of care despite resource obstacles, confidentiality concerns, cultural issues, extended roles, and overlapping relationships.

CASE SCENARIOS

- A school counselor in a very small community in Idaho develops a serious problem with alcohol. The nearest treatment center is located 200 miles away.

- A woman tells the physician assistant that she has felt suicidal. The clinic receptionist is her next-door neighbor.

- The only therapist in an Alaskan village must purchase all of his essential goods from patients or family members of patients.

- A scientist working for a government laboratory is afraid to seek treatment for a recurring cocaine problem. He informally asks the occupational health physician, whom he trusts, for the name of a psychiatrist. Fearful of losing his security clearance, he asks that the occupational health physician make no mention of his request to anyone and that the physician not document the referral in his records.

- The only doctor in a remote community believes that one of his patients is developing postpartum psychosis. Because he does not feel competent to treat her, he calls the nearest university medical center to see if he can arrange a consultation.

9

Veterans

Honor Hsin, M.D., Ph.D.

Laura Weiss Roberts, M.D., M.A.

Since classical antiquity, the citizen-soldier has played a pivotal role in society. In the United States, there are over 20 million veterans of the armed forces, approximately three-quarters of whom served during an era of active war (Government Accountability Office 2011; Roberts 2015b). Veterans deserve respect given their personal sacrifices for the country, and society has a reciprocal obligation to provide former service members with access to high-quality care and benefits. As patients, veterans possess unique mental health needs, with recent estimates of about 2 million veterans receiving mental health care from the U.S. Department of Veterans Affairs (VA) alone; an increasing percentage of these individuals served in the recent combat theaters of Afghanistan and Iraq. According to VA estimates, approximately 22 veterans die from suicide per day (Kemp and Bossarte 2012). Mental health clinicians, therefore, have an ethical duty to treat veterans with special care, in recognition of both their service to the nation and their distinct clinical circumstances.

In this chapter we begin with a broad overview of the veteran population and special demographic considerations, followed by a discussion of the veteran-patient's unique mental health vulnerabilities and resiliencies related to military service. We then examine how these issues might complicate the standard practice of care. We also describe potential explicit and implicit sources of conflict that a mental health provider may face while caring for veterans. Empirical findings related to these topics are introduced where appropriate, although further research in many areas is sorely needed. In the chapter's conclusion, we summarize an ethical approach to the mental health care of veterans, by applying the principles of respect for persons, autonomy, beneficence, fidelity, nonmaleficence, confidentiality, veracity, and justice.

UNIQUE DEMOGRAPHICS OF THE VETERAN POPULATION

As veteran health care draws increasing national and political attention, epidemiological research in this area has become a burgeoning field. While caring for veterans, mental health clinicians should be aware of three key demographic trends, which are highlighted briefly in this section: 1) the population is at high mental health risk and high suicide risk, contributing to an important public health problem; 2) the population is shaped by preservice selection bias that may influence mental health risk factors; and 3) the population bears a disproportionate share of socioeconomic burdens that may perpetuate mental health conditions.

From 2006 to 2010 approximately one-third of all veteran-patients at the VA received mental health care for a diagnosed condition; in comparison, one-quarter of the U.S. general population is estimated to carry a mental health diagnosis per year. The most prevalent diagnostic categories at the VA are adjustment reaction disorders, which include posttraumatic stress disorder (PTSD) (~11% of all VA users); depressive disorders (~10%); episodic mood disorders, which include severe depression or mania (~8%); neurotic disorders, which include phobias, obsessive-compulsive disorders, and somatoform disorders (~7%,); and substance use disorders (~7%), with significant co-occurrence of disorders (Government Accountability Office 2011). Veterans of wars in Iraq and Afghanistan (Operation Enduring Freedom and Operation Iraqi Freedom [OEF/OIF]) are a growing population of VA patients and currently comprise 10% of mental health users within the VA. In the OEF/OIF patient subpopulation, a dramatic sixfold increase was found in the number of veterans diagnosed with a mental health condition at the VA, from 6% in 2002 to 37% in 2008 (Seal et al. 2009). Prevalence of PTSD is significantly higher in OEF/OIF veterans (22%) than in veterans of all other eras combined (~8%) or in the general population (4%). These numbers do not include veterans who have not accessed VA health services, approximately three-quarters of all living veterans.

Suicide risk is also of paramount concern in veterans. From 2001 to 2009, the estimated suicide rate among VA patients ranged from 34.4 to 39.8 suicides per 100,000 person-years (Kemp and Bossarte 2012). Suicide mortality among VA patients is significantly higher than that for the general U.S. population. Vietnam-era veterans remained the age group at greatest risk of suicide from 2000 to 2007 at the VA (Blow et al. 2012). Among active-duty military members, however, the number of suicides increased rapidly during the OEF/OIF period to an all-time high of 350 deaths in 2012 alone, surpassing the number of combat deaths that year (Dao and Lehren 2013). Tragically, the suicide rate in the U.S. Army exceeded that of the civilian population by the year 2008 (Schoenbaum et al. 2014). It remains uncertain what the long-term consequences of this trend will be as more active-duty soldiers enter the veteran population, but safety is clearly an essential aspect of veteran mental health care.

The veteran population is demographically unique due to the historical composition of the military. In 2013, veterans were overwhelmingly male (91%) and white (83%) and predominantly elderly (55% over age 60), characteristics that alone are well-known risk factors for suicide in civilians (Nock et al. 2013; U.S. Department of Veterans Affairs 2014). In contrast, education can be a protective factor in comparison with the general population, because few service members have attained less than a high school diploma (1%–2%). Most service members also identify themselves as religious (75%), another attribute that may protect from self-harm. Although the military has vigorous health screening processes in place, recent data suggest that one-quarter of active-duty personnel meet criteria for a mental health diagnosis and that most (77%) of these cases began before enlistment (Kessler et al. 2014). Several of these preenlistment disorders are significant risk factors for subsequent suicide attempts, including panic disorder, PTSD, and intermittent explosive disorder (Nock et al. 2014). Therefore, preservice characteristics may play an important role in veteran mental health and safety risk.

Homelessness and unemployment can impact veterans' well-being and mental health recovery after they separate from the service (Tsai and Rosenheck 2015). Veterans constitute 16% of homeless adults in the United States but account for only 10% of the entire adult population. It is also believed that veterans are more likely than nonveterans to be homeless for chronic periods. Although unemployment in the veteran population is lower than in nonveterans (5.5% vs. 6.4% in 2013), the unemployment rate of OEF/OIF veterans is much higher (7.3%; U.S. Department of Labor 2015). Although these issues are likely influenced by the presence of mental health disorders (especially substance use), they nonetheless may perpetuate a vicious cycle of continued social isolation and inadequate access to care.

It is important to note that the veteran population is a highly dynamic one and that new demographic developments may bring new mental health concerns. As discussed in this section, the subpopulations of active-duty soldiers and OEF/OIF veterans are rapidly setting new trends that may impact veteran mental health in the future. Female veterans, for example, constitute a growing group that has served mostly in the OEF/OIF era. The VA estimates that the proportion of female veterans will nearly double to 17% of the total veteran population by 2043 and that the percentages of minorities will rise as well (U.S. Department of Veterans Affairs 2014). Mental health clinicians should be aware of the evolving nature of veteran demographics, which may impact future patient needs.

VULNERABILITIES AND RESILIENCIES RELATED TO MILITARY SERVICE

In their military service, veterans experience unique problems that may affect mental well-being. In this section we provide an overview of some of the special vulnerabilities and resiliencies derived from military experience (Table 9–1), with the caveat that the salience of each characteristic may differ from patient to patient.

The lifestyle and major events of military experience can cause significant stress and may even precipitate mental health problems when individuals return to civilian life. Specifically, an extended military deployment involves considerable disruption to the daily routine and social network of a service member and is a known risk factor for suicide in active-duty soldiers (Cabrera and Benedek 2014; Schoenbaum et al. 2014). Deployment can last a year or longer, recur in multiple cycles, and involve exposure to combat and/or violent acts (Hamaoka et al. 2014). With severe exposure comes the risk of mental and physical trauma, including PTSD and traumatic brain injury (TBI) (Cabrera and Benedek 2014). PTSD can also result from military sexual trauma, which has gained increasing attention in recent years. Although the military has expanded training for some service members to include resiliency skills and cognitive restructuring exercises as a preventive measure, the effect of these interventions on mental health outcomes remains under investigation.

Military culture and values are also unique and may affect access to mental health care (Meyer 2015). In that the primary mission of the military

TABLE 9–1. Unique characteristics of military service

Characteristics of military service	Factors contributing to mental health vulnerabilities or resiliencies
Military lifestyle and events	Deployment
	Combat/violence exposure
	Trauma (mental, brain, physical, sexual)
	Training
Military culture and values	Collective identity
	Projection of strength
	Hierarchy
	Stigma
	Leadership and unit cohesion
Military skill	Firearms

is to provide the armed forces needed to protect national security, the organizational culture is one of collective identity, self-sacrifice, and projection of strength. Hierarchy is also necessary, to establish a clear chain of command. Unfortunately, some of these cultural characteristics (in addition to other factors, such as male gender and preservice values) may contribute to stigma against mental health problems and treatment. Examples of stigmatizing concerns include potential harming of careers, being labeled as crazy, experiencing ostracism from peers, and projecting weakness, all of which may pose a significant barrier to seeking care. In contrast, some aspects of military culture may decrease stigma and facilitate access to care, including strong officer leadership and unit cohesion.

Military service members are trained to use deadly force when necessary and are skilled in the operation of firearms. Lethal means can exacerbate the impact of self-harmful intent, and access to firearms is a known suicide risk factor. The majority of military suicides (61%) from 2008 to 2010 involved firearms (17% by military-issue firearm), a greater proportion than among civilian suicides (Bush et al. 2013). Lethal skills acquired through military service are therefore important safety considerations in the veteran-patient.

ETHICAL ISSUES IN STANDARD OF PRACTICE

The unique risks, vulnerabilities, and resiliencies of veterans suggest areas of possible tension in the ethical practice of mental health care. Key examples include the standards of informed consent, confidentiality, therapeutic alliance, harm reduction, and disability assessment. In each of these areas, practice of care may be affected by a patient's military experience, culture, or skills.

Informed consent relies on the components of information disclosure by the provider, decisional capacity of the patient, and voluntarism of patient choice (see Chapter 4, "Informed Consent and Decisional Capacity"). For veterans steeped in the hierarchy of military culture, the ability to make autonomous decisions may be impacted by perceptions that a clinician has higher status than a patient. In the military, officers possess legal authority to order medical evaluations and certain procedures (e.g., vaccinations) for service members under their command. Veterans who are accustomed to this structure of care may feel deference toward their providers or pressure to consent to treatment, perhaps more strongly if they depend on the clinical organization for care. Further research exploring this possibility is needed. Alternatively, the cultural emphasis on projection of strength may compel some veteran-patients to decline mental health treatment, as observed in studies of military stigma. Voluntarism of veteran-patients, therefore, may be subject to a variety of military influences. The ethical clinician should be aware of these influences and anticipate their effects whenever possible.

Information sharing during the informed consent process may also be colored by military experience. In 1998, the Department of Defense sought to vaccinate service members against anthrax, a decision that sparked controversy over the vaccine's safety and adverse effects (Government Accountability Office 2002). Further investigation revealed that the majority (60%) of surveyed Air National Guard and Air Force Reserve members were dissatisfied with the accuracy and completeness of information provided about the program and vaccine. It is conceivable that military experience may affect expectations of an objective dialogue for information sharing. Without clear dialogue, consent is no longer informed. An early empirical investigation of veterans who consented to participate in medical research found that 28% of patients did not know they were part of a study, despite having signed the consent forms (Riecken and Ravich 1982). Although there seemed to be very little perception of coercion, cases of unaware patients were often associated with problems in information provision (length of consent form, or identity of person obtaining consent). To prevent such inappropriate outcomes, it is prudent for mental health providers to share information accurately and completely with veterans.

After informed consent to treatment is obtained, the expectations of confidentiality during care may be different for veteran-patients. In the military, disclosure of mental health and medical information to commanding officers is indicated when a patient's safety or work performance may be compromised. Officers may also issue a command referral to mandate evaluation of a service member, in which case some clinical information will be disclosed to the requesting officer. A low expectation of confidentiality may contribute to the fear that seeking mental health care could potentially harm military careers. In fact, a focus group study of OEF/OIF veterans found that subjects were concerned that potential government employers may be able to access VA mental health records (Vogt 2011). Clinicians have an ethical duty to uphold confidentiality, and special attention to this duty should be given to veteran-patients who may have preconceived notions of privacy.

This concept ties closely with the importance of the therapeutic alliance between provider and veteran-patient, because low expectations of confidentiality in a military setting may impair the strength of the therapeutic relationship. Other contributing factors may include emotional detachment stemming from a military culture that gives emphasis to mental toughness and anger as adaptive responses. Mental health clinicians may need to pay special attention to establishing trust with veteran-patients, exploring concerns of mental health treatment with patients, and providing appropriate psychoeducation when needed.

Harm reduction—that is, a policy of minimizing potential negative consequences of behavior—has been used in cases of substance use disorder (see Chapter 14, "People Living With Addictions"). The premise is to trade the goal of complete mental health recovery, which may be very difficult to achieve, for more attainable goals of reducing harmful outcomes. For veteran-patients with unique safety concerns arising from military training, another example would be to reduce easy access to firearms (a highly lethal means of self-harm), even if the patient declines mental health treatment. In fact, there is mounting evidence from various statewide programs that implementation of firearms barriers is associated with a reduction in suicide rate and only partial substitution of suicide by other deadly means (Nock et al. 2013; Swanson et al. 2015). Some individuals may view this counsel as conflicting with a constitutional right to bear arms, creating a possible tension between the clinician's ethical duty to protect patients from harm and a patient's inherent values (Swanson et al. 2015). Mental health providers, however, are uniquely poised to discuss the health consequences of gun ownership proactively with veterans. For patients who are at elevated risk of self-harm, clinicians should engage in an open dialogue about the safety concerns of firearm possession and provide appropriate safety recommendations to minimize or eliminate access when indicated.

Another important issue is that clinicians may find themselves in the position of providing disability assessments for veterans. The VA processes over 1 million disability claims each year. In this setting, the veteran is a claimant instead of a patient, and the assessment is written primarily for claims administrators rather than treatment team members. The VA compensation and pension assessment process may elicit tension between two competing clinical values: the desire to advocate vigorously for resources that may benefit a patient's individual circumstances and the need to allocate disability benefits appropriately and justly across an entire patient population. In the clinician's role as examiner, however, the primary obligation is to ensure truthfulness and confidence in the disability assessment. Clinicians should abide by the appropriate standards of practice and credentialing process for these types of examinations, including obtaining informed consent, encouraging and documenting patient effort, and adhering to rating guidelines. Clinicians should also be aware that accuracy of symptom self-reporting may be limited by traumatic injury, as in cases of PTSD or TBI, so appropriate validity measures should be used. These safeguards will help ensure that an assessment is honest so that benefits can be fairly distributed across all veterans.

POTENTIAL SOURCES OF CONFLICT FOR THE VETERAN CARE PROVIDER

In caring for veterans, mental health clinicians may interact with various organizations invested in veteran health. On occasion, these stakeholders may have priorities that conflict with the clinician's goal of providing the best possible care for a patient. Practice within the VA, for example, occurs in the context of a large health service organization with a federal mandate to deliver care efficiently to a population of patients. A focus group of VA clinicians identified resource distribution within this organization as a key ethical challenge, with specific concerns about how resource limits may affect quality of care (Foglia et al. 2009). A nonformulary medication exemption for a patient's clinical needs, for example, allocates resources away from other veterans. Although some providers may argue for a cost-effective approach to resource distribution, there may be situations in which societal or moral obligations are transcendent, as in supporting community-based treatment programs for patients with severe mental illness. These issues remain the subject of wide debate. One viewpoint is that VA clinicians hold dual obligations as providers to patients and as stewards of organizational resources—suggesting that clinicians ought to participate in resource discussions to ensure an inclusive and consistent process of allocation, in addition to providing the best standard of care for their own patients (Foglia et al. 2009).

For health providers who treat active-duty service members, the military can be another possible source of conflict. The mission of medical care in the military is to conserve service members' fighting strength and ensure their fitness for duty, a directive that may be at odds with patient welfare. Redeploying a soldier recovering from PTSD, for example, may not be in that individual's best interest. Clinicians working with service members outside the military setting (including VA providers) do not have an obligation to sustain the military mission but may feel pressured (by the military or their patients) to return service members to active duty or even a combat theater. In these situations, mental health clinicians should perform their fiduciary duty to the patient and advocate for the best possible environment that will ensure patient well-being. When patients wish to return to active service against their best clinical interest, the clinician can frame the discussion as one of informed consent to refuse treatment recommendations.

Some VA hospitals and clinics are affiliated with academic institutions, and consequently some clinicians hold dual appointments as veteran health providers and academic faculty. The latter role may involve additional obligations of education and research, which may draw clinicians away from patient contact (see Chapter 19, "Innovation in Psychiatry," and Chapter 20, "Clinical Training"), but academic positions are critical for training future generations of clinicians and furthering clinical knowledge. Jointly appointed clinicians are in a unique position to balance these roles and to ensure they remain aligned with a common goal of advancing veteran care.

Mental health of veterans can occupy a unique spotlight in the national media, especially on the heels of publicized military conflicts. Clinicians caring for veterans may feel uniquely judged by civil stakeholders, such as political establishments, religious institutions, nonprofit organizations, or the general media. There may be cases in which these stakeholder values conflict with goals of care, such as when an institution disagrees with appropriate standards of care or objects to specific wars. In these situations, the ethical clinician will place the needs of the veteran-patient first and foremost, similar to how pressures from the military would be managed in clinical care.

Values may be personal as well; some mental health clinicians may hold private views about the military or particular wars, leading to implicit biases against treating former service members. To provide proper care to veterans, clinicians need to be aware of their preconceptions about military service. Table 9–2 lists self-assessment questions that can assist mental health

TABLE 9–2.   Self-assessment questions for implicit biases of the veteran health provider

What are my preconceived notions about military culture?

What stereotypes do I have about the military?

What are my beliefs about the military and its role in the country?

How were my beliefs about the military and its role in our country formed?

What are my beliefs about the people who join the military?

How do I feel about the current conflicts?

Regardless of my feeling about the current conflicts, negative or positive, can I separate these feelings from how I feel about those who serve?

Source.   Reprinted from Hamaoka D, Bates MJ, McCarroll JE, et al.: "An Introduction to Military Service," in *Care of Military Service Members, Veterans, and Their Families.* Edited by Cozza SJ, Goldenberg MN, Ursano RJ. Washington, DC, American Psychiatric Publishing, 2014, p. 17. Copyright © 2014 American Psychiatric Publishing. Used with permission.

providers in this regard. Continued reappraisal of these internal beliefs, with clinical supervision as appropriate, may help minimize potential conflicts with the treatment of veterans.

Caring for veterans, especially for those with trauma or PTSD, can be personally taxing and challenging to clinicians. Secondary traumatic stress, whereby the health care provider develops posttraumatic symptoms from clinical exposure to a patient's trauma, has been associated with burnout (Voss Horrell et al. 2011). Mental health clinicians should be aware of this possible outcome, which may interfere with their ability to provide high-quality care. Adequate training, support, and supervision have been suggested as possible means to prevent or neutralize the impact of transmitted trauma. Clinicians who become unable to care for patients adequately due to acquired secondary traumatic symptoms are well advised to seek treatment themselves.

Providers should also be aware of other potential contributors to burnout, including "difficult" patient characteristics such as irregular appointment attendance or aggressive behavior. Caring for veterans who are suspected of malingering or who have comorbid personality disorders may also be associated with clinician burnout and negative perceptions of quality of care (Garcia et al. 2015). Mental health clinicians should be cognizant of these situations and the implicit effects that certain patient behaviors or characteristics may have on their capacity to provide effective care (see Chapter 13, "Difficult Patients").

CONCLUSION

In this chapter, we discussed various important topics and concerns in the ethical care of veterans. In Table 9–3, these issues are summarized and re-organized in relation to the core ethical principles from which they are derived—principles that drive the components of everyday ethical practice.

Veterans are unique as a population and as individuals, standing in special relation to others in society by virtue of their service to the nation. Respect for persons in the care of veterans acquires this additional meaning and behooves clinicians to recognize the unique mental health risks, vulnerabilities, and resiliencies of veterans. Patient autonomy may also need to be accorded special attention by clinicians working with veterans, because veterans may be more accustomed to a military culture of interdependence and hierarchy that could impact voluntarism in treatment settings. The clinician's duty of beneficence involves not only providing the best possible care to veterans but also fidelity to treatment goals in the face of potential conflicts from external organizations and/or implicit biases. The clinician's duty of nonmaleficence can be applied to the important issue of veteran safety and taking appropriate steps to "do no harm" in a patient population with high risk of self-harm. Special consideration also extends to patient confidentiality, a principle that is upheld differently in military settings. Veracity necessitates accuracy and completeness in the sharing of clinical information with veterans and also with the VA in disability assessments. Finally, the duty of justice encompasses efforts toward fair access and distribution of mental health resources to all veterans. Together, these principles and their applications can assist the ethical clinician in navigating complex mental health issues of veterans.

TABLE 9–3. Approaches to care: ethical principles applied to the care of veterans

Ethical principle	Application to care of veterans
Respect for persons	Regarding all veteran-patients with respect given their service to the country, and recognizing their unique mental health risks, vulnerabilities, and resiliencies
Autonomy	Protecting patient autonomy, and recognizing that voluntarism may be shaped by military culture
Beneficence, fidelity	Providing the highest standard of care to veteran-patients, and recognizing possible external and implicit pressures that may conflict with this value
Nonmaleficence	Reducing harm by promoting patient safety, and recognizing that veteran-patients have unique safety concerns
Confidentiality	Building trust in patient confidentiality, and recognizing that such trust may be shaped by military culture or experience
Veracity	Sharing information accurately with patients and the VA, and recognizing that this value may conflict with military culture or experience
Justice	Ensuring equitable access to mental health care and benefits for all veterans, and recognizing that VA organizations have a unique burden of distributing resources in a fair and just manner

Note. VA=U.S. Department of Veterans Affairs.

CASE SCENARIOS

■ A 60-year-old male Vietnam-era veteran with insomnia agrees without question to any treatment his physician recommends.

■ A 73-year-old male Korean War veteran suffering from PTSD does not accept his diagnosis because he is "stronger than that."

■ A 32-year-old female OEF/OIF veteran is afraid to receive therapy for military sexual trauma, because she believes her former peers will find out.

■ A VA clinician performs a compensation and pension eligibility examination of a 25-year-old male OEF/OIF veteran with TBI and feels sympathetic to the client's lack of financial resources.

■ A psychiatrist who opposed the Vietnam War learns that his patient, a 64-year-old male Vietnam-era veteran, participated in gruesome acts of combat during his deployment.

10

People From Culturally Distinct Populations

Daryn Reicherter, M.D.

Emily Yang Liu, B.A.

Laura Weiss Roberts, M.D., M.A.

The marked population increase of individuals of non-European origins, as a result of both births in and immigration to the United States, is transforming the social and demographic landscape. Should this present rate of change continue, it is believed that by the year 2042, the country will truly be a multigenerational, culturally pluralistic society. As this shifting demographic occurs, psychiatrists and other mental health providers must recognize and adjust knowledge, attitudes, and skills related to multiculturalism. Cultural awareness and attunement will become even more crucial to the provision of competent mental health care.

Although traditional standards of ethics and professionalism will certainly endure as the population changes, cultural plurality will create new, complex, and quickly evolving expectations for psychiatrists and their colleagues across the health professions. Nuances in the application of ethical principles are not likely to be universal. For example, whereas the notion of *respect for persons* may be held across cultures, the definition of *personhood* may not be consistent. Physicians may encounter very different views of their ethical obligations in the doctor–patient relationship when caring for people of different ages; ethnic, racial, and cultural backgrounds; faiths; and socioeconomic strata. With greater cultural diversity, basic assumptions around Western medicine may be challenged and challenged more forcefully than in the past. Medical professionals now find themselves in the interphase between traditional ethical standards of the West and the standards that will emerge, and be tested, in the future.

People living with mental disorders can be rendered vulnerable because of the symptom and disability burdens of their health conditions. For people from distinct cultural backgrounds who become ill, other factors may further heighten this potential for vulnerability, such as being away from supportive family, speaking a different language than the majority culture, learning how to navigate novel systems of clinical care, having legal or immigration status issues, having lessened access to religious or spiritual advisors, or having few economic resources. As a consequence, although cultural diversity is not necessarily associated with vulnerability, the astute clinician will remain thoughtful about the additional challenges experienced by people from culturally distinct backgrounds who are seeking or receiving care in settings where they may feel they are in the minority.

MULTICULTURALISM AND CLINICAL CARE

Multiculturalism refers to the concept that human behavior and the lived reality of diverse cultural groups cannot be conceptualized singularly (McLoyd 1998; Sholevar 2007). Within this framework, mental health care providers are asked to critically reflect on the consideration that each individual has a unique story and contemplate how culture and meaning are interwoven into that story and that individual.

Involved in any clinical encounter are at least two distinct cultures: that of the patient and that of the clinician. Patients come to the encounter with culturally shaped biases, assumptions, and beliefs that are not always apparent or accessible to the provider but that can affect the expectations and desired outcomes of the patient. Specifically, the patient's expectations of the physician, reason for treatment, explanation of symptoms, and adherence with treatment plans can all be influenced by the patient's cultural background. The second culture to consider is that of the clinician, whose socioeconomic status, demographics, life experiences, personal beliefs, and professional training will influence the interaction and communication with patients. For example, in the United States, most medical providers are white, whereas certain groups (e.g., African Americans, Latinos, and

Native or Indigenous peoples) are historically underrepresented within the U.S. health care workforce (Association of American Medical Colleges 2012). Even when there are apparent similarities between patient and clinician in race, ethnicity, age, socioeconomic status, or religious background, differences are inevitable and may present themselves in subtle and surprising ways. Consequently, how patients, families, physicians, and other health care professionals regard each other may vary depending on the dominant culture in a given environment.

Differences in worldview between patient and clinician may affect their ability to establish and sustain a therapeutic relationship. These differences may present barriers not only for understanding mental health concerns and creating treatment plans but also for some of the ethical considerations necessary for appropriate treatment. Patients and physicians may have different perceptions of the relative benefits and harms of certain psychiatric diagnoses, for example, or about treatment because of concerns related to stigma.

There may also be negative effects on the therapeutic relationship that derive from overt or implicit kinds of stereotypes and bias. Men from some cultures, for example, may be very uncomfortable with the idea of women physicians. Malebranche et al. (2004) examined negative perceptions of physicians regarding HIV-positive black men who have sex with men. These researchers found that "[p]hysician-negative perceptions of [this patient population of] African Americans as less educated, less intelligent, and less pleasant influence their expectations of these patients to engage in risk behavior and follow medical advice" (pp. 97–98). These attitudes adversely affected the physicians' willingness to educate these patients on risky behavior and to initiate certain kinds of treatment plans. Although accommodations based on background and worldview may be necessary to attain optimal patient care outcomes, such accommodations may be very difficult to arrange in many circumstances, and an argument could be made that such accommodations could be reinforcing negative stereotypes, which has ethical implications as well.

Other studies indicate that significant disparities in the accessibility and quality of mental health services produce poorer outcomes for immigrants and racial and ethnic minorities. Examples include underutilization of psychiatric services as well as poor treatment engagement and retention due to negative encounters with (e.g., racial discrimination, cultural stereotypes, bias) and feelings of distrust toward mental health services and providers. Data from a national survey demonstrate that among adults with mental health or substance abuse problems, 37.6% of white patients were receiving treatment in comparison with only 22.4% of Hispanic patients and 25.0%

of African American patients (Wells et al. 2001). Given the crucial role of the therapeutic relationship in mental health care, where physician–patient interactions serve as the foundation for many interventions, the possibility of such bias must be confronted with courage and addressed proactively.

Attention to attitudes affecting services for individuals from distinct backgrounds is all the more urgent given that specific immigration-related factors have been shown to negatively impact patients' mental health. For example, many new immigrants to the Unites States are refugees or asylum seekers in distress. In 2008 alone, the United States granted asylum to 20,500 individuals and resettled approximately 60,200 refugees (U.S. Committee for Refugees and Immigrants 2009), who were forced to leave their countries due to war, persecution, and human rights abuses. Experiences of torture and trauma, lower education, social isolation, unemployment, and chronic pain have all been identified as strong predictors of emotional and mental distress (Carlsson et al. 2006). For example, refugees resettled in Western countries are approximately 10 times more likely to develop post-traumatic stress disorder than other age-matched populations in those countries and are at high risk for developing other psychiatric comorbidities (Fazel et al. 2005). Moreover, a population-based survey of immigrants by Rousseau and Drapeau (2004) revealed high rates of trauma exposure even among independent and sponsored immigrants (48% of independent and 42% of sponsored).

Although it is important that physicians know about culture and culturally related factors that might influence health outcomes, the encounter between physician and patient should be focused on the individual patient rather than based on generalities, prejudices, and assumptions. For instance, a clinician about to meet a Haitian patient who recently immigrated to the Unites States may make several assumptions: that the patient speaks only Creole, believes in voodoo, is poorly educated and likely uninsured, and will have difficulty with treatment adherence. Assumptions like these are unhelpful at best and may be inaccurate, offensive, and even harmful, given the great diversity that exists even among individuals who share a racial or ethnic heritage. It is important to remember that education and literacy levels, socioeconomic status, length of residency in the United States, degree of assimilation, and specific region of origin all influence how larger cultural considerations play out on an individual level.

Consequently, knowledge about cultural beliefs, customs, and practices and the typical circumstances involved with immigration may be helpful in establishing a therapeutic dialogue between provider and patient in this scenario. Listening carefully and understanding the life circumstances of the individual patient are essential for the clinician to be exceptionally attentive to the problems of conscious and unconscious bias in the care of this person, as a matter of clinical competence and professional ethics.

UNIVERSALITY VERSUS NONUNIVERSALITY OF ETHICAL CONCEPTS

The main ethical values that serve as the foundation of contemporary bioethics are respect for persons, beneficence, nonmaleficence, and justice. Features of these four bioethics principles appear across a spectrum of cultures and are therefore often assumed to be universal; but to the extent that ethics and culture are intertwined, they are culturally mediated and expanded (Table 10–1) (Hoop et al. 2008). In addition, these values appear as rules, regulations, and requirements within the U.S. health care system, lending further support to this notion and also providing additional considerations as to how these values might be interpreted and implemented by health care professionals.

Of these four principles, respect for persons is the concept that presents the greatest cultural value bias because it is most closely associated with Western culture's valorization of the individual separate from his or her role within the community. The formulation of respect for persons through privacy, confidentiality rights, and informed consent documents and protocol reflect this fundamental interpretation, emphasizing full, direct, and confidential disclosure of medical information to patients to facilitate their self-determination in their clinical care. Such an interpretation creates a challenge for universal application, however, because of the existence of alternative values and beliefs. For example, this strong emphasis on the individual might conflict with the value placed on family and community, especially within collectivist cultures such as those found in Japan, China, Korea, Taiwan, Argentina, Brazil, and India. Family members of patients from these cultural traditions may claim a right to confidential medical information as well as a primary role in the decision-making process.

For instance, the direct disclosure to a patient of his or her terminal diagnosis might be considered inappropriate, disrespectful, or even dangerous within some Hispanic, Chinese, and Pakistani communities in which family members actively shield terminally ill patients from knowledge of their condition and assume near complete control over the patient's medical decisions and care (Searight and Gafford 2005). Dealing with an issue such as this is more fully explored in Chapter 6, "Confidentiality and Truth Telling," but full disclosure of "facts" to the patient, meant to be respectful and truthful, represents a commonly encountered example

TABLE 10–1. Bioethical principles in cross-cultural mental health settings: expanded definitions and potential problems encountered

Ethical principles	Expanded definition	Potential problems
Respect for persons	Acknowledgment of and respect for cultural differences	Values differences related to individualism, autonomy, collectivism, and confidentiality; considerations of linguistic support
Beneficence and nonmaleficence	Minimization of negative consequences resulting from cultural differences	Transference and countertransference; cultural stigma of mental illness; underdiagnosis or misdiagnosis
Justice	Maintaining a fair and equitable standard of care despite cultural differences	Modesty versus thoroughness; standards of care versus alternative medicine; standards of care versus culturally sanctioned practices

of how values assumed to be universal throughout medical practice in the United States might not hold in light of the specific cultural dynamics of a doctor–patient encounter. Additional concerns specific to the realm of psychiatry include the possible harms that could befall patients receiving a psychiatric diagnosis due to cultural stigma attached to these conditions, which could significantly affect ethical considerations of beneficence and nonmaleficence. Moreover, there may be tension between maintaining standards of care and being respectful of cultural beliefs and practices when discussing alternative medicine.

Our discussion of such cautions is not intended to suggest that physicians should not uphold these principles in situations involving patients from other cultures. In fact, *it is always the duty of the physician to uphold ethical standards*. Such principles, however, must be appropriately translated to the specific cultural context of each encounter. Because of the possible violations and harms that can occur to patients in these situations, clinicians need to give these principles special consideration as they would in caring for individuals from other potentially vulnerable populations.

CONTRIBUTION OF CULTURAL DIVERSITY TO POTENTIAL VULNERABILITY

Vulnerability refers to individuals in need of special care, support, or protection because of age, disability, or risk of abuse or neglect. More specifically, within health care and health policy, vulnerable populations are understood to be those at greater or special risk of poor physical, psychological, and/or social health. Under this definition, public health institutes like the U.S. Centers for Disease Control and Prevention have identified racial, ethnic, and cultural minorities as potentially vulnerable populations for reasons related to their relative inability to access quality medical care. Many barriers exist, such as inadequate insurance coverage, limited resources, lack of transportation, difficulty navigating an unfamiliar and complicated health care system, language differences, and feelings of distrust and hostility toward health care institutions in the United States due to previous negative encounters such as cultural stereotypes and institutional racism. Specific to mental health, concerns of stigmatization may deter help-seeking behaviors, particularly among Asian Americans due to the strong cultural emphasis placed on the avoidance of shame.

Concerns about vulnerable populations within clinical care and research also come from bioethics and are reflected in the Belmont Report (National Commission for the Protection of Human Subjects of Biomedical and Behavioral Research 1979) and the Common Rule, which together frame and codify the basic ethical principles for human research (as discussed in Chapter 18, "Psychiatric Research"). Both the report and the policy give special consideration to vulnerable populations, here referring to individuals at increased risk for harm and exploitation and limited capacity for autonomy in their encounters with the research enterprise.

Although the context, setting, and aims of medical research involving human participants are decidedly different from those involved in the provision of mental health services, the underlying principles of respect for persons, beneficence, nonmaleficence, and justice invigorate both. As such, applying concepts of vulnerability from bioethics to mental health care settings is appropriate, even critical, for encouraging a more profound appreciation of the significant harms that could befall vulnerable populations, not only in terms of quality and accessibility of care but also in its ethical provision. Many of the barriers identified by providers, policy makers, and scholars—difficulty navigating the health care system, language differences, and the like—that disproportionately affect racial, ethnic, and cultural minorities also place them at increased risk of harm or exploitation. These factors also stand to compromise patient autonomy within mental health care settings.

For example, countertransference occurs when mental health care providers project their feelings and unresolved conflicts onto patients. As Comas-Díaz and Jacobsen (1991) noted, "Ethnicity and culture can touch deep unconscious feelings in most individuals and may become targets for projection by [the] therapist" (p. 392). Therefore, patients from racial, ethnic, or cultural minorities can be affected by inappropriate countertransference reactions. This pattern of reactions can disrupt the therapeutic process, and there is a risk that the patient's interests and well-being will be hurt. Negative countertransference can create instances wherein the provider misattributes cultural explanations to actual pathology, resulting in great harm to the patient.

Case Example 1

A newly graduated psychiatrist is hired to work at an urban hospital, whose patient population includes many Muslim immigrants from Indonesia and Pakistan. To educate herself on Muslim religious beliefs and practices, the clinician reads books and consults with local spiritual leaders within the community. In the course of a visit, she learns that one of her patients, a female Pakistani graduate student, has not eaten in the past 8 days. Because it is the time of Ramadan, the therapist immediately attributes this behavior to religious fasting and fails to recognize signs and symptoms of an eating disorder.

Another risk of poor understanding of a culture and unmonitored countertransference could be transgression of therapeutic boundaries. A clinician may accept an expensive gift from a patient for fear of appearing culturally unaware or insensitive because refusal could be a grave cultural offense, but this acceptance—especially if continued—raises concerns of exploitation.

The patient–physician power differential is especially exacerbated in instances in which physicians not only possess privileged medical knowledge and control over resources but also belong to a mainstream culture to which their patients do not. Patients from cultural minority groups whose values and beliefs are foreign to the society in which they live are at risk of having their perspectives uniformly dismissed, misinterpreted, or unaddressed in clinical care decisions and practices. These concerns are all the more prevalent within mental health care settings, given the predominantly American and European focus of much of psychology and psychiatry. This focus may have significant implications for professional ethics and fiduciary obligations.

An important consideration regarding informed consent specific to mental health care contexts relates to potential differences in the understanding of mental illness. As discussed by Hoop et al. (2008), "Both the clinician's concepts...and the patient's concepts of illness are influenced by their cultural heritage and, in the clinician's case, by the culture and theoretical orientation of his or her training" (p. 361). Cultural misunderstandings or gaps in knowledge not addressed during the clinical encounter may compromise information sharing and hinder the patient's ability to provide informed consent. Obtaining informed consent often will require additional time and consultation. This process will also help ensure that the clinician fully understands the patient's mental health concerns and will facilitate the creation of more appropriate and patient-centered treatment plans.

Case Example 2

A 5-year-old Yemeni boy presents to the psychiatrist with his mother following a diagnosis of autism spectrum disorder. The mother and son immigrated to the United States a year ago from Yemen. The mother is not fully fluent in English but declines a translator. The psychiatrist details a care plan involving various behavioral interventions, and the mother appears to understand and consents. Later, when the boy is undergoing therapy to encourage social behaviors such as direct eye contact, his mother is confused by what is occurring and the reason for the intervention. She is upset that the psychiatrist did not explain the diagnosis and treatment plan to her. In the ensuing conversations, it is revealed that in many parts of her home country, there is little understanding of autism spectrum disorder, and many of the behaviors identified by the psychiatrist as pathological were not recognized as such by the mother.

This scenario illustrates how the principles that inform the ethical practice of medical care might be complicated and compromised in cross-cultural mental health care settings. Previously identified factors (e.g., language barriers, unfamiliarity with the U.S. health care system) that render racial, ethnic, and cultural minority people potentially vulnerable from the perspectives of health care and health policy also do so from a bioethical standpoint. Thus, applying considerations of vulnerability from bioethics empowers providers to identify and improve practices, helping to ensure that professional and ethical standards of care are met.

RELATING CULTURAL DIVERSITY TO CORE ETHICAL PRINCIPLES

Case Example 3

A Japanese American inpatient psychiatrist treats a Native American man hospitalized for grave disability. The patient was admitted to the hospital after living outdoors and presenting with disorganized thinking to an outpatient mental health provider at a homeless clinic. The outpatient physician suspected schizophrenia. The patient reported thought-sharing with animals and auditory hallucinations. He had no reasonable plan to provide himself with food, shelter, or clothing and was placed on an involuntary commitment.

Dismissing the outpatient physician's suspicions, and despite her training, the inpatient psychiatrist does not discuss the possibility of schizophrenia or any other psychiatric disorder with the patient. She worries that to do so would pathologize a culturally appropriate phenomenon. In her limited knowledge of Native American culture, she is aware of communication with totem animals as an important expression of cultural belief. She is also aware that in the patient's culture, speaking openly of negative things, such as the possible diagnosis of major mental illness, would likely be culturally inappropriate. For both reasons, she feels comfortable giving the patient reassurance that the phenomena seen by the outpatient psychiatrist did not indicate a psychotic disorder. The patient is released from his involuntary commitment and not treated with antipsychotic medications. Six weeks later the patient presents to the homeless clinic again, disorganized and psychotic. He has been living on the streets and is unbathed, undernourished, and dehydrated.

In this case, the psychiatrist's limited understanding of Native American culture, resulting potentially from inadequate knowledge, constitutes a stereotype. The fact that she did not verify her cultural assumptions not only placed the patient at grave risk of harm but also resulted in substandard care, violating the principles of beneficence, nonmaleficence, and justice. In addition, the psychiatrist's failure to discuss a psychiatric diagnostic differential with the patient on the basis of assumptions about the patient's communication preferences prevented the patient from providing informed consent, further compromising his autonomy. This case illustrates how the four core bioethical principles—respect for persons, beneficence, nonmaleficence, and justice—can arise in a single physician–patient interaction and provides a lens to examine the specific kinds of cultural sensitivities that should inform these principles when applied in cross-cultural mental health care settings.

In cross-cultural settings, acknowledgment of and respect for cultural differences (i.e., respect for persons) become crucial. Culture is understood as an essential aspect of personal identity; failure to recognize and attend to the role of culture in patient–physician interactions, especially during the informed consent process, could result in a significant violation of respect for persons. For example, mental health care providers who neglect to address cultural understandings of mental illness or who fail to navigate cultural practices related to shared decision making could compromise patient autonomy within these encounters.

Additionally, more comprehensive definitions of both beneficence and nonmaleficence in cross-cultural mental health care settings would include specific mention of the minimization of negative consequences resulting from cultural differences (Paasche-Orlow 2004). These consequences may manifest not only as overt racial biases, stereotypes, or prejudices but also as subtler kinds of countertransference. In a routine clinical interaction, being surprised that a patient's father is not educated or that a patient's sibling is unemployed, for example, could be a signal to the clinician that assumptions are being made about a patient's background. Harm may also result from the stigma attached to certain psychiatric diagnoses and the possibility of underdiagnosis of culturally bound syndromes and behaviorally defined conditions that may be perceived and understood differently within different communities. Concepts of justice ought to emphasize maintaining a fair and equitable standard of care despite cultural differences. Accommodations from providers (e.g., translators) may be required in some cases, but any accommodations should be made with sensitivity and care to ensure that overall standards of care are still met and also to minimize negative repercussions (e.g., stigma of receiving "special treatment").

CONCLUSION

Racial, ethnic, and cultural minorities are potentially vulnerable populations in need of special considerations so that they receive clinically and
ethically sound care. Psychiatrists and other mental health professionals
must consider specific cultural sensitivities alongside existing ethical standards for mental health specialists. Cultural competency is an overarching
model for identifying and addressing cultural tensions that arise within
daily practice and an emerging ethical obligation for physicians, given an
increasingly multicultural patient population.

Of the various definitions of cultural competency that exist, Tseng and
Streltzer's (2004) definition is recognized as one of the most comprehensive
and particularly well-suited for mental health care settings due to its strong
emphasis on cultural issues in psychotherapy. They define *cultural competency* by three main characteristics:

1. Cultural sensitivity: a recognition and appreciation of diverse cultures
2. Cultural knowledge: the factual understanding of basic anthropological
   knowledge about cultural variation (via reading and research, expert
   consultation, meaningful interactions with community leaders/individ-
   uals of diverse backgrounds, and so forth)
3. Cultural empathy: the ability to engage emotionally with a patient's cultural perspective

Central to this model of culturally competent care is physician insight
into how cultural issues affect therapeutic role and relationships. Culturally
competent providers should practice what Tseng and Streltzer (2004) describe as cultural guidance, which involves thoughtfully assessing the potential relationship between cultural factors and the patient's present
medical condition when designing and discussing appropriate therapeutic
interventions. Nie (2012) notes, "main features of this paradigm...include
resisting a variety of cultural stereotypes and stereotyping; highlighting the
great internal plurality, richness, dynamism, and openness of medicine and
morality in any culture; acknowledging cultural differences as well as common humanity; and searching for more appropriate methods of generating
genuine and deep cross-cultural dialogue" (p. 343).

Given the intercultural and intracultural complexities that inform each
patient–physician interaction, what it means to behave in a culturally competent manner in a bioethics context will vary depending on the specifics
of the situation. Nevertheless, these are essential considerations that should
be thought of in most, if not all, situations to promote the provision of cul-

turally sensitive and ethical care. Cultural differences might create challenges but do not change the fact that fulfilling standards of bioethics remains imperative in the service of the well-being of the patient.

CASE SCENARIOS

- An anorexic Hispanic patient develops hypokalemia and cardiac arrhythmias but refuses hospitalization or intravenous nutrition.

- A Native American medical student is seen in the university health center for "stress." She sees a therapist weekly, and she asks that the therapist make no mention of her concerns, academic challenges, or newly discovered pregnancy in her medical record.

- A 15-year-old runaway girl has just been the victim of a rape. She is terrified of the pelvic exam and other invasive aspects of the evaluation.

- A 40-year-old Hispanic male veteran with major depressive disorder and previous suicide attempts believes it is his constitutional right to continue owning firearms.

- A third-year resident attends services at a Buddhist temple. He gathers up the informational material about the temple and its programs and places it in the waiting room of the community mental health center.

11

People Living With HIV/AIDS

Lawrence M. McGlynn, M.D.
Laura Weiss Roberts, M.D., M.A.

In March 1981, at least eight cases of an aggressive form of Kaposi's sar-
coma were identified in gay men in New York City. Three months later, the
Centers for Disease Control and Prevention (CDC) in Atlanta reported on
five cases of men presenting with pneumocystis pneumonia in Los Angeles.
Within the next 2 years, the virus causing these mysterious illnesses would
be identified, and the era of a global epidemic known as HIV/AIDS began,
characterized by not only aggressive physical illness but also debilitating
mental illness. Although the cause of the disease, a retrovirus, became
known and identifiable by laboratory tests, many could not help but recognize the demographic distribution early in the course of the epidemic—gay
men and intravenous drug users—and thereby assign blame and immorality
to those infected. As a result, stigma has had profound implications not only
for those living and dying with HIV/AIDS but also for the HIV-negative
members of the high-risk groups. The fear of HIV/AIDS, and of those potentially infected, took on a life of its own. People would become ostracized
from their families and communities and face discrimination in housing and
employment.

Ethical issues in caring for people living with HIV/AIDS are challenging. Although the virus is not spread through casual contact, it remains con-

tagious and thus the health of the public must be considered. At the same time, strict confidentiality must be maintained to protect the rights of individuals living with the virus. Issues surrounding reproductive choices, end of life, and treatment are also significant. Decisional capacity may need to be considered in those with HIV-associated neurocognitive disorders. Clinical research using human volunteers must consider these issues but also maintain respect, beneficence, and justice. Finally, medications are now available to treat HIV/AIDS and help prevent infection. Although on the surface these medications would seem to be a clear benefit, ethical issues surrounding treatment and prevention remain subjects of passionate debate; these issues become even more complicated in the context of psychiatric and behavioral health.

HIV/AIDS AND MENTAL ILLNESS

The human immunodeficiency virus is the organism that causes HIV infection and AIDS and enters the body through the introduction of blood, semen, vaginal fluid, or breast milk. HIV infects specific cells in the immune system. The CD4+ T cells are one of its targets, and as the number of these protective cells drops, so does cell-mediated immunity, and ultimately the body becomes vulnerable to opportunistic infections. The CD4 lymphocyte count is a quantification of the body's ability to fight against HIV-associated illnesses. Viral load, another important measure in people living with HIV, refers to the quantity of virus in a given sample of blood. When a patient's virus is well controlled, the viral load may be undetectable or below detectable limits. When the immune system is not under good virologic control, such as when a patient is not yet taking medications or not adherent to prescribed medications or when a pattern of resistance has developed, the viral load may be quantifiable.

Soon after infection, HIV crosses the blood-brain barrier and initiates a cascade of immune and inflammatory processes within the central and peripheral nervous systems. Psychiatric illness is not uncommon in patients with HIV/AIDS, and may include mood, anxiety, and psychotic disorders. These illnesses may be the result of the HIV itself, the inflammatory response to HIV, or other causes (Table 11–1). The psychiatric illness may also precede the HIV.

Despite the availability of medications to treat HIV/AIDS, approximately 50% of those living with the virus develop some level of cognitive impairment (Heaton et al. 2010). Most of these patients are asymptomatic and do not notice a decline in their ability to function in their day-to-day

TABLE 11–1. Common causes of psychiatric disorders in HIV

HIV	CNS inflammatory response secondary to viral presence in the brain
Opportunistic infections	CNS toxoplasmosis, cryptococcal meningitis, Kaposi's sarcoma (human herpesvirus 8 [HHV-8]), CNS lymphoma (Epstein-Barr virus), and progressive multifocal leukoencephalopathy (JC virus)
Medications	HIV antiretrovirals, antibiotics, interferon, chemotherapy, steroids, opioids, benzodiazepines
HIV-related disorders	Hypogonadism, nephropathy, polyneuropathy
Other comorbidities	Hepatitis C, neurosyphilis, substance use disorders, primary (preexisting) psychiatric disorders
Psychosocial stressors	Rejection, homelessness, loss of work, financial troubles, death of loved ones

Note. CNS=central nervous system; JC virus=virus named using the initials for John Cunningham, a patient with the virus.

lives. Others may go on to develop impairments in their ability to function, ranging from minor to severe, as in HIV-associated dementia. Central nervous system and systemic illnesses may lead to the waxing and waning pattern of delirium. In addition, imaging studies investigating the impact of HIV on the brain have implicated the involvement of frontostriatal circuitry (Melrose et al. 2008), thus providing a possible explanation for cognitive and behavioral changes seen in some HIV-positive patients. These disorders—psychiatric, neurocognitive, and behavioral—play a central role in many of the ethical issues of HIV/AIDS.

HIV TESTING

One in eight Americans with HIV do not realize they are infected with the virus. It is estimated that this group accounts for one-third of HIV transmissions in the United States (Gardner et al. 2011). Testing for HIV can be a very emotional experience. Until the early 2000s, test counseling and written consents were considered important components of the HIV testing process. Recognizing the urgent need for more people to be tested, the CDC issued recommendations in 2006 (Branson et al. 2006). Very importantly, unlike nearly all clinical testing procedures, these guidelines stated that opt-out testing without written consent should be integrated into routine health care. In opt-out testing, the patient is notified that the test is normally performed but that he or she may still elect to decline or defer the testing. Some jurisdictions continue to impose more stringent requirements in areas such as counseling and written consent, recognizing that opt-out testing does not in itself eliminate the need for informed consent (Loue and Pike 2007; Moser et al. 2002). The risks of HIV testing clearly extend beyond the risks of a blood draw. A positive result may lead to significant consequences for the individual, including social rejection, loss of employment, homelessness, and disclosure to the local public health department. Rigorous debate has surrounded HIV opt-out testing protocols and informed consent. Some ethicists argue that a patient's silence in opt-out testing cannot be interpreted either as assent or as informed consent (Hanssens 2007).

Testing for HIV requires careful consideration of issues facing the individual as well as the community. On one hand, those who may be more vulnerable, such as those with severe mental illness, may not have the voice to decline opt-out testing even if they do not feel ready to receive the results. Reasons and consequences for testing should also be considered in vulnerable individuals. Some may be coerced into getting tested by an abusive partner. A positive result may lead to dire consequences. On the other hand, rates of HIV infection and transmission among those with severe mental illness are as much as 76 times higher than in the general population (Loue 2012; Moser et al. 2002). Not testing, therefore, could lead to even worse outcomes.

Asylum seekers represent another vulnerable group (François et al. 2008). They may be victims of violence suffering from posttraumatic stress disorder and coming from countries where the economy, politics, and social climate are unstable or unsafe. Many may be unsure of their rights and the ramifications of HIV testing, including whether or not they will have access to HIV medical care in the host country. Some may avoid testing for fear of being deported to their country of origin. The World Health Organization recommends expanded HIV testing and counseling but does not endorse mandatory testing for asylum seekers. Ultimately, leaders making the decision whether to enact testing for those seeking asylum (or immigrants in general) must consider both 1) protecting the host country by identifying and controlling diseases and 2) limiting the introduction of diseases that might cripple a nation's health care system. At the same time, care providers involved in testing must recognize the life and well-being of the individual asylum seeker, including identifying those who are HIV-positive and linking them to treatment.

Individuals in corrections facilities make up another population that demonstrates increased risk for HIV infection (Kondo et al. 2014; Rich et al. 2011). Understandably, inmates are hesitant to be tested due to stigma and concern that confidentiality will not be maintained. HIV-positive inmates may be housed in protective custody units. The CDC recommends that HIV screening of an individual be provided upon entry into prison and before release and that voluntary HIV testing be offered periodically during incarceration. By offering comprehensive medical care, including treatment for those with HIV/AIDS, a facility has the opportunity to identify those infected with HIV, initiate medications and education, and ultimately provide linkage to care on release.

In general, facilities offering opt-out testing need to consider the availability of resources for the person who tests positive for HIV and be able to answer the question, "What are we going to do with a positive result?" It is important to ensure access to and integration of medical, mental health, substance use, and reproductive planning services. HIV testing programs should be able to link HIV-positive patients with adequate services.

DISCLOSURE OF HIV STATUS

Once an individual has been diagnosed with HIV, the issue of disclosure must be considered. Forty-one states and the District of Columbia have enacted specific laws, regulations, or directives that require laboratory reporting of all levels of CD4$^+$ T-cell counts and viral loads (detectable and undetectable) of all HIV-positive individuals (CDC 2015). Depending on the jurisdiction, partner notification may be voluntary or involuntary. The CDC (2009) recommends that partner notification should be voluntary and noncoercive. Some states require individuals who test positive for HIV to notify past sexual contacts. Other states require doctors and public health officials to inform known sexual contacts of patients who have tested positive for HIV (Galvin and Crooks 2014; Hanssens 2007). In clinical practice, psychiatrists ideally will encourage individuals who are HIV-positive to engage in safe-sex practices, as with other patients, and to provide support when individuals who are HIV-positive disclose their status to others, including intimate partners.

Issues surrounding disclosure are not limited to personal relationships. Questions have arisen regarding a health care provider's responsibility to disclose his or her positive HIV status in certain professions and the right to privacy of dentists and surgeons—as well as the safety of their patients. Some argue that a patient cannot provide informed consent to an invasive procedure when the HIV status of the health professional is not disclosed. In 1991, the CDC created recommendations—guidelines that have not yet been updated—addressing the issues of disclosure for health care workers:

- [Health care workers] who are infected with HIV...should not perform exposure-prone procedures unless they have sought counsel from an expert review panel and been advised under what circumstances, if any, they may continue to perform these procedures. Such circumstances would include notifying prospective patients of the [health care worker's] seropositivity before they undergo exposure-prone invasive procedures.
- Mandatory testing of [health care workers] for HIV antibody...is not recommended. The current assessment of the risk that infected [health care workers] will transmit HIV...to patients during exposure-prone procedures does not support the diversion of resources that would be required to implement mandatory testing programs. Compliance by [health care workers] with recommendations can be increased through education, training, and appropriate confidentiality safeguards.

Disclosure statutes should balance the health care worker's right to confidentiality with the safety and health of their patients and others in the community, while at the same time not creating a climate in which recommendations around prevention, testing, and treatment are feared or ignored.

At least 34 states and two U.S. territories have criminal statutes or sentencing enhancements authorizing prosecutions for various acts involving HIV-positive individuals, including nondisclosure and engaging in acts that lead to HIV exposure or transmission. Some argue that HIV-positive individuals should be punished for not disclosing their status to sexual partners and that criminalizing the behavior would ultimately promote public health and prevention strategies (Newman 2012). Opponents counter that these policies and laws increase the stigmatization and fear of people living with HIV, and ultimately undermine public health goals.

INFORMED CONSENT
FOR RESEARCH AND TREATMENT

The process of informed consent for research or treatment asks for adherence to specific criteria for the protection of the subject or patient and the investigator or provider, as well as the integrity of the work. The Nuremberg Code of Ethics lays out preconditions for an individual to provide consent (Katz 1996). In addition, basic bioethical principles are commonly called upon as research protocols are developed and informed consent variables are considered (see Chapter 18, "Psychiatric Research").

HIV/AIDS is associated with stigma worldwide. People with the virus, in the absence of any other condition, are vulnerable. Given that HIV/AIDS not uncommonly occurs with some level of mental illness, the stigma is increased even more. As the clinician considers stigma and a patient's ability to exercise free power of choice, many factors must be considered when attempting to obtain informed consent, such as in the following examples: in some countries and cultures, women are not seen as self-determining people but rather as property; some individuals may only be able to access health care by enrolling in a clinical trial; cognitive impairment is seen frequently in patients with HIV/AIDS (as mentioned earlier in the section "HIV/AIDS and Mental Illness"), and the pattern of deficits may involve frontostriatal circuits and dopamine dysregulation; delirium may also be a component for individuals with more severe illness. Because of the potentially fluctuating or waxing-waning nature of cognitive impairment in HIV-associated neurocognitive dysfunction, HIV encephalopathy, and delirium, researchers may need to obtain multiple consents during the course of the study.

Finally, randomized placebo-controlled studies contributed invaluably to the early body of literature in HIV/AIDS. Informed consent in research involving potentially fatal illnesses, such as HIV/AIDS, must clearly convey a thorough understanding of the risks involved in both the treatment and placebo arms of the studies. Given the success of antiretroviral medications in treating HIV/AIDS, an institutional review board would no longer approve the use of an ineffective placebo in a study. Even for studies of preexposure prophylaxis (see the section "Preexposure Prophylaxis" later in this chapter), the use of placebos has been the topic of ethical debates (Kuhn et al. 2011).

PREVENTION AND PREEXPOSURE PROPHYLAXIS

HIV prevention historically has focused on education, counseling, and behavioral interventions, such as the use of condoms and clean needles. New to prevention campaigns is the use of antiretroviral medications, because studies reveal that HIV-positive individuals whose immune systems are well controlled with antiretroviral medications are significantly less likely to infect other individuals than if they were not being treated with antiretrovirals (or not fully adherent with the treatment). The concept of treatment as prevention involves offering antiretroviral medications to HIV-positive people, in some cases before they would normally need treatment. This practice has been adopted in many jurisdictions and clinics and may be useful for HIV-positive individuals, such as those who are actively using methamphetamine or who have cognitive impairment and do not consistently adhere to traditional prevention methods. Some providers, however, continue to follow other standards of care (e.g., not offering antiretroviral medications until the patient's CD4+ T-cell count has dropped below a certain threshold). Treatment as prevention may be challenged on the basis of concerns that responsibility may become reframed, beneficial sexual norms may be eroded, and resources may be wasted on those who do not yet need the antiretroviral medications. Finally, antiretroviral medications have many potential side effects, including renal failure, fat redistribution, metabolic syndrome, and mental status changes. Thus, any debate surrounding the ethics of treatment as prevention must consider whether this policy respects the well-being of the individual.

In 2014, the U.S. Public Health Service released the first comprehensive clinical practice guidelines for a new HIV prevention tool, preexposure prophylaxis (PrEP). The White House Office of National AIDS Policy (2015) released the updated National HIV/AIDS Strategy for the United States, highlighting the effectiveness of PrEP as part of the overall goal of reducing new HIV infections. PrEP consists of two medications used in combination: tenofovir disoproxil fumarate (TDF) 300 mg and emtricitabine (FTC) 200 mg. When taken consistently, PrEP can reduce the risk of HIV infection in people who are at high risk by up to 92%. The CDC led the development of the federal guidelines, collecting input from providers, HIV patients, partners, and affected communities. In addition to developing prescribing guidelines, the group underscored the importance of counseling on adherence and HIV risk reduction, including the encouragement of condom use for additional protection. The protocol also recommends regular monitoring of HIV infection status, side effects, adherence, and sexual or injection risk behaviors.

TDF belongs to a class of antiretroviral drugs known as nucleotide analogue reverse transcriptase inhibitors. It is commonly used as a component in treatment regimens designed to fight HIV in humans and also is used to treat hepatitis B virus infections. FTC, in the class of nucleoside reverse transcriptase inhibitors, is also used as a component in fighting HIV infection in humans. Although commercial insurance and employee benefits programs have defined policies for the use of these medications in treating HIV infection, some have yet to consider their use in PrEP. Public insurance sources also vary in their coverage. The company that manufacturers the TDF/FTC combination has established a PrEP medication assistance program for patients who do not have health insurance, whose insurance does not cover PrEP medications, and whose personal resources are inadequate for out-of-pocket payments.

Although PrEP would appear to be a welcome weapon in the war against HIV/AIDS, some ethical concerns have been raised (Haire and Kaldor 2013). Some argue that PrEP may encourage an increase in risky sexual behaviors for certain individuals. Some also worry that the adherence necessary to protect an individual may not be possible and that HIV infection may therefore still occur. From a resource allocation standpoint, prioritizing the use of TDF/FTC for PrEP rather than for the treatment of HIV/AIDS (including for treatment as prevention) represents an ongoing ethical question.

CONCLUSION

Tremendous advances have been made in the diagnosis and treatment of HIV/AIDS and have led to changes in local, national, and global policy. Many ethical dilemmas continue to challenge health care providers and administrators, directly affecting those living with HIV/AIDS. Some policies may fail to fully integrate the core ideals of autonomy, beneficence, nonmaleficence, and justice. HIV/AIDS and other stigmatized conditions may create feelings of discomfort and fear for not only the patient but also the community as a whole. Policy makers are encouraged to reflect on their fears and feelings as they face the difficult ethical issues in HIV/AIDS so that policy recommendations serve the interests of all individuals in society.

CASE SCENARIOS

- An older HIV-positive man has presented with recurrent sexually transmitted illnesses, including syphilis. He was started on a selective serotonin reuptake inhibitor for depression and now reports erectile dysfunction. The patient requests a prescription medication to treat erectile dysfunction.

- A 27-year-old HIV-positive man in Africa learns of a new medication to treat HIV, offering the potential for a more robust therapy with fewer side effects. To obtain the medication, he must enroll in a clinical research trial.

■ A 41-year-old man grew up in rural Mexico and came to the United States to live openly as a gay man, but his life is limited because he is undocumented. He is HIV-positive with a very resistant viral profile, which necessitates that he take an elaborate mixture of HIV antiretroviral medications, some of which are new and not readily available to HIV-positive individuals in countries with limited resources. The patient fears he would not be able to get this mixture of medications in Mexico if he were deported.

■ A 32-year-old married woman is pregnant. She is HIV-positive, but her husband's status is unknown. She has yet to disclose her status to him but repeatedly promises the doctor that she will. She admits that she fears his family will hurt or even kill her if she tells him. She is worried for herself and her pregnancy.

■ A year ago, a man with a history of HIV and intravenous substance use pursued treatment for a hepatitis C infection. The 3-month treatment course cost over $80,000, and he completed the treatment, achieving a sustained virologic response. A year later he has become reinfected with hepatitis C. He admits that he has had frequent relapses on methamphetamine but denies any sharing of needles and refuses to attend addiction treatment.

12

People at the End of Life

Laura Weiss Roberts, M.D., M.A.

The inevitability of death is one of the central features of existence. Although the certainty of eventual death applies to all living things, human beings uniquely have the ability to reflect on this reality. Even so, the certainty of death is a truth that people tend not to keep in consciousness but rather to repress, forget, or even deny. Ensuring that explicit conversations about end-of-life care occur is an important task for all clinicians, especially given the impact of modern technologies and health care systems on the occurrence and process of death.

From a mental health perspective, psychological suffering before death may be immense, and psychiatric disorders may distort decisions in the dying process. Death may trigger significant psychiatric symptoms among grieving loved ones. Psychiatrists, psychologists, nurses, therapists, counselors, and other mental health clinicians may have particularly important roles in preparing patients for death, safeguarding dying persons, and helping those who grieve.

SIX DOMAINS FOR CAREFUL ATTENTION

Psychiatrists may find it valuable to organize their thinking about end-of-life care for their patients in relation to six domains: diagnosis, comfort,

capacity, clarity, controversy, and collaboration. Table 12–1 presents some
of the issues and questions relevant to each of these domains, which are discussed more fully in the subsections that follow.

Diagnosis

It is crucial that clinicians seek to understand key aspects of the dying person's
physical illness and remain vigilant for signs of a psychiatric disorder, which
may greatly affect the patient's care and decision making. The primary care-
giving clinician should have a working understanding of the nature and
course of the patient's medical condition, and engaging a psychiatric consultant may be very helpful in recognizing mental health issues.

To provide optimal care, several questions should be clear in the clinician's mind: What is the anticipated course of the illness? Are there features
of the illness that will cause physical pain, psychiatric and/or cognitive disturbances, or specific forms of disability? If the illness is a form of cancer,
for instance, is it especially likely to cause physical pain? Is it likely to spread
quickly or slowly? Is it locally invasive, or does it spread to distant sites, including the brain, which may affect the person's cognitive and emotional
functioning? Does the dying person have evidence of a psychiatric disorder,
such as delirium, major depression, anxiety, or psychosis? Have causes of
symptoms—ranging from adjustment issues, disease-related issues, adverse
effects of medications, and preexisting illnesses—been carefully established? Is the main clinician aware of the potential impact of the medical
condition on the patient's psychological well-being and psychiatric status?
Has appropriate treatment been initiated for the medical condition or for
primary or secondary psychiatric processes that coexist?

Comfort

Beyond accurate diagnosis and appropriate treatment, comfort is an imperative in caring for dying persons. Pain is what many fear most about the dying process. Making every effort to help the person have some control over
pain is a positive contribution to the care of a dying patient. Toward this
goal, physical and psychological pain should be carefully assessed, with both
subjective and objective measures, and then clearly documented for all clinicians involved in the care of the patient. This evaluation may include formal tools, such as measures of quality of life. A number of comfort measures
should be planned and put in place for the future care of the patient. More
than this, however, the patient should understand these measures and the
extent to which they are in his or her direct control. Specific steps to facilitate communication about the need for enhanced treatment for pain

TABLE 12–1. Six domains for consideration by mental health clinicians in end-of-life care

Diagnosis	What is the dying person's medical condition? What is the anticipated course of the illness? Are there features of the illness that will cause physical pain, psychiatric and/or cognitive disturbances, or specific forms of disability? Does the dying person have evidence of a psychiatric disorder, such as delirium, major depression, or anxiety? Has appropriate treatment been initiated?
Comfort	Have diligent efforts to assess the physical and psychological pain been undertaken? What comfort measures are in place and are planned? Does the dying person understand what pain control measures are in his or her direct control? Have clear approaches to "stepping up" the pain control been discussed, so that the patient can request this?
Capacity	What is the decisional capacity of the dying person? What is the voluntarism capacity of the dying person? Has every reasonable effort been made to improve the patient's capacities when he or she is making key treatment decisions (e.g., through careful efforts to address physical pain, to minimize use of unnecessary psychotropic medications)?
Clarity	Are the patient's values and wishes clear regarding end-of-life care? Is there appropriate documentation to assist all clinicians and family members involved in the care of the patient?
Controversy	Have the tough issues been addressed with the patient and his or her loved ones? Are the views of the patient, of key decision makers (e.g., family members), and of other individuals involved (e.g., the clinical care team, community members) known? If there are sources of controversy, have these been addressed carefully, with specific roles, boundaries, and decision-making processes and options clearly laid out?
Collaboration	For the benefit of the dying person, have all of the people— loved ones, multidisciplinary clinicians, community members—been appropriately included? Do other people or resources need to be invited in to help the patient?

Source. Reprinted from Roberts LW, Dyer AR: *Concise Guide to Ethics in Mental Health Care.* Washington, DC, American Psychiatric Publishing, 2004, pp. 186–187. Copyright © 2004 American Psychiatric Publishing. Used with permission.

should be addressed early and remembered explicitly together in the care of the dying person. Psychiatrists and palliative care experts, available in many settings, can help with goals of care conversations, strategies for pain relief, and overall care planning.

The mental health clinician has a special role in tracking the internal experience of the dying person. For one patient, this may mean helping to dismantle barriers to requesting help and pain medications. For another patient, it may mean working through loss, anger, and existential issues. For yet another patient, it may mean helping other clinicians to see the culturally sanctioned comforts valued and needed by the patient. The mental health clinician should remain attentive to psychological, cultural, and social issues from the perspective of the patient. Helping the patient to communicate with family members and ensuring that goals of care are embraced by loved ones can be an important role for the mental health professional as well. Ultimately, the mental health clinician serves as both an advocate and a healer in seeking and providing comfort for dying persons.

Capacity

Formally assessing decisional capacity in the context of end-of-life care is a vital role of the consultation-liaison and general adult psychiatrist. Chapter 4, "Informed Consent and Decisional Capacity," provides a detailed discussion of the systematic assessment of decisional and voluntarism capacities. Therapists and counselors working with dying persons will need some sense of patients' strengths, deficits, and ability to make crucial clinical care decisions; clinicians will also need an understanding of when to talk with the main clinical team about concerns regarding the patients' changing status.

In thinking about the care of a dying person, the mental health clinician ideally will ask a series of questions: What is the set of overall strengths and deficits of the patient? What is the patient's decisional capacity, as assessed along the four dimensions of communication, understanding, reasoning, and appreciation? What is the patient's capacity for voluntarism, as assessed along the four dimensions of developmental, illness-related, psychological and cultural, and contextual factors? Has every reasonable effort been made to improve the patient's capacity when he or she is making key treatment decisions? Answering these questions includes a wide set of activities, such as careful efforts to diagnose and treat overlooked psychiatric conditions; relieve physical pain; address grief and psychological pain; include family, spiritual, and/or culturally appropriate supports; and minimize use of unnecessary psychotropic medications.

Clarity

As clinicians who are committed to understanding the experiences and the ability of patients to make meaning of their experiences, mental health care providers have a special responsibility to ensure that the dying person's values and wishes are clarified regarding end-of-life care. Some dying persons will have thought a great deal about these issues and have a sophisticated understanding of the kinds of decisions required in modern medical situations. Some other patients will not have thought about these issues, for many reasons that may relate to psychological defenses, emotional distress, education level, and geographic isolation, for example. Tools such as the Values History Form (University of New Mexico Health Sciences Center Institute for Ethics 2015) and the FICA Spiritual History Tool (Puchalski and Romer 2000) are excellent resources for facilitating discussions of these issues with patients, their families, and their caregivers.

This approach allows the voice and preferences of the dying person to be identified and honored, not presumed or usurped. And it allows dignity and personhood to be preserved in the face of great fear and loss. Toward this aim, a crucial task is to ensure that appropriate documentation of the patient's values and preferences exists and is available to assist all clinicians and family members involved in the patient's care. With the permission of the patient, clinical advance directives and other formal legal documents should be prepared, and multiple copies should be distributed to all appropriate clinicians, health care facilities, and family members.

Controversy

The experiences of loss are often accompanied by controversy and controversial decision making, and dying is no exception. The psychiatrist, as part of a larger multidisciplinary team, can help anticipate the complex, controversial issues that may arise so that they may be acknowledged and worked on explicitly, respectfully, and with appropriate "rules of engagement." Every practicing physician has experienced a situation in which, just after a constructive, supportive plan has been developed to provide care for a dying person, a late-arriving sibling, an estranged spouse, a beloved child, or a nephew—who has not been involved in the therapeutic planning process— will cry "Wait, how can you do this?!" In part motivated by fear of litigation, the process comes to a halt, and the positive work of supporting the dying patient can come completely undone. Intensive, prospective efforts to identify key individuals involved, immediately or more remotely, in the patient's life and to identify potential areas of disagreement or controversy are extraordinarily helpful in this process. It is important to note that the personal views of the mental health clinician figure into this process as well, and considerable self-understanding of his or her own preferences (and biases) regarding palliative care and difficult topics such as rational suicide, assisted death, and euthanasia is essential.

The clinician therefore should consider the following questions: Have the tough issues been addressed with the patient and loved ones? Are the views of the patient, key decision makers (e.g., family members), and other individuals involved (e.g., the clinical care team, community members) known? If there are sources of controversy, have these been addressed carefully, with specific roles, boundaries, and decision-making processes and options clearly laid out?

Collaboration

The dying person's needs should be the ultimate consideration. It is important for the mental health clinician to determine whether consultation with other people—including loved ones; clinicians from other disciplines; attorneys; rabbis, priests, or other spiritual leaders; and community members—should be pursued for the benefit of the dying person. It may help to mobilize other resources as well, such as palliative care experts and hospice clinicians.

EMERGENT ETHICAL QUESTIONS IN END-OF-LIFE CARE

Beyond these six domains of immediate importance to mental health clinicians in providing end-of-life care is the societal context in which that care is provided. Modern technology has altered how death is understood—what it is and when it occurs. Social thought leaders have challenged medicine to examine the interplay between what are characterized as scientific and spiritual goals of health care at the end of life (van der Steen et al. 2014). The recognition that there could be such a thing as a good death has indeed been a constant tension throughout the history of medicine. As described by Reuben (2010), "In medicine there are 3 do's: the can do, the actually do, and the should do" (p. 467). The "can do" category is boundless—"more [intervention] is always better"—whereas the "should do" category is delimited by "medical evidence" and "personal, societal, and ethical values" (p. 467).

The Hippocratic Oath admonishes physicians to "neither give a deadly drug to anybody if asked for it, nor make a suggestion to this effect." The American Medical Association (2001) code of ethics explicitly forbids physician-assisted suicide and euthanasia, stating that such activities are fundamentally incompatible with the trusted role of the physician in society. Heinous examples of euthanasia with disabled (not dying) individuals, including people with mental illness and no other physical health condition, reinforce the importance of examining the issue of the physician's role and the heterogeneity of acceptance for assisted death and euthanasia practices throughout the world. In the United States, however, most states have passed legislation focusing on "death with dignity." These laws do not support physician-assisted suicide or euthanasia practices per se but permit physicians to provide comfort care, even though it may hasten death as a "second effect." In other words, physicians can make things better for patients, alleviate suffering, sometimes cure disease, and forestall—but not directly induce—death as a primary objective. Most legislation related to death with dignity includes provisions for psychiatric evaluations to determine whether the individual is capable of making health care decisions and is in need of care for underlying conditions such as depression or delirium. The international debate on the ethical acceptability of assisted death practices—encompassing physician-assisted suicide and euthanasia—is intense, and people of goodwill exist on all sides of these controversial issues (Gopal 2015).

Many psychiatrists have expressed concern about the emergence of assisted death practices in light of what is understood about the clinical phenomena of suicide and important empirical work on attitudes toward assisted death practices. Psychiatric diseases such as depression and delirium and their symptoms and signs (e.g., negative cognitive distortions, hopelessness, difficulty with concentration, despair) may greatly influence a request for assisted death, just as it has been shown that severe, treatable physical pain will prompt this same request in oncology settings (Roberts et al. 1997). Psychiatrists are also very cognizant of the complexities of obtaining informed consent for major health care decisions in the context of very serious or terminal illness and of how vulnerable patients with great suffering can be. Just as ethical palliative care is based on diagnosing and addressing sources of suffering, ethical mental health care at the end of life has the same imperatives.

Intriguing empirical work suggests the importance of these issues. Studies of people with advanced cancer reveal that the preference for assisted death is not common, although, importantly, it is an accurate marker of treatable major depression (Emanuel et al. 1996). Interest in assisted death practices as expressed by 378 persons with HIV in another study was determined by lack of emotional support, psychological distress, and symptoms of mental illness rather than physical illness determinants (Breitbart et al. 1996). In a classic study of elderly psychiatric inpatients, the most severely depressed and hopeless patients overestimated the risks and underestimated the benefits of medical care at end of life (Ganzini et al. 1994). With appropriate mental health treatment, these beliefs reversed, and the patients changed their end-of-life care preferences to allow for more intensive therapeutic interventions. A series of early studies suggested that as medical students, residents, and physicians advance through training, their acceptance of assisted death practices decreases and that psychiatrists are significantly less supportive of assisted suicide and euthanasia than are physicians in other specialty areas. This work also indicated that clinicians are more comfortable with the performance of assisted death by others than being engaged in these activities themselves. This finding has important implications related to moral agency within the clinical professions. More recent empirical work on suicide requests continues to demonstrate that insufficient pain relief is a strong factor for many individuals at the end of life. Since the 1990s, relatively little empirical work on assisted death practices has been conducted, although legislative measures have accelerated as the elderly population grows.

CONCLUSION

Debates about the rights and wrongs of end-of-life issues travel from the courts to the bedside and back to the courts and legislatures. Clearly, death is distinctly personal and profound in a manner that cannot be comprehensively captured by the impersonal proceedings of courts and laws. End-of-life conversations touch on the most inner, subjective aspects of the meaning of life and death. Psychiatrists who can help keep this focus will do much to serve their dying patients and help families, caregivers, clinicians, and other care providers.

CASE SCENARIOS

- An 80-year-old retired technician with metastatic lung cancer refuses further chemotherapy because, he says, "there is nothing it can fix." His children become very upset and demand that he receive psychiatric treatment for depression.

- A 67-year-old career military officer whose wife has advanced Alzheimer's disease is diagnosed with colon cancer. He tells his son it would be better if "both of us were out of the way."

- Before undergoing quadruple bypass surgery, a very active 72-year-old woman fills out an advance directive assigning power of attorney for health care to her husband.

- A 54-year-old woman with progressive multiple sclerosis is wheel-chair bound and unable to perform any tasks of daily living for herself. She asks the psychiatrist who is treating her for depression if he could arrange to give her "too many sleeping pills."

- A 75-year-old farmer who is filling out an advance directive indicates that he does not want to "depend on any machines."

13

Difficult Patients

Laura Weiss Roberts, M.D., M.A.

There are patients, and there are patients. The difficult ones can be perceived as demanding, noncompliant, whiny, entitled, or manipulative. They can be too different from or too similar to the clinician, too seductive, too unclean, too smart, too fat, too thin, or too anxiety provoking (McCarty and Roberts 1996). Difficult patients require special attention because their care is very complex and invites significant ethical pitfalls. Recognizing what makes some patients difficult, understanding that "being difficult" is a clinical sign that warrants diagnostic interpretation, identifying the special ethical problems arising in the care of the difficult patient, and responding therapeutically are the key elements of ethically sound care for these challenging patients.

RECOGNIZING DIFFICULT PATIENTS

Often it is obvious who is or who is going to become difficult: the patient who is perceived as drug seeking, the patient who is notorious for not taking medications, the patient who engages in frequent self-mutilating behavior, the patient who seems to complain incessantly, the patient who threatens violence toward clinic staff, the patient who demands discharge from the hospital, the patient who "just has a personality disorder," the patient who seems never to get better—these are the tough cases.

Sometimes, however, the difficult patients can be more subtle in presentation. The patient with a professional background who is utterly bright and engaging may end up being very difficult because he or she relates to the clinician as a friend from whom the patient requests "favors" of prescriptions and laboratory tests. Similarly, the care of a patient who is also a clinician may become especially complex, for several reasons. For example, the patient may feel ashamed to reveal health issues to a professional colleague, and meanwhile the care provider–clinician may assume that the patient-clinician needs less support and reassurance than other patients. The care provider–clinician may also fail to explore the possibility of the patient-clinician self-diagnosing and self-prescribing. Other subtly difficult patients include individuals who omit or obscure important details when providing their histories and those who, along with their multiple medical and psychiatric symptoms, have multiple doctors and multiple ongoing treatments.

Recognizing the difficult patient, then, involves identifying those individuals who are unusual in one of two ways: 1) they evoke powerful feelings in clinicians or 2) they demonstrate an atypical pattern of clinical service use.

Patients Who Evoke Powerful Feelings

First, some patients are difficult because of the special intensity of feelings (i.e., countertransference) they evoke in the clinical care team. For example, the patient whom a clinician is especially tempted to "rescue," identify with, or feel awed by is likely to be difficult. The victimized child, the physician-patient, the parish priest, the local television news anchor, and people who look like the clinician's uncle, cousin, or fifth-grade teacher may all fit into this category. Worse yet are patients who actually *are* the clinician's uncle, cousin, or fifth-grade teacher; having such patients is not unusual for clinicians working in small towns or small health care systems. The patient who is also a litigation attorney may be a particularly intimidating—and therefore challenging—patient for any clinician. The patient who has extraordinarily severe symptoms may be perceived as a difficult patient if he or she evokes feelings of distress or inadequacy in the clinician.

Other patients who evoke intense feelings are those whose experiences and illness processes are so tragic that they engender very powerful feelings of empathy and pain in their clinicians—for example, the young mother dying of cancer, the military colonel who gradually succumbs to Alzheimer's disease, the newly quadriplegic motorcycle accident victim, the survivor of wartime torture and trauma, the child who has been raped, the college student who attempts suicide during his first psychotic break. These are the patients whom clinicians carry with them, over whom clinicians lose sleep, whom clinicians always remember. They are also the patients whom clinicians and clinical trainees may find very overwhelming and for whom they may find it extraordinarily difficult to provide effective care.

Patients who trigger unusually strong negative feelings ("gut reactions") from members of the staff are also likely to present special challenges. These reactions may be due to the patients' particularly problematic feelings and conduct (e.g., anger, emotional lability, inconsistency, indifference, repeated suicide threats, self-mutilating or self-defeating behaviors) and psychological defenses (e.g., denial, projection, reaction formation). The reactions may also be related to uncomfortable or stigmatizing elements of a patient's life history, such as the gang member who has served time in prison, the father whose careless driving resulted in the death of his child in an accident, or the pregnant woman who uses methadone. An unusual physical appearance—such as obesity, cachexia, exceptionally poor hygiene, congenital abnormalities, or regions of infection—may also trigger such feelings in clinicians. In some instances, the clinical care team will react to a given patient with disinterest and detachment. Although less overt than other negative reactions, such detachment likewise is an indicator of a problematic patient. The clinician who is well attuned to his or her emotional responses, and those of the patient care team, will thus be well prepared to identify these difficult patients. As social attitudes become more accepting and progressive, overt biases may be eliminated, although the stain of unconscious bias may persist and negatively shape a patient's care (Haider et al. 2011; Hannah and Carpenter-Song 2013; Teal et al. 2012).

Patients Who Demonstrate an Atypical Pattern of Clinical Service Use

A second cue in recognizing difficult patients is their atypical pattern of clinical service use. Care providers may experience as difficult those patients who appear to seek prescription medications from many sources, to be overly insistent about clinic appointments and specialty referrals, or to obtain care repeatedly through emergency or urgent care facilities. Patients who appear to emphasize physical symptoms in mental health care settings and mental health symptoms in physical health care settings are particularly apt to stymie their clinicians. These patients often suffer from several comorbid physical and mental illness processes, giving rise to this kind of service utilization pattern. In contrast, the "underutilizers" of clinical services, such as individuals who present late in the course of illness for treatment, demand discharge from the hospital against medical advice, do not take their medications, miss their scheduled appointments, or do not pursue necessary preventive care (e.g., parents who do not arrange for their children to receive vaccinations) will also pose special challenges and arouse strong emotions in clinicians. Such individuals have been described as "help rejecters" (Robbins et al. 1988). Clinical syndromes may be the direct "cause" of these impaired care-seeking behaviors, as in the case of the patient with social phobia or the patient with negative symptom–dominant schizophrenia who misses numerous appointments. Similarly, the cardiac patient with an unrecognized alcohol problem may place care providers in clinical and ethical binds by insisting on leaving the hospital prematurely as withdrawal symptoms become hard to tolerate.

UNDERSTANDING THE PREVALENCE AND ATTRIBUTES OF DIFFICULT PATIENTS

Because difficult patients have so many varied characteristics, their numbers are challenging to estimate accurately. In medical settings, clinicians commonly acknowledge encounters with difficult patients. In one study of 500 patients, 15% were identified by their primary care providers as difficult; these patients were more likely to have mental disorders, more than five somatic symptoms, more severe symptoms, poorer functional status, less satisfaction with care, and higher use of health services (Jackson and Kroenke 1999). In this study, physicians with more negative psychosocial attitudes, as measured on the Physician's Belief Scale, were significantly more likely to experience patient encounters as difficult. This work suggests that "difficult" is, to some extent, an attribute that resides in the "eye of the beholder," or at least reflects a problem of "fit" between a clinician and patient. In an earlier study of 293 patients presenting for care in medical and surgical clinics, consultants identified 22% as leading to difficult encounters, primarily due to medically unexplained symptoms, coexisting social problems, and severe, untreatable illness (Sharpe et al. 1994). Difficult encounters were associated with greater patient distress, less patient satisfaction, and heightened use of services.

Individuals with personality disorders are often experienced as difficult in patient care settings. A survey study involving 113 patients found that psychosomatic symptoms, at least mild personality disorder, addiction, and major psychopathology (e.g., affective or anxiety disorders) characterized difficult patients, but demographic characteristics, provider characteristics, and most diagnoses were not correlated with a higher score on the Difficult Doctor–Patient Relationship Questionnaire (Hahn et al. 1994). Not surprisingly, in another study of 43 patients (21 identified as "difficult" and 22 control subjects), structured diagnostic evaluation revealed that a greater number of the difficult patients (7 of 21 vs. 1 of 22) had personality disorders. Five of the difficult patients with personality disorders met criteria for dependent personality disorder from the *Diagnostic and Statistical Manual of Mental Disorders*, Fourth Edition, Text Revision (American Psychiatric Association 2000), although none had been previously diagnosed with this psychopathology (Schafer and Nowlis 1998). In a study that echoed these results, borderline personality disorder was found to be present in patients at an urban primary care clinic at 4 times the prevalence found in community populations (Gross et al. 2002). Half of these patients had received no mental health treatment, and 43% had not been accurately diagnosed in their primary care clinic. Other factors that may contribute to difficult patient encounters, such as perceived deception by patients, have been studied only minimally. One interesting study assessed patient encounters of 44 family practice residents and attending physicians; findings indicated that clinicians commonly doubted the truthfulness of their patients' disclosures (Woolley and Clements 1997).

Analogous data have not been collected recently or systematically in mental health care settings. Suggested causes of difficult encounters in psychiatric settings include treatment resistance and nonadherence, very heavy use of mental health services, severe psychopathology due to personality disorders or psychotic disorders, and comorbid disease. The prevalence of difficult patient encounters is likely to be significantly higher in mental health care than in traditional medical settings because of the specific nature of psychiatric illness and its care. Psychiatric patients have illnesses that affect behaviors, personal attitudes, mood symptoms, insight and motivation, and decision making. They have complex psychosocial issues, and the sicker patients often are poor and have limited abilities and/or opportunities to improve their socioeconomic circumstances. Patients with personality disorders who ultimately are referred for mental health treatment tend to be very seriously disturbed, and their care poses immense challenges. Patients with a constellation of medical and mental health symptoms who are referred for psychiatric consultation also tend to be very distressed, to pose diagnostic enigmas, or to have especially overwhelming psychosocial issues. For these reasons, mental health practitioners may feel that every patient encounter will potentially become a difficult one.

With newer thinking in medicine—focusing on improving the patient experience and more fully demonstrating compassion and respect for patients—the topic of the difficult patient is less discussed. Challenging patients have not gone away, however, and a concern is that issues that had been explicit have now become implicit in the health environment. Psychiatrists may play an increasingly important role in helping multidisciplinary teams to reflect on the challenges of caring for certain patients and helping teams to develop positive treatment planning strategies.

RECOGNIZING "BEING DIFFICULT" AS A CLINICAL SIGN

The clinician's first duty in the care of the difficult patient is to understand that the aspects of the patient's presentation that make him or her difficult are, in essence, clinical signs—that is, observable manifestations of the patient's underlying health and of factors affecting his or her health status. In other words, generating a differential diagnosis list is important for patients who are difficult. The patient who exhibits threatening behavior toward clinic staff may in fact be experiencing irritability, fear, and psychotic symptoms early in the course of a manic episode. The patient could also have a head injury or be delirious or intoxicated. The frustratingly "noncompliant" patient with unremitting symptoms may hold different religious beliefs about acceptable healing practices, may have experienced unpleasant side effects of pills, may not have insight about the need for treatment, or may not have the resources to purchase prescription medications or obtain transportation for clinic appointments. Moreover, because traumatized individuals often tend to relive their past experiences in present contexts, the patient who behaves seductively in the therapeutic relationship, for example, may have been sexually exploited in the past. Rather than expressing authentic romantic feelings for the clinician, this patient manifests core psychological issues for the clinician, who has the duty to understand this clinical phenomenon. Such difficult behaviors should be understood in a dispassionate, nonjudgmental manner. They are observable clinical signs.

Clarifying the reasons why patients appear to be undermining their health and health care is therefore an important responsibility of the clinician. Patients' behavioral cues should be explored and interpreted clinically, not superficially or too concretely. Just as the seductive patient should not be taken at face value, the angry patient also should not be viewed as intentionally acting out in order to create trouble. In sum, all elements of the patient's presentation are important clinical data, and clinicians must remain within their professional roles and uphold their professional duties when dealing with the challenges of the difficult patient.

IDENTIFYING ETHICAL PITFALLS
IN THE CARE OF DIFFICULT PATIENTS

Difficult patients are at risk of receiving care that deviates from usual ethics standards in several respects. First, therapeutic abandonment of patients is much more likely when patients are unlikable, frustrating, apparently non-compliant, extraordinarily tragic, or otherwise atypical. Efforts to preserve the therapeutic alliance and obtain appropriate informed refusal of treatment may be minimal, for instance, with a patient who is perceived as medication seeking or who demands discharge against medical advice. The clinician may pay less attention to carefully diagnosing the multiple clinical problems of the patient whose interpersonal manner and use of health services are seen as inappropriate. Important medical issues that merit exploration may be dismissed as psychiatric, such as in the situation of a medical student with undiagnosed Crohn's disease whose symptoms are attributed to exam-related stress and poor coping skills. Gradual, quiet disengagement from the persistently suffering patient, although not legally problematic, is another subtle form of therapeutic abandonment that may occur.

Second, professional boundaries may erode in the care of difficult patients, resulting in ethically compromised care. When patients are difficult because they resemble their clinicians by having similar backgrounds, professions, or interests, the clinician and patient may begin relating to one another in a manner more congruent with a friendship than a professional relationship; for example, the clinician may disclose aspects of his or her personal life, accept financial advice, or make social plans in the course of talking with the patient. Personal-professional boundaries are crossed in such situations, and the ethical foundation of the relationship—trust and absolute dedication to the well-being of the patient—may be seriously jeopardized. Informed consent processes may suffer, because clinicians in such cases may provide insufficient information about clinical care alternatives or suggest only those treatment options that they personally would consider. Clinicians who overly identify with their patients may also be tempted to document clinical issues inaccurately or not comply with mandatory reporting duties when stigmatizing issues arise. Splits within treatment teams may occur when some clinicians become closer to difficult patients for whom they have warmer personal feelings, whereas other members of the team do not. Clinicians may act unprofessionally in subtle ways by providing undocumented prescriptions or samples of medications. They may also act unprofessionally in more overt ways by becoming intimately involved with patients who give sexualized behavioral cues or who are otherwise vulnerable to the approaches of a person they perceive as powerful.

Third, confidentiality breaches may occur when a clinician discusses a difficult patient's case in relatively public settings, a behavior fueled by strongly held and hard-to-contain feelings. The temptation to discuss a case is especially acute when the patient is an aggravating individual about whom the clinical team has passionate complaints, but it is also an issue when, for example, the patient is a celebrity or a celebrity's relative who suffers from a serious mental illness and/or substance problem. It is often difficult for clinicians to manage their natural curiosity, even voyeurism, and their desire to discuss the patient with colleagues and friends in such cases.

The challenges in caring for difficult patients therefore affect every ethically important aspect of clinical practice. Maintaining attentiveness to the patient's clinical signs and symptoms, building and sustaining the therapeutic alliance, respecting the patient's autonomy through sound informed consent and refusal-of-treatment processes, upholding the law, and maintaining appropriate confidentiality safeguards may all be adversely affected.

RESPONDING THERAPEUTICALLY

Ensuring that difficult patients receive clinically and ethically sound care is no small task, yet it is an important health disparity issue. The most critical step in responding therapeutically is to recognize the discomfort and problems that difficult patients generate as a clinical sign. Monitoring one's reactions and responding with professionalism and thoroughness to the symptoms and behavioral presentations of these special patients are the keys to providing good care in potentially taxing clinical situations. Responding therapeutically may entail building a sense of empathy for the unlikable or otherwise off-putting patient; or it may entail assuming a more professional, objective stance with the especially charming or intriguing patient. Table 13–1 lists important tasks involved in managing difficult patients.

Experienced clinicians have proposed several core elements of treatment for the difficult patient (Drossman 1978; McCarty and Roberts 1996). These include maintaining a nonjudgmental interest in the patient's reports; keeping personal and professional roles straight; reflecting on one's attitudes and biases; taking a complete history and accepting (not arguing with or discounting) the patient's symptoms; performing or referring the patient for a thorough physical examination; avoiding patronizing or inappropriate reassurance (e.g., "it's just stress"); refraining from prematurely intervening with medications or aggressive treatments; setting up regular

TABLE 13–1. Steps in managing difficult patients

Step 1. Understand yourself.

Be aware of your biases and responses.
Understand why certain types of patients upset you.
Realize you're not a "bad" doctor if you have negative feelings about some patients.
Recognize that everyone has trouble managing some patients.

Step 2. Understand your patient.

Every difficult behavior is a form of communication.
Every difficult patient is trying to express real fears and needs.

Step 3. Think, don't react.

Remember your duty to help and not harm.
Focus on medical and psychiatric issues you can treat.
Strive to be empathic, consistent, and stable.

Step 4. Form an alliance.

Find something you can agree on.
Educate the patient about your limits and responsibilities.
Reinforce positive behavior, and don't reward negative behavior.

Step 5. Treat whatever is treatable.

Screen for medical conditions.
Screen for mental disorders.
Use therapy and medication to treat problems.

Step 6. Avoid traps of wanting to…

Save the patient and be idealized.
Reject the patient and not be hurt.
Punish the patient.
Do anything to help the patient so the patient won't hurt himself or herself.

Step 7. Get help.

Seek consultation.
Foster team consensus.
Encourage patient to participate in support groups.

Step 8. Handle your emotions.

Find constructive ways of venting frustration.
Prepare yourself for seeing difficult patients.
See managing difficult patients as a clinical skill to master.

Acknowledgment. Cynthia M.A. Geppert, M.D., M.A., M.P.H., M.S., D.P.S., provided assistance in preparing this table.
Source. Adapted from Roberts LW, Dyer AR: *Concise Guide to Ethics in Mental Health Care.* Washington, DC, American Psychiatric Publishing, 2004, p. 162. Copyright © 2004 American Psychiatric Publishing. Used with permission.

visits and being interpersonally predictable and consistent; remaining alert for new developments; clearly presenting therapeutic options to the patient; preparing for a protracted course of treatment; communicating all findings and treatment plans to the clinical care team before, during, and after their discovery or implementation; and educating oneself about the biopsychosocial aspects of the patient's disease process.

It is also important to accept one's limitations in dealing with the countertransference and ethical issues presented by difficult patients, as noted in Chapter 3, "The Tradition of the Psychotherapeutic Relationship," and to seek out appropriate professional venues for clarifying these issues. For example, thoughtful discussions with members of the clinical care team about strategies for responding to the frustrations encountered in a particular patient's care may be highly valuable. Comparing and double-checking one's perceptions with those of trusted team members will be a helpful step in this process. Seeking out additional clinical, ethical, and legal expertise from knowledgeable colleagues and supervisors is especially important.

Use of humor when discussing highly problematic patients with clinical team members is controversial ethically. Humorous remarks occur almost inevitably in the care of difficult patients. As a marker of distress and anxiety, humor can be observed explicitly and then put to constructive use in illuminating the more troublesome features of the patient's case and highlighting the powerlessness or frustration felt by members of the clinical team. As long as there is an abundance of manifestations of respect toward the patient and faithfulness to the ethical principles of beneficence and nonmaleficence in the patient's care—and a thoughtful discussion of the treatment issues—the team leader may interpret the humor in a manner that contributes positively to the care of a patient with multiple problems. With more progressive views about respectfulness toward team members and patients in medicine and a newly emerging dialogue about hostility and microaggression in the workplace (Levy and Jones 2013; Yearwood 2013), psychiatrists will need to help ensure that humor does not become weaponized or weaponizing in discussions of difficult patients.

CONCLUSION

One final consideration in the challenging process of working with difficult patients is the importance of examining the lessons learned in the course of caring for these patients. The clinician can learn, for example, from the unexpected diagnosis of the patient, the unexpected strengths of a team member, the unexpected impact of a miscommunication, the unexpected community resource, or the unexpected resilience of the family caregiver.

Paying attention to these valuable lessons will help address the natural exhaustion felt by many clinicians and also help expand their repertoire of skills and abilities for their next patient encounter, which may or may not pose special difficulties.

CASE SCENARIOS

- A young man with self-mutilating behavior presents to the psychiatric emergency room, having chewed and swallowed glass after being stopped by police for driving while intoxicated.

- A young woman with a history of sexual trauma and abnormal menstrual bleeding calls her primary care physician to request a gynecological examination. Although she has missed her last two appointments, the office schedules an appointment later in the week. The patient arrives late, says "I'm pregnant," appears distraught, and tells the nurse that she "just took a lot of pills." She is taken to the emergency room.

- A senior medical student approaches his supervisor, an attending physician, for antidepressant and sleeping medications. He states that he is under tremendous stress but does not wish to seek formal care because he "can't afford to get a mental health record" if he wants to "get into a residency program."

- An elderly man who ordinarily lives in a motel for transients in a poor neighborhood presents to the psychiatric emergency room on a cold winter night, with all of his possessions in a large plastic bag. He demands admission to the hospital, stating that he will kill himself if he is sent to a shelter. The staff note that the patient's pattern is to come to the emergency room toward the end of the month, when he has run out of money and is unable to stay at his motel.

- A recently retired man with mild hypertension and arthritis whose parents died from cancer seems to fill every appointment by reciting complaints and worries. Each time the physician tries a different treatment, the patient returns, complaining of its lack of efficacy. The patient frequently discontinues medications prematurely because of "side effects." He often calls the doctor's office and is known for his pattern of frequent visits to urgent care and walk-in clinics.

14

People Living With Addictions

Michael P. Bogenschutz, M.D.
Laura Weiss Roberts, M.D., M.A.

Addictions are best conceptualized as disorders similar to other chronic psychiatric and medical conditions. Like their physical counterparts, addictions and comorbid disorders are prevalent and severe and lead to great suffering and societal burden. All of the major bioethics principles, such as respect for persons, justice, autonomy, and confidentiality, apply to addictions (Table 14–1). Although the ethical issues that arise in addictive disorders are similar to those that arise in physical disorders, they differ in emphasis and in particulars (Geppert and Roberts 2008). Ethical issues in addiction psychiatry, moreover, are made more complex by the role of stigma.

PREVALENCE AND SERIOUSNESS OF ADDICTION AND COMORBID DISORDERS

In the *Diagnostic and Statistical Manual of Mental Disorders*, Fifth Edition (DSM-5; American Psychiatric Association 2013a), substance use disorders comprise diagnoses for each major class of substance, including alcohol; caffeine; cannabis; hallucinogens; inhalants; opioids; sedatives, hypnotics, and anxiolytics; stimulants; and tobacco. In DSM-5, gambling is also explicitly identified as a behavioral addiction. Addictive disorders may be understood

TABLE 14–1. Ethical principles and issues in addiction

Respect for persons	Stigma carries with it disrespect and discrimination, which are major considerations in diagnosis and treatment intervention with addiction and comorbid disorders.
Justice	Parity or equitable treatment for addiction and comorbid disorders represents the need for social justice in the allocation of resources for these conditions, which affect millions of people and pose significant burden.
Autonomy and personal responsibility	These are key concepts in addiction because of the fundamental nature of the illness and because addiction may involve use of substances that are unlawful to possess or use.
Confidentiality	Special protections exist in relation to confidentiality and safeguarding privacy because of the risk of discrimination toward people with addictive disorders.
Truth telling	Stigma and legal consequences of addictions may generate conflicts around truth telling for patients and clinicians.
Therapeutic alliance	Because clinicians have access to substances that may be requested by patients with addictive disorders and because addictive disorders are characterized by periods of relapse, establishing trust in the therapeutic alliance may be especially difficult.
Beneficence and nonmaleficence	Treatment of addiction requires a paradigm of seeking harm reduction through periods of remission or reduced use of addictive substances and efforts to balance risks and benefits in minimizing the negative consequences of addiction.

Source.   Adapted from Roberts LW, Dyer AR: *Concise Guide to Ethics in Mental Health Care.* Washington, DC, American Psychiatric Publishing, 2004, p. 138. Copyright © 2004 American Psychiatric Publishing. Used with permission.

as having core elements, such as impaired control, social impairment, risky use, and certain physiological criteria.

In 2014 in the United States, adults age 25 and older had significant lifetime use of alcohol (88%), cigarettes (68%), and illicit drugs of any kind (51%), including marijuana (47%), cocaine (17%), hallucinogens (16%), lysergic acid diethylamide (LSD; 11%), methamphetamines (6%), and heroin (2%) (National Institute on Drug Abuse 2016). Nonmedical use of psychotherapeutics reached 27% lifetime use in young people ages 18–25 years and 21% in adults age 26 and older. In 2013, more than 20,000 people (more men than women) died from overdoses associated with prescription medications, and from 2001 to 2013, there was a 2.5-fold increase in deaths related to prescription medications (National Institute on Drug Abuse 2016). Tragically, misuse of prescribed narcotics and narcotic-related overdoses, as well as benzodiazepine abuse and overdoses, have become a recognized threat to public health.

Lifetime prevalence of alcohol use disorder in the United States is estimated at 17.8% (Hasin et al. 2007); for drug use disorders, the lifetime prevalence is 9.9% (Grant et al. 2016). Patients with substance use disorders have elevated rates of most psychiatric disorders; conversely, patients with most psychiatric disorders have elevated rates of substance use disorders. SAMHSA's 2014 National Survey on Drug Use and Health (Center for Behavioral Health Statistics and Quality 2015) reported that approximately 44 million (18%) people in the United States who are ages 18 years and older have experienced mental illness. More than 20 million adults (8%) had a substance use disorder, and among these, 8 million people had co-occurring mental and substance use disorders (Center for Behavioral Health Statistics and Quality 2015). Certain subpopulations are at special risk for addictions; for example, medically ill and incarcerated groups are disproportionately affected by opioid use disorders (Ludwig and Peters 2014).

The costs in human suffering and economic impact of substance use disorders are staggering. People with substance use disorders die at markedly elevated rates. Overall mortality ratios (relative to the general population) are 2:1 for individuals with alcohol use disorders, 6:1 for persons dependent on opioids, and anywhere from 2:1 to 21:1 for persons with other drug use disorders. Ratios for unnatural death (suicide, homicide, and accidents) are substantially higher than those for total mortality, and such ratios tend to be particularly high in women (e.g., 18:1 for women with alcohol abuse or dependence relative to women in the general population) (Harris and Barraclough 1998). Decades ago, the total economic costs of substance use disorders were estimated at $428.1 billion: $175.9 billion for alcohol, $138 billion for nicotine dependence, and $114.2 billion for other drugs (Rice et al. 1991). These costs included lost productivity due to crime, illness, and death, as well as added costs for health care and involvement in the criminal justice system. In 2015, the National Institute on Drug Abuse cited an annual cost of $700 billion annually in relation to crime, lost work productivity, and health care due to abuse of tobacco, alcohol, and illicit drugs.

STIGMA

Stigma is a negative social value associated with a personal attribute that has consequences in thoughts, emotions, and/or behaviors (e.g., ascribing blame, feeling shame or embarrassment, being shunned and avoided by others). Many psychiatric and medical conditions carry stigma. Stigma affects the perception and treatment of addiction at multiple decision points, including legislative, judicial, and clinical. Stigma primarily involves the ethical principle of respect for persons, but it becomes a fairness issue when it affects decision making.

The stigma associated with having an addiction is of a particular kind, owing to the fact that addictive behaviors look like, are believed by many to be, and in some (but not all) respects are voluntary behaviors (Table 14–2) (Geppert and Roberts 2008). A close parallel in medicine to apparent voluntariness is overeating and obesity. To the extent that a behavior is held to be a voluntary choice made by a free individual (and thus preventable), the individual may be held responsible or blamed for the behavior and its consequences.

Another major element of the stigma associated with addiction is that substance use itself is often considered morally wrong in certain cultures and is often illegal. This element of moral condemnation is also active in the stigma associated with medical disorders such as HIV/AIDS, in that having the disorder implies or suggests behavior that some people consider immoral (e.g., high-risk sexual behavior and/or intravenous drug use). Addiction is associated with a number of other behaviors that are considered morally wrong by many or most people because the behaviors may also cause harm to others (e.g., violence, theft, prostitution, drunk driving, other forms of irresponsibility and negligence). Although many individuals with addictions do not engage in any of these behaviors—and many persons without addictions may engage in all of them—people tend to make assumptions about the character of individuals with addictions on the basis of either accurate or exaggerated knowledge of these associations.

A major source of stigma also arises from the negative affective responses that people may have to individuals with addictions. These feelings are highly individual and may include reactions such as fear, anger, and avoidance, depending on the individual's psychological makeup. Again, such feelings are aroused by many other medical and psychiatric disorders as well as addiction.

TABLE 14–2. Sources of stigma in addictions

Individuals and society may judge addiction to be fully voluntary; therefore, questions about moral accountability arise.

Use of illicit substances or misuse of legal substances has legal implications and is considered immoral by many in society.

Addictions are perceived to be associated with other stigmatized conditions, such as having HIV/AIDS or hepatitis, being homeless, and engaging in criminal activity or prostitution.

Addictions are associated with negative health consequences that carry heavy societal burdens, such as sexually transmitted and infectious diseases, liver failure, heavy use of emergency services, and suicidal or self-destructive acts.

Addictions are associated with negative behaviors or stressors, such as driving under the influence of substances, domestic violence, unemployment, school dropout, and theft.

Addictions evoke negative cultural and psychological responses, such as fear, disgust, and rejection.

Source.   Adapted from Roberts LW, Dyer AR: *Concise Guide to Ethics in Mental Health Care.* Washington, DC, American Psychiatric Publishing, 2004, p. 140. Copyright © 2004 American Psychiatric Publishing. Used with permission.

HEALTH PARITY AND HEALTH DISPARITIES

Parity refers to equitable treatment and access to health care resources according to consistent criteria and thus is primarily related to the ethical principle of fairness. There is room for debate about the requirements of fairness in health care. There are several approaches that different people might consider fair. For example, the following models address resource allocation:

1. Health care resource allocation may be based on ability to pay (for insurance or directly for services). In this case, health care is seen as an industry governed by market forces, with minimal government involvement.
2. Resource allocation may occur according to need (severity, acuity).
3. Resource allocation may derive from the utilitarian principle of maximizing benefit to individuals and to society.

The present system in the United States embodies elements of all three of these models without a single coherent organizing principle. Many public and private health plans provide limited or no coverage for treatment of addictions. Such discriminatory policies have been justified by pragmatism: it is argued that full coverage would be prohibitively expensive or politically impossible. Nevertheless, substance use disorders represent valid, treatable disorders that often have a genetic basis. Health care costs should not be controlled by arbitrarily excluding treatment of particular disorders. It would be just as irrational to exclude treatment of diabetes to contain costs.

Returning to the three possible models of fair allocation of health care, in the first model, market forces may in part determine whether a person has health insurance and his or her overall level of coverage; however, such forces generally have little to do with the particulars of the coverage or the question of parity. Consistent application of either of the other two models (need-based and utilitarian) would lead to appropriate resource allocation for addiction services. In terms of acuity and severity, addictive disorders cause morbidity and mortality comparable to those of mental illnesses such as depression. The morbidity caused by substance abuse is immense; an estimated 40 million illnesses and injuries each year are attributable to substance addiction (McGinnis and Foege 1999). A Canadian study found that use of alcohol, tobacco, and illicit drugs accounted for 22.2% of years of potential life lost and 9.4% of admissions to hospitals (Single et al. 2000). Shield et al. (2013) reported that alcohol was responsible for 9% of all deaths in 2005 and more than 1.2 million potential years of life lost. Smyth et al. (2007) evaluated heroin addicts 33 years after treatment and determined that they lost 18.3 years (SD=10.7) of potential life before age 65 from causes including heroin overdose (22%), chronic liver disease (14%), and accidents (10%). Finally, in utilitarian terms, addictions are clearly treatable, frequently demonstrating large treatment effects that compare favorably with those of treatments of medical illnesses such as diabetes or hypertension, with benefits to individuals and to society.

Treatment of addiction is not more expensive than treatment of other illnesses, and cost offsets (e.g., from increased productivity and decreased crime and medical costs) are substantial and, according to some studies, considerably greater than the cost of treatment. For example, a study involving 150,000 members of a California health plan found that every $1 spent on substance abuse treatment saved taxpayers $7 in future costs (Gerstein et al. 1997).

Given the clear severity of addictive disorders and the relative efficacy of addiction treatment, the only remaining argument against parity for addiction treatment is that addictions are not valid disorders in the same way that major depression and cancer are. This kind of logic usually views substance use as a voluntary behavior and therefore simply a matter of personal responsibility.

PERSONAL RESPONSIBILITY

Although choice certainly plays a role in addictive behavior, important factors beyond personal choice are clearly involved. There is overwhelming evidence that addictive disorders have a biological basis, including genetic inheritance of risk, neurochemical correlates of risk and of active addiction, brain reward neurophysiology, and craving states. Many other disorders similarly involve behaviors that seem to be voluntary but must be addressed as symptoms of the disorder or determinants of illness (e.g., diet and medication adherence in diabetes, suicidal behavior in depression). Categorizing behavior as purely voluntary or involuntary does not correspond to observed reality and distracts from the primary treatment goal of reducing harm.

Personal responsibility is a perplexing issue in behavioral health treatment because practitioners frequently must grapple with the questions of how much to hold a patient accountable for his or her actions and how much to attribute those actions to the patient's illness. Part of the defining character of addiction is the relative loss of control. One useful strategy is to recognize that responsibility is ultimately an attribution rather than an observable phenomenon. Whether to hold a person responsible is a value judgment based on explicit or implicit values and psychological theories. For clinicians with the primary goals of treating illness, reducing or preventing harm, and/or maximizing wellness, the most appropriate criterion for attributing responsibility is the therapeutic one: attributing responsibility on the basis of therapeutic effect on the patient. They need to consider whether it will be helpful to the patient to be held responsible for his or her actions, and if so, to what degree. This criterion can address issues such as limit setting and treatment contracts. Of course, the issue of potential harm to others must also be considered. Therefore, beneficence, fairness, and respect for persons are all involved in the ethical attribution of responsibility.

CRIMINAL JUSTICE INVOLVEMENT, TRUTH TELLING, AND CONFIDENTIALITY

Patients with substance use disorders have particularly high rates of involvement with the criminal justice system. Psychiatrists become involved in a number of roles, including but extending beyond usual clinical caregiving roles. Ethical issues arise in treatment that are most effectively dealt with by remembering that the clinician has a primary responsibility to try to help the patient and an additional responsibility to try to prevent harm to others. Beneficence (toward both the patient and society) and respect for the patient must be balanced in situations in which the patient has already lost some civil rights.

Patients who are involved with the criminal justice system may be adjudicated, may have a parole or probation officer without a specific treatment participation requirement, or may be involved in treatment pretrial. In any of these cases, information may be requested from the clinician (e.g., by parole or probation officers, judges, pretrial supervisors) regarding the patient's substance use, participation in treatment, psychiatric status, and the like. Because truthful reporting of information may have negative consequences for the patient, the clinician may experience tension among the conflicting demands of truth telling, confidentiality, and beneficence (see Chapter 6, "Confidentiality and Truth Telling"). One helpful way to think about this dilemma is to recognize that the patient's autonomy and confidentiality are generally compromised primarily by involvement in the criminal justice system and only secondarily by involvement in treatment. In the United States, people who have violated the rights of others through criminal behavior may lose some of their civil rights. Truthful reporting requirements in fact usually have significant positive consequences for the patient. Given that documentation of treatment adherence is often a condition of release, such contact can literally keep the patient out of jail. The patient would be unable to receive and benefit from treatment if the reporting requirements were not met. Such requirements, moreover, serve as a strong, albeit coercive, incentive for the patient to participate in treatment. Patients in court-ordered treatment clearly benefit from such treatment.

At the outset of treatment of patients who are in the criminal justice system, it is particularly important for the clinician to discuss with both the patient and any applicable authorities the limitations to autonomy and confidentiality that may apply. The patient, even if adjudicated, must provide informed consent to treatment. This consent has a limitation: treatment may be to some degree coerced and is therefore not fully voluntary. Still, the patient does have the option of refusing treatment and suffering the consequences (e.g., incarceration). The potential risks of treatment (e.g., a report of nonadherence resulting in incarceration) should be discussed, and if the patient is willing, consent for sharing of specific information with the parole or probation officer or other authority should be obtained. In general, if the form of treatment for the patient is negotiable, the clinician should attempt to limit reporting to the patient's adherence, attainment of general treatment goals, and violent or dangerous behavior. This agreement should be clear to the patient, the applicable authorities, and the clinician. By allowing the clinician honestly to withhold certain information that could be detrimental to the patient's legal status, such an agreement decreases the potential for conflict between the principles of truth telling and beneficence. In particular, reporting of specific substance use should be avoided, because such a requirement encourages the patient who is using a substance to lie to the clinician. The parole or probation officer, for example, can take responsibility for monitoring substance use by regularly obtaining urine drug screens.

A variety of other situations exist in which truth telling and beneficence can come into conflict in the treatment of patients with addictions. Some of these entail the obligations of compliance with law—for example, reporting an airplane pilot with serious addiction issues or a patient who insists on driving away from the clinic while intoxicated. Other situations involve the intersection of therapeutic and justice issues—for example, the temptation to refrain from accurately documenting and assessing a candidate for a liver transplant who continues to drink alcohol or inject drugs.

NONMALEFICENCE

Another issue relating to beneficence is the physician's concern about causing harm by prescribing medication, causing or enabling addiction, or causing dangerous interactions with substances of abuse. The idea of providing access to addictive substances challenges physicians' basic sense of their caregiving role, particularly when physicians prescribe these substances for patients who have substance use disorders. The rationale for such prescribing is evidence driven and essentially pragmatic: the physician does it if it helps. For example, for patients with opioid addiction, methadone treatment clearly does much more good than harm. Psychiatrists frequently avoid prescribing benzodiazepines for anxiety disorders in patients with a history of substance use disorder out of concern that these agents carry a high risk of addiction in such patients. This belief is grounded in ideology rather than data, however—there is little empirical evidence that such patients are at elevated risk of benzodiazepine addiction (Posternak and Mueller 2001). Although a review of pharmacotherapy for patients with addictions is beyond the scope of this chapter, an important consideration is that treating psychiatric disorders in the presence of active substance use disorders is generally possible—and even advisable. The primary goal is to reduce morbidity of the psychiatric disorder. Treatment of comorbid psychiatric disorders may improve the outcome of the substance use disorder in some cases and also serve as a bridge to addiction treatment. Although effective pharmacological treatments are currently available only for alcohol, opioid, and nicotine dependence, medications are frequently used for symptomatic treatment of intoxication and withdrawal from a wider range of substances. Decisions about the use of these medications should be made by applying the same kind of risk-to-benefit analysis and informed consent process used for any other medication. There is no evidence that any of the approved medications enable addiction or compromise recovery.

HARM REDUCTION

The concept of harm reduction has engendered considerable controversy among those who believe that abstinence is the only acceptable goal of addiction treatment. The term *harm reduction* has been applied to a wide range of interventions and strategies that aim to decrease substance use or the harmful consequences of use rather than focusing on abstinence. From an ethical perspective, the reduction of harm clearly is inherently good unless it secondarily causes other harms. In that case, the secondary harm might be a reduction of the probability of the more highly valued outcome of total abstinence. On one hand, the concept of harm reduction is an empirical question: there is no evidence that harm-reduction programs such as needle exchange decrease rates of abstinence. On the other hand, it is an ideological question relating to the value of abstinence versus various levels of substance use. Clinicians will come to different conclusions if they see recovery as black and white (i.e., either using or abstinent) than if they assign a continuum of values to a continuum of outcomes (Geppert and Roberts 2008; Järvinen and Miller 2014).

PSEUDOADDICTION AND PAIN MANAGEMENT

Management of analgesic addiction in the context of pain syndromes requires heightened sensitivity to ethical considerations, an awareness of the importance of clinician bias, avoidance of stigma, and conscientiousness to the duty of thorough evaluation and careful documentation. A patient seeking drugs because she enjoys them and a patient seeking drugs because she is in pain look and behave much the same. Physicians must be as careful not to induce difficult power struggles related to medication seeking by undertreating pain as they are not to cavalierly dispense addicting substances simply because states license them to do so. In every community, certain doctors are more quick to prescribe, sometimes with no more rationale than the patient's request for a particular medication. Conversely, however, there are also doctors who refuse to prescribe pain medication or who undertreat pain for fear of creating addiction. As standards of care regarding practices such as mandatory drug testing evolve, the heterogeneity of physician practices should narrow and evidence regarding outcomes should be far easier to ascertain.

Adequate treatment of pain syndromes requires spending enough time with a patient to understand the sources of both emotional and physical pain and having the ability to tell the difference. For example, patients with coexisting mood disorders frequently find that they can better tolerate pain when their depression is adequately treated, and vice versa. By the same token, patients often find that when they can give voice to emotional hurts, tolerating physical pain becomes easier. It is irresponsible to treat either pain or addiction as an all-or-none phenomenon (i.e., by prescribing enough medication "no questions asked" to eliminate the pain or by refusing altogether to prescribe addictive medications). In light of the national crisis surrounding overprescription and overuse of narcotics in the United States, vigilance and new medical evidence are both needed.

EMPIRICAL ETHICS STUDIES

Although many of the ethical considerations involved in treating addictions—such as the importance of respect, fairness, and minimizing harm—are conceptual, many issues could be clarified through empirical data. For example, to what extent can people struggling with addiction provide informed consent at different stages of illness? How does substance dependence affect decisional capacity and voluntarism? Does the effect vary by type of substance? What problems are experienced in protecting the confidentiality of people with addictions? How does stigma alter the practices of clinicians who work with individuals with addiction and comorbid disorders? How does stigma affect the attitudes of medical students and residents who might consider career paths in the field of addiction treatment?

Nevertheless, very few empirical studies exist of ethical issues in addiction treatment. A study that examined informed consent practices among federally funded clinical investigators in the drug and alcohol field (McCrady and Bux 1999) found that two-thirds of the 91 respondents (51% response rate) who completed the survey reported using objective methods to determine participants' ability to provide informed consent. Less than half indicated that they routinely informed study participants of limits to confidentiality in situations of suicidality, homicidality, or child abuse. A substantial minority of the investigators reported experience with these situations in conducting research. Studies of college students have suggested that moral beliefs about substance use influence substance use behavior and that the degree of consistency between moral views and substance use increases with increasing moral maturity within Kohlberg's hierarchy (Abide et al. 2001). A qualitative study has outlined ethical dilemmas arising in work with intravenous drug users (Buchanan et al. 2002). A study of patients entering cocaine treatment found that coercive pressures were pervasive and that "informal psychosocial pressures" were more important than pressures from the legal system in stimulating the request for treatment (Marlowe et al. 1996). In a semistructured interview study, economically disadvantaged New York City residents living with addiction applied moral principles to hypothetical addiction research ethical dilemmas; the study suggested that these individuals view themselves (and researchers) as moral agents and responsible for their acts (Fisher 2011). Clearly, there is a need for much more empirical work on the ethics of addictions treatment and research.

CONCLUSION

The field of addiction treatment requires psychiatrists and other mental health clinicians to deal with a number of complex ethical issues. Although some of these issues are particularly prominent in addiction treatment, most of them are significant in other fields as well. The underlying ethical principles of beneficence, fairness, respect for persons, and truth telling are the same in all areas of medicine.

CASE SCENARIOS

■ A patient with bipolar disorder and severe alcohol use disorder fills out an advance directive stating that if he stops taking lithium and relapses, he wants to be placed back on medication and hospitalized if necessary.

■ A middle-aged man omits information related to his personal mental health and his past use of illicit substances from his application when looking for a job with a new employer.

■ A 13-year-old boy in counseling for oppositional defiant disorder tells the counselor that he has experimented with alcohol and marijuana but asks that his parents not be told.

■ A veteran with comorbid mental and addictive illnesses is admitted to a psychiatric inpatient unit. Four days into his hospitalization, he is allowed to take a walk with his brother and sister-in-law on the grounds of the VA facility. He returns 10 minutes late, walking unsteadily and speaking rapidly and in an animated fashion.

■ A 25-year-old journalist mentions to her physician that she has a family history of bipolar disorder and substance addiction. She does not want this history recorded in her electronic medical record.

Evolving Topics

15

Integrity and the Professional Roles of Psychiatrists

Laura Weiss Roberts, M.D., M.A.

Alan K. Louie, M.D.

Integrity *is a word* that means completeness. In recent years, it has come to mean the full alignment of a professional's behavior with the values and ethical guidelines of his or her field—a kind of professional "wholeness." Integrity, as noted by Miller-Keane and O'Toole (2003), is "a virtue consisting of soundness of and adherence to moral principles and character and standing up in their defense when they are threatened or under attack. This involves consistent, habitual honesty and a coherent integration of reasonably stable, justifiable moral values, with consistent judgment and action over time."

Implicit to the concept of integrity is that the values and guidelines of the profession are "right" or "good," and thus moral judgment and ethically important actions are involved. A degree of intentionality or volition is assumed in that the practitioners consciously decide to conform their behaviors to these "good" values, suggesting that this does not always come naturally, automatically, or easily. The intimation is that people, left to their natural instincts, might not always follow these values, especially when the values dictate a self-sacrifice on the part of the practitioner. Thus, professional integrity involves practitioners disciplining themselves to obey standards set forth by their profession, usually with the intention of contributing to a greater good and being in accordance with a moral good.

Although these comments are relevant to clinician-practitioners across the mental health professions, for the sake of simplicity, the focus in this chapter is on the professional standards of psychiatry. Professionals have been privileged with a certain body of knowledge and skills that others do not have, and in psychiatry, practitioners have studied medicine and the medical subspecialty of psychiatry—giving them access, when licensed, to the use of psychoactive medications, psychotherapy, somatic therapies, and other treatments for mental disorders and related conditions. The expertise and tools of psychiatrists represent a resource that may be helpful to many who are in great need and may benefit from them. The psychiatrist has something the patient may find helpful, and even when that something is provided, the patient still may lack knowledge of whether it is done properly—in the right way, at the right time, and for the right reasons. In these respects, as with any relationship between a professional and an individual in need of professional services, an inequity in power affects the relationship between the psychiatrist and the patient. For these reasons, trust in the psychiatrist–patient relationship is fundamental.

In some instances and professions, the required level of trust is said to be especially high. Sometimes the term *fiduciary relationship* or *duty* is invoked, in which the practitioner has an unusually high duty to protect the interests of the beneficiary. In psychiatry, patients at times may not be capable of making decisions or caring for themselves, because of the effects of delusions, dementia, extreme emotions, and other symptoms, for example. With legal safeguards in place, society allows psychiatrists to insist that patients remain in safe surroundings and even to administer medications or other treatments to ensure that patients and others are protected from danger. Certainly, such situations must carry the highest fiduciary duty to do what is right for the beneficiary, because what may be at stake are not merely worldly possessions but the civil liberties and life of the person.

The wide variety of fiduciary relationships outside of health care do not usually include compassion as a defining characteristic, but it is a core, or *the* core, requirement of a practitioner in medicine. *Compassion* implies an awareness of, empathy for, and joining in the patient's anguish. The practitioner's attempt to alleviate that anguish is the driving force for professional behaviors. Despite the tremendous emphasis and time put into developing the cognitive skills of a psychiatrist, the emotional ones supporting compassion are at the heart of the profession—perhaps the raison d'être for medicine. Because of the nature and prevalence of mental disorders and their severity, sensitivity, and stigma, many have argued that psychiatrists must both uphold the highest fiduciary duties and demonstrate the deepest levels of compassion.

SELF-SACRIFICE AND INTEGRITY

Professional integrity in psychiatry involves clinicians looking out for the best interests of their patients in the context of a compassionate desire to alleviate pain and suffering. One of the greatest challenges to integrity is when looking out for a patient's best interest requires some self-sacrifice on the part of the psychiatrist. In general, like other types of professionals, psychiatrists are duly compensated monetarily for their services and efforts. Nevertheless, caring for a patient may unavoidably run counter to the best interest of the provider, and in those instances the psychiatrist is expected to put the interests of the patient above his or her own. In these instances, the psychiatrist is asked to go beyond what would be reasonably expected for the professional fee offered, beyond the call of duty, and beyond what most people outside the profession would be willing to do. For instance, psychiatrists may be called on to treat patients who are violent. Despite taking standard precautions in an inpatient unit or outpatient clinic, a risk remains that the psychiatrist may be attacked and injured. The psychiatrist must draw on his or her sense of purpose and compassion for ill individuals to accept this risk. A long tradition of sacrifice exists in medicine; of historical note are the physicians who treated people during epidemics and plagues, risking the contagion of infectious diseases rather than abandoning their patients. Taking such risks closely aligns with altruism.

The question arises as to whether self-sacrifice is really necessary to provide compassionate care to others. Although self-sacrifice may not occur on a daily basis and may not be a necessity, it is eventually unavoidable given the unpredictable and extreme nature of illnesses; it is so unavoidable, in fact, that self-sacrifice is part of the values and expectations for physicians. Many authors have written about self-sacrifice or putting the needs of the patient first as part of the professionalism of physicians, but of great note are relevant parts of the guidelines from professional organizations. The American Medical Association (AMA) has published since 1847 a code of medical ethics to guide the ethical behaviors of physicians in the United States. For example, the AMA Council on Ethical and Judicial Affairs (2014) includes an opinion on the patient–physician relationship in the

AMA's *Code of Medical Ethics* 2014–2015 edition: "The relationship between patient and physician is based on trust and gives rise to physicians' ethical obligations to place patients' welfare above their own self-interest and above obligations to other groups, and to advocate for their patients' welfare" (Opinion 10.015). The AMA also publishes separately its Principles of Medical Ethics, which is included in its *Code of Medical Ethics*. One of the principles states, "A physician shall, while caring for a patient, regard responsibility to the patient as paramount" (American Medical Association 2001). In 2013, the American Psychiatric Association added this principle to its text *The Principles of Medical Ethics With Annotations Especially Applicable to Psychiatry*, noting that if "outside relationships" of the psychiatrist conflict with patient care, resolution should benefit the patient.

In day-to-day practice, most psychiatrists do not feel they are risking their lives in the care of patients, and self-sacrifice is infrequently dramatic. More often, the public associates the professionals who risk their lives in the service of others as firefighters, police officers, and soldiers, who take on their risk with special gear and weapons. The public is more likely to consider the sacrifices of physicians to involve years of medical training and long working hours with high levels of responsibility. The most common sacrifice, however, results from daily stress that accumulates, incrementally and insidiously. The effects of this stress have been studied and quantified as physician burnout and/or poor mental health (see Chapter 17, "Clinician Well-Being and Impairment"). According to the American Foundation for Suicide Prevention (2016), the suicide rate for physicians is more than twice that of the general population, and each year the number of physicians who commit suicide in the United States (approximately 400) is equivalent to the number of all the graduates from two to three medical schools. However, comprehensive, present-day studies are needed to better understand suicide among physicians and the larger health care workforce.

Perhaps the most frequent and even important ethical issue, then, relates to the small sacrifices that practitioners must decide to make every day. Sometimes these decisions are clear. For instance, taking the time to elicit a complete history about trauma may be clearly indicated and so the psychiatrist will do so. Then again, the psychiatrist may wonder if the first visit is too soon to explore the trauma, even though the patient seems quite willing and ready to do so, tearfully saying he has never told anyone else about the experience. The psychiatrist questions whether his own reluctance is based on the patient's needs—a therapeutic alliance has not yet been established for this type of trauma work—or whether he is feeling time pressure because he will surely be late to pick up his child at daycare if he extends the interview. Such decisions are hard enough, but conflicting emotions and motivations that may cloud the clinician's thinking, which are typical of life, add more stress and self-doubt. In this example, the risk to the patient of delaying the trauma interview and the sacrifice to the psychiatrist of picking up his child late lack the drama of life-and-death scenarios, yet this and higher-stakes examples constitute a whole continuum of ethical challenges up to life-and-death ones that psychiatrists must navigate regularly as part of professional integrity.

The data on physician burnout has led to some questioning about self-sacrifice in the profession. Self-sacrifice continues to be embraced as a basic tenet, as in the AMA's *Code of Medical Ethics* opinion quoted earlier, but the profession now considers whether a well physician—in contrast to an over-stressed physician and certainly an impaired one—is better able to serve the interests of patients, with better patient outcomes (Grepmair et al. 2007; Halbesleben and Rathert 2008). Thus, physician wellness has become a goal, as has mitigation of the negative effects of self-sacrifice. This effort has in spirit followed the measures in other professions, such as being sure that airline pilots are well rested when on duty to decrease pilot errors. For instance, since 2011, the Accreditation Council for Graduate Medical Education (ACGME) has limited the number of hours that a resident physician may work to 80 hours per week. This requirement and other duty-hour regulations are meant to address the previous practice of resident physicians working continuously for 36 hours—that is, working all day, all night, and all the next day. Most likely resident physicians are less sleep deprived with these revised regulations. Mitigating the adverse effects of self-sacrifice is not easy, however. Studies suggest that the duty-hour regulations may not reduce medical errors (Cedfeldt et al. 2009). Another concern is that although the hours on duty have been reduced, the amount of work expected has not, so the resident physician has to compress the same amount of work into fewer hours (Ludmerer 2010). Sleep deprivation may be lessened, but paradoxically, stress on the job may be increased.

ROLE CONFLICTS AND INTEGRITY

Beyond the individual relationship between a psychiatrist and a patient is the relationship of the discipline of psychiatry—as a specialized field within the profession of medicine—with society at large. As noted in the previous section "Self-Sacrifice and Integrity," the AMA's *Code of Medical Ethics* references "physicians' ethical obligations to place patients' welfare above their own self-interest and above obligations to other groups." The inclusion of the words "other groups" is relevant to role conflicts of the psychiatrist, because the psychiatrist may have a role in another group that conflicts with his or her role as a psychiatrist for a patient. In other words, a conflict of interest may arise from having multiple roles. A psychiatrist may have conflicting roles as a practitioner and, for example, as an owner of an imaging facility. A conflict of interest arises when the psychiatrist tells a patient to go to that imaging facility for testing. Does the fact that the psychiatrist will profit from the patient having the test done at that facility influence his or her judgment about whether the patient needs the test? Even if the bias is only on an unconscious basis, it is an ethical concern.

Role conflicts involving physicians and the pharmaceutical industry have increasingly become major issues as the number of medications and medication prices have escalated in recent times. Most patients assume that a visit to a doctor will result in a prescription, and that the physician chooses the medication in the best interest of the patient. Physicians have often prided themselves on this choice being an independent one that is based on their ample fund of scientific knowledge and considerable experience with prescribing over the years. In fact, physicians are probably far more influenced than they are aware by pharmaceutical marketing campaigns and the selective information they receive about medications. The influence of a pharmaceutical company may be even greater if the physician is a speaker for the company, a member of its consulting board, or a researcher studying its medication. These are examples of roles that might conflict with being a patient's psychiatrist. The psychiatrist may believe that the medication in question is indeed the very best one for a specific patient, but a potential for conflict of interest must still be examined.

In a 2015 series on conflicts of interest in the *New England Journal of Medicine*, Rosenbaum stated, "Suggestive data may be worse than no data at all. Studies seeking evidence of industry influence usually find it, providing us with well-publicized associations. Some 94% of physicians have relationships with industry, though these interactions most often involve activities such as receiving drug samples or food in the workplace" (Rosenbaum 2015, p. 1959). She added, "These associations are probably valid. But they don't answer the key question: Are any of these interactions, or efforts to curtail them, beneficial or harmful to patients?" (p. 1959). One of us (L.W.R.) made the same argument regarding the issue of potential conflicts of interest of individuals serving on institutional review boards (IRBs).

> Why do COIs [conflicts of interest] matter? Differing and overlapping roles, and therefore potential COIs, are common for professionals. Indeed, it is expected and correct that professionals will use their expertise as physicians, investigators, educators, consultants, leaders, and policymakers to

best serve society. These roles are sometimes paid; sometimes influential; sometimes involved with private, public, and academic partners; and often generate tensions and divided loyalties. The salient issue is whether decisions made by professionals...will be biased and their judgments distorted by these role conflicts, thus endangering study volunteers and the public trust. (Roberts 2015a, p. 1507)

Nevertheless, examples of conflicts of interest are commonplace, including physicians who prescribe more expensive medications rather than less expensive and equally effective medications due to the impact of advertising and physicians who work for speakers' bureaus and use prepared materials provided by the drug manufacturer (DeAngelis 2015).

Conflict of interest is thus not an all-or-none issue. If every physician who had anything to do with a pharmaceutical company were not allowed to prescribe that company's products, then his or her patients would be at risk of not getting an appropriate drug. If physicians were not allowed to work for pharmaceutical companies, furthermore, drug development would lack a clinical, real-world perspective. Medicine is inextricably related to the pharmaceutical industry, and isolating the two from each other would not make sense. Therefore, safeguards need to be in place that assess degrees of conflict of interest and protect the welfare of patients. These safeguards need to be evidence based, effective, and efficient.

Safeguards are essential for all types of role conflicts (see Figure 15–1), not only roles with pharmaceutical companies but also with various other organizations related to health care, such as hospital boards, medical research institutes, and consulting groups. The professional behaviors of the psychiatrist, whether prescribing medications, delivering a lecture about medications, or conducting pharmaceutical research, should be open to examination as a safeguard against bias resulting from the potential conflict of interest. For instance, if a psychiatrist has a role in a pharmaceutical company and is going to speak at a continuing medical education (CME) symposium, his or her role in the company must be declared in the printed materials of the symposium, and a director of the symposium, without conflicts, must review the speaker's talk to ensure that it is not biased and that the information is balanced and fairly represented. This safeguard practice of disclosure is now part of CME rules across most academic institutions (Jibson et al. 2015).

Consider the example of clinical research and the integrity issues that are operating at the level of the investigator and the institution itself. An IRB is entrusted with helping to ensure the rights and well-being of research subjects, who are often also patients. The investigator who leads a

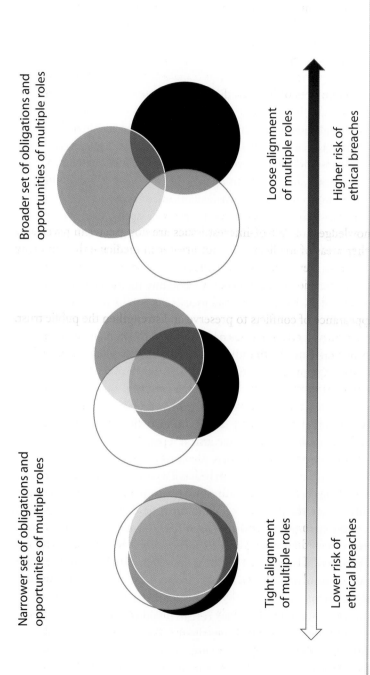

FIGURE 15–1. Ethical risk associated with multiple roles.

Source. Copyright © 2015 Laura Weiss Roberts, M.D., M.A. Used with permission.

clinical research protocol may have a dual role (as a clinician and a scientist)—or perhaps a more complex role as an owner of a company whose product is being tested in the clinical trial. Interestingly, as noted earlier, even IRB members may have conflicts of interest, which also require disclosure and management, and the institutional leadership may have conflicts because of financial investments associated with clinical research.

Managing conflicts of interest thus involves the safeguarding practices of recognition and awareness, communication and disclosure, oversight, financial limits, and recusal and role separation. For example, an IRB committee deciding on the safety of a device used in surgery would ask a committee member who has investments in the device's company to withdraw from the discussion and decision making of the committee, and literally leave the room. Financial limits are useful to draw attention and oversight to potential conflict with decisions involving large sums of money. To our knowledge, conflict-of-interest issues are not greater in psychiatry than in other areas of medicine and not greater in medicine than in many other professions. Nevertheless, given the potential vulnerability of patients and the recent attention to conflicts of interest in the media and federal legislation, it is prudent for psychiatrists to be especially vigilant to conflicts and the appearance of conflicts to preserve and strengthen the public trust.

Lastly, a growing area for role conflict relates to the evolving commercialization of medicine. In the nineteenth century, medicine centered on the doctor visiting the patient at home—all those who could afford care at home stayed away from hospitals. Because remedies were limited, much of the treatment was in the physician–patient relationship. Patients paid what they could. Since then, medicine has become much more complicated. Advances in science and technology have led to a proliferation of medications, surgeries, imaging, devices, and other therapies—all of which have added to the cost of care. Concurrently, the academic medical center, the National Institutes of Health, Medicare, Medicaid, and the medical insurance industry developed. Now the physician and patient are not alone—third parties, such as insurance companies and health care organizations, intrude on their relationship. More than ever, physicians are employees or contractors of some organization. Therefore, they have both the role of being the patient's physician and the role of being an employee of the organization. Conflicts of interest may result when the physician advises a patient not to pursue a treatment—one that would be costly for the organization. In this context, the question arises whether the physician's decision is influenced by the fact that the employer will save money; in many cases of early managed care in the United States, the physician was rewarded for such a decision (see Chapter 21, "Population Health and Evolving Systems of Care").

The commercialization of medicine also means that health care appears to have become more of a business transaction than an act of human care-giving. This transactional quality detracts from, or even threatens, the trust and compassion that are fundamental to the physician–patient relationship. Physicians have less time to spend with patients because they spend more time filling out insurance forms and dealing with business aspects of their practices. More physicians work on shifts, resulting in patients being handed off from one team to another around the clock. Even when the physician is with the patient, a computer may be between them in the examination room, because records are now computerized. Lastly, health care organizations are focused on populations of patients. Financial considerations may emphasize making better health care decisions for the population than for the individual patient. Because resources are limited, the most cost-effective decisions may favor screening a population over intensive treatment of one individual. In the end, the population may be better off at the expense of the individual; this ethical issue is very different from what the nineteenth-century physician had to weigh.

MEDICAL TRAINING AND INTEGRITY

Medical educators are interested in how to teach professional integrity (see Chapter 20, "Clinical Training"). Such teaching is often thought of rather simply as the curriculum regarding humanism in medicine. Highly knowledgeable, skilled, and humanistic practitioners are critically needed—but how are these qualities developed? One strategy is to provide more education during medical school about ethics and the behavioral and social aspects of medicine and to fortify the long tradition of the bond between physician and patient. This kind of exposure is also extending to premedical education. The Medical College Admission Test includes a section about behavioral and social science knowledge. Perhaps this section will assist in screening applicants on this type of knowledge, in addition to motivating applicants to take college courses in these subjects. We do not know, however, whether increased knowledge in these areas, including ethics, actually results in greater valuing and practice of compassion and self-sacrifice. Nevertheless, there is clear evidence that core ethical skills can be taught, such as how to obtain informed consent sensitively and in a manner that fulfills the ideal of optimal communication, clear decision making, optimal support for voluntary choices, and minimal external coercive pressures (Roberts et al. 1999b, 2003a; Walker et al. 1989).

The development of professional integrity must proceed in earnest after graduation from medical school. At that point, during graduate medical education or residency, the ACGME oversees the training programs of the vast majority of all psychiatrists and other physicians in the United States. The ACGME (2011) core program requirements for professionalism in all residency training programs, including psychiatry, state, "Residents are expected to demonstrate responsiveness to patient needs that supersedes self-interest" (p. 13). This expectation resembles the professional virtue of self-sacrifice. As discussed previously, this requirement has been counterbalanced by regulations that restrict duty hours for residents and that are meant to protect the wellness of residents. The training director is tasked with making residents aware of the decisions they make that may be biased by their self-interests, even unconsciously, every day. Once aware, residents need to monitor themselves to be sure that their behavior adheres to the profession's values, guidelines, and standards of care. Thus, professional integrity has a learning curve. Early-career physicians must learn to be aware, to monitor themselves, to make their behaviors adhere to correct standards, and to learn what the professional values, guidelines, and standards of care are in each patient situation. This developmental maturity takes several years with supervision from experienced physicians who themselves model professional integrity.

Because the calling and practice of medicine set a high bar not just for intellect, knowledge, and medical skill—but also for character—professional integrity that the physician begins to learn in medical school is built on a foundation of personal integrity that influences all spheres of an individual-physician's life. The concepts and practice of medical ethics may seem particularly unnatural and difficult to value as one's own when a personal ethical foundation has not already been established to some degree, even as all physicians and individuals have the potential to value and practice ethics in greater degrees of maturity.

Therefore, in medicine, physicians are not born with professional integrity, it is not all or none, and it is not learned overnight. Some individuals, however, as a result of temperament or development, may be more or less inclined to the medical values of compassion and self-sacrifice. Some would argue that these factors suggest that not everyone is suited to becoming—or living the life of—a physician. This observation leads to a difficult question: Should medical schools screen applicants to determine who is more inclined to these ethically important values? Indeed, admissions committees have been trying to do this for a long time, mainly on the basis of individual interviews. In this regard, however, interviews are not highly reliable or perhaps even valid. Attempts are being made to better assess applicants with techniques such as the Multiple Mini-Interview, first published in 2004, which includes ethical dilemma questions (Eva et al. 2004a, 2004b, 2004c). It is hoped that this and other approaches will prove valid and practical.

Research has suggested that prediction in medical schools of future unethical behaviors in physicians is hard. Despite best efforts, some people will be accepted into medical school who will have difficulty assimilating the values of compassion and self-sacrifice. Many students who have to leave medical school do so because of issues with professionalism and/or interpersonal skills (Dyrbye et al. 2010b). Medical schools should do their best to find these students early on and provide remediation. If remediation efforts fail, the school's faculty and leadership must have the courage to pursue appropriate dismissal proceedings with due process. Medical schools are loath to dismiss students, because so much time and so many resources are invested in the training of a medical student. It is natural that every school would work toward graduation for every student, but justified dismissals are, in fact, part of the professional integrity of the medical school.

THE PURSUIT OF EXCELLENCE

Following the values and guidelines of the profession of psychiatry is not as simple as blindly following rules. The AMA's *Code of Medical Ethics* indicates that ethical behavior includes a proactive quality to better oneself and the profession—to pursue excellence. The code states that the physician should "study, apply, and advance scientific knowledge" (Principle V; American Medical Association 2001). Consistent with this, physicians are required by most state licensing boards to obtain CME credits each year. Most boards that certify physicians in various specialties and subspecialties are beginning to require Maintenance of Certification activities. Beyond continuous study, physicians are directed to further knowledge in medicine. The AMA's *Code of Medical Ethics* also states that physicians should participate in the "improvement of the community and the betterment of public health" (Principle VII; American Medical Association 2001). Today's physician needs to think about the whole population, systems of health care delivery, and public health needs. Physicians are called on to take leadership roles in health care, to advocate for patient care, and perhaps even to influence health policies. The pursuit of excellence entreats physicians to make medicine more than a job or career and to live it as a calling.

CONCLUSION

The concepts of professionalism and integrity are strongly related and particularly salient in psychiatry. Professionalism assumes a wholeness and consistency in conduct and beliefs, and these serve as the foundation of professional integrity. In psychiatry, patients, who are at times dependent and vulnerable, need to be able to trust that their psychiatrists are knowledgeable, skilled, and compassionate and will put the patients' interests before their own self-interests. At times, psychiatrists must make sacrifices to serve their patients' best interests. This is unavoidable in practice, and psychiatrists are expected to make such sacrifices while monitoring that their performance is not impaired by decreased well-being secondary to the sacrifice (e.g., sleep deprivation). Most certainly, they must eschew conflicts of interest that compromise the care of patients, especially resulting from dual roles as a psychiatrist as well as an investor, business owner, board member, researcher, and so on. Safeguards need to be put in place to manage conflicts of interest, including those that unexpectedly arise or are not in the physician's conscious awareness, and may include monitoring for risky situations, disclosure of additional roles, oversight, financial limits, recusal from decision making, and role separation. Not only do psychiatrists need to avoid harm, but they should also do good, by advancing the field and the health of society and always pursuing excellence in the profession of psychiatry. Meeting these aspects of calling requires that psychiatrists have education, training, discipline, and years of practice.

CASE SCENARIOS

- The chair of psychiatry at an academic medical center receives a call from the chief executive officer of the university hospital, requesting mental health treatment for her mother-in-law and follow-up reports.

- The lone psychiatrist in a rural area is treating a patient with borderline personality disorder. The patient is verbally abusive, saying the doctor is terrible, insulting his family, and cursing at him. Nevertheless, the patient wants to continue psychotherapy. The psychiatrist finds the sessions extremely stressful but views the patient's behavior as part of the disorder, which he alone is trained to treat.

- A psychiatrist's spouse is very supportive of her career, but her long hours on duty have threatened their marriage. They hardly see each other, have stopped being intimate, and are on the verge of divorce. Couples therapy has not helped. At their tenth wedding anniversary dinner, one of her long-time patients calls in crisis and says he does not want to see the covering psychiatrist.

■ The psychiatrist works for a health maintenance organization that needs its physicians to carry large patient loads to stay profitable. One patient would benefit from more frequent visits, but the psychiatrist's schedule is booked for 2 months. He could give her a new patient slot, but this would make his access metrics worse. He is trying to decide how much the patient "really" needs to come in and what to tell the patient.

■ A psychiatrist exclusively prescribes one antidepressant for her patients with depression, even though most psychiatrists prescribe various available antidepressants that are of similar efficacy depending on a patient's history. The psychiatrist truly believes that the antidepressant she prescribes is a great medication, and she owns stock in the pharmaceutical company that manufactures it.

16

Patient Care Ethics Committees and Consultation Services

Tom Townsend, M.D.

Laura Weiss Roberts, M.D., M.A.

Many ethically important decisions rest on the shoulders of individual professionals. Depending on the nature of the patient care situation, however, other stakeholders, such as members of the profession or colleagues within the organization, may share in the responsibility of making, enabling, enacting, or overseeing decisions. Patient care ethics committees and consultation services are examples of resources that help in highly important and ethically complex clinical situations. These resources are so important that each hospital is required to provide these patient care ethics resources as part of its formal accreditation.

The formal, structural requirement to provide ethics resources reflects broad recognition that individual professionals may not be sufficiently equipped to deal with all the different kinds of ethics questions that arise, even though they may be individuals with great knowledge, skill, and conscience. Furthermore, because there may be legitimate differences in values, preferences, and judgments between patient and clinician, between family and patient, and among health care professionals, some social and administrative mechanism is needed—short of judicial review—to air, clarify, and find common ground among these differences so that actions may be taken in caring for patients. Patient care ethics committees and consultation services represent one approach to this need. Psychiatrists and other mental health professionals are important participants in these committees and services. This chapter reviews the development of these organizational ethics resources and their application in clinical practice.

RISE OF PATIENT CARE ETHICS COMMITTEES

It is helpful to review some reasons for the claim that decisions by committees (and clinicians in conjunction with guidance provided by consultative services) in hospitals have moral significance. Whereas the modern bioethics movement had its origins in the 1960s, the last half of the twentieth century saw the recognition and buttressing of global civil rights—not just the rights to guarantee racial fairness, but the rights of all groups at risk: children, women, those with mental illness or handicaps, and, almost by definition, the medically ill. These individual rights were developing at the same time that modern medicine was developing technologies to prolong life and reduce suffering. These interventions changed practice, for example, in the care of premature newborns in the neonatal intensive care unit, of permanently unconscious patients, and of patients with advanced renal failure. Concurrently, controversies related to dubious research practices, definitions of legal and clinical death, abortion rights and legislation, and new strains on access to health care arose. Responses to these events led to a new mechanism for critical thinking about making difficult, ethically laden choices—in this case, decision by committee.

Historical Background for Medical Research Practices

The most direct antecedent of the hospital ethics committee was the institutional review board (IRB), which arose out of the national response to reports of abuses of human subjects in research in which moral claims for informed consent were severely breached (see Chapter 18, "Psychiatric Research"). Many examples of such abuses were listed by Beecher (1966) in his landmark article "Ethics and Clinical Research," forever changing the consciousness of medical scientists in the United States. Katz's (1972) monumental text, *Experimentation With Human Beings*, provided an in-depth catalogue of exploitative human research practices. The exploitation of people with mental illness paled in comparison with that of elders, people with intellectual disabilities, children, and individuals at the end of life, as revealed over the next several years. Of special concern was that these exploitative research practices in the United States occurred in the aftermath of the 1946 Nuremberg Trials of Nazi physicians, which revealed that involuntary "research" had been done on human beings, resulting in tremendous suffering and often death. The worldwide outrage in response to these discoveries in the Nuremberg Trials led to the development of the Nuremberg Code of Ethics (U.S. Department of Health and Human Services 1949), which contained 10 ethical requirements for experimentation on human participants. This code of ethics was intended to recognize and guarantee the rights of each subject as an individual, as well as protect the participants' welfare (Katz 1996). Regrettably, this rather simple and unassailable goal was not to be achieved in the United States for several decades.

Three U.S. incidents are presented here as examples:

- In 1963, elderly patients with chronic illnesses living at the Jewish Chronic Disease Hospital in Brooklyn were injected with live cancer cells to see if the cells would survive in ill patients without cancer. Although the researchers apparently did not believe that the cells would remain viable or induce cancer, they did the experiment without any forewarning and without obtaining consent from the patients or their families.
- Earlier, in 1932, the U.S. Public Health Service began research on African American men in impoverished rural Tuskegee, Alabama, to discover the natural course of tertiary syphilis. Patients were followed closely with examinations and blood tests but were provided no therapy, even after penicillin became available in the 1940s. Some invasive tests (e.g., lumbar punctures to study spinal fluid) were even presented as therapy. The study continued until reported to the public in a newspaper article in 1972. That article prompted a review by the U.S. Department of Health, Education, and Welfare, which concluded that the study had been "ethically unjustified" from its inception.
- Finally, in 1967, it was discovered that ongoing research at the Willowbrook State School in New York had been exposing institutionalized children with intellectual disabilities to hepatitis to observe the course of the disease. Although this so-called research occurred at a time when hepatitis was not well understood and a vaccine was not yet available— and during an era when many institutionalized individuals contracted hepatitis—it emerged that the institution's admission policy accorded preference to children whose families had "volunteered" them for the research (Fletcher et al. 1997).

Once revealed, these and other research debacles prompted Congress to create the National Commission for the Protection of Human Subjects of Biomedical and Behavioral Research in 1974. The commission subsequently developed *The Belmont Report: Ethical Principles and Guidelines for the Protection of Human Subjects of Research* (National Commission for the Protection of Human Subjects of Biomedical and Behavioral Research 1979). From the commission's work and the Belmont Report came a recommendation that any research involving human subjects be reviewed locally by IRBs. IRBs were to include not only researchers but also, importantly, lay members to contribute vital community perspectives that might otherwise be overlooked. This important addition to committee membership modeled the way that hospital ethics committees would be constituted.

Early Forms of Hospital Ethics Committees

Compelling patient care issues that propelled the development of health care ethics committees in the 1960s and 1970s often involved moral dilemmas created by the difficult decisions of how to use developing technologies most effectively. For instance, hemodialysis for chronic renal disease was developed in the 1930s by Willem Kolff and used after World War II, but there was not a technology that allowed repeated use until Belding Scribner, a physician in Seattle, made an artery-to-vein shunt that could be reused. Scribner's first patient, Clyde Shields, lived for 11 years after Scribner's discovery. Although the new technology represented an astonishing advance for individuals previously doomed to uremia (renal toxicity) and death, it initially was available only in Seattle. This meant that despite the immediate demand for the machines, access was limited. In fact, a patient had to live in Washington State to receive dialysis in the University of Washington hospital where Scribner worked.

To guide the decision of rationing use of these scarce and expensive "artificial kidney machines," the hospital recruited an anonymous committee of lay members from the community to review candidates and determine whether to offer the procedure, depending on the committee's judgment about the relative social worth of the individuals. The committee, colloquially known as "the God Committee," became notorious after an article describing its deliberations appeared in *Life* magazine. Although the article was favorable toward dialysis, the committee's role led to considerable controversy and increased media attention to medical ethics issues in general.

In 2002, Kolff and Scribner (at ages 91 and 81 years, respectively) received the Lasker Award for Medical Research for their work with the early dialysis units. The award citation stated that dialysis not only transformed kidney failure from a fatal disease to a treatable one but also spawned the discipline of medical ethics (Altman 2002).

In 1967, Christiaan Barnard successfully performed organ transplantation with a human heart in South Africa. This event signaled substantial changes in medicine and health care ethics attitudes. Its significance for institutional ethics committees became clear within a year, when the Ad Hoc Committee of the Harvard Medical School to Examine the Definition of Brain Death (1968) published its work to establish the criteria that would be used to pronounce death in patients being kept on respirators until their organs could be retrieved for transplantation. Subsequent legislation derived from the President's Commission for the Study of Ethical Problems in Medicine and Biomedical and Behavioral Research, established by Congress (1978–1983), included a Uniform Determination of Death Act. Thus, the prior work of the Harvard ethics committee successfully addressed the very difficult issues of delineating death and determining who should receive organ transplantation. This committee was entrusted with acting responsibly within a health care institution to influence national policy without waiting for persons or organizations outside medicine to develop such policies.

In 1976, the New Jersey Supreme Court heard the case of Karen Ann Quinlan, a young woman in a coma who required ventilator support to live. The significance of this case for bioethics was immense. In their decision, the justices were clearly impressed by an article stating that "many hospitals have established an ethics committee...which serves to review the individual circumstances of ethics dilemma[s]" and act in an advisory capacity to the clinical team (Teel 1975, pp. 8, 9). In their decision on whether to allow disconnection of the respirator at the request of the family, the justices ruled that if Quinlan's attending physician determined that there was no reasonable chance that she would ever return to a "cognitive, sapient state" and if the hospital ethics committee (they called it a "prognosis committee") agreed with that prognosis, the family's request for withdrawal could be granted. The court's decision suggested to the medical community that end-of-life health care issues needed to stay out of the judicial system when possible.

In 1983, the President's Commission for the Study of Ethical Problems in Medicine and Biomedical and Biobehavioral Research published "Deciding to Forgo Life-Sustaining Treatment." The commission recognized that the many difficult treatment decisions surrounding life-prolonging therapies offered to adults with compromised decisional capacity and to seriously ill newborns would require committees to protect the interests of incapacitated patients. The members of the commission understood that these ethics committees could not fully safeguard patients against potential harm, but they believed that attempts to educate, recommend policy, and review cases would increase the likelihood that these tough decisions would be made locally and without repeated forays into court; in fact, the commission hoped to see the courts used only as a last resort.

EVOLVING ROLES OF PATIENT CARE ETHICS COMMITTEES AND CONSULTATION SERVICES

Most professional practice organizations call for health care institutions to have some sort of ethics resource. Very importantly, since 1991, the Joint Commission on Accreditation of Healthcare Organizations (now called The Joint Commission), which sets standards and regulates the health care industry, has required a mechanism for considering ethical issues arising in the care of patients. This mechanism, most commonly a patient care ethics committee or consultation service, must also provide education to clinicians and patients on ethical issues in health care. The Joint Commission requirement was later changed to entail a "functioning process to address ethical issues" in patient rights and organizational ethics. This broader language permits diverse forms of ethics activities to fulfill institutional ethics requirements.

From the very start, the inclusion of a psychiatrist, psychologist, or other expert in mental health was recommended for patient care ethics committees, services, and programs. Consultation-liaison psychiatrists, now referred to as psychosomatic medicine physicians, historically have played a critically important role in the evolution and conduct of hospital ethics committees and services.

Ethics committees and consultation services have been a part of the decision-making landscape in U.S. health care for decades; however, debate continues about what is expected of such resources and how they can be evaluated.

CORE FUNCTIONS

Both health care ethics committees and consultation services are customarily expected to play three important roles—ethics education, policy formulation and review, and case consultation—in the institution and the community they serve. (These core functions are discussed further in this section.) The American Society for Bioethics and Humanities has prepared a resource document updating the core competencies and emerging standards for health care ethics consultations (Tarzian and ASBH Core Competencies Update Task Force 1 2013).

Health care ethics committees and consultation services perform the following activities:

- Host educational programs on salient medical ethics topics.
- Create a venue for discussion of biomedical-ethical issues in the institution.
- Provide advice and resources on patient care decision making.
- Conduct reviews of ethically important cases or decisions.
- Offer guidance on institutional policies related to bioethical issues.

Within an institution, the committee or consultation service both educates and advises, which makes it imperative that the ethics program be available and visible.

Ethics Education

Education is essential to any ethics program, regardless of the institution's size. Education on issues of ethics and health care law should be continuously offered to health care professionals, staff, and the lay community. Ethics education for clinicians and ethics committee members in the form of ethics rounds in hospitals, particularly in intensive care units, has been shown to have a beneficial effect. In some situations these educational activities can function proactively to obviate the need for a full ethics consultation.

Educational opportunities led by the ethics committee or consultation service may serve to further educate members of these teams—a form of "on-the-job" training. It is also useful to have new ethics team members join the committee simultaneously. This shared transition period offers a kind of orientation phase in which knowledge about the history and theory of bioethics may be imparted. In addition, new members can become comfortable engaging in honest—and occasionally quite candid—moral discourse with others on the committee. Acquiring and practicing ethics skills may be enhanced by reviewing current cases, studying landmark or paradigmatic cases in the literature, role-playing of important cases, and participating in general discussions of applied ethical theory. It is not difficult to engage staff or laypersons in the compelling topics of clinical and research ethics that appear in the news.

Programs just getting started usually do well to have some form of organized reading program, in which motivated members lead conversations about specific issues they have identified and about outside regional resources and networks (including recently developed Web sites). Such a program might begin by reviewing in greater depth the general history of ethics committees, as outlined briefly in this chapter, and especially the publications of the various governmental bioethics commissions. Several in-depth introductory texts (American Medical Association 2001; American Psychiatric Association 2013b; Beauchamp and Childress 2012; Bloch and Green 2009; Council on Ethical and Judicial Affairs 2014; Jonsen et al. 1998) offer more support to interested learners who have had limited exposure to the literature of bioethics. Although the case-based consultations provided by ethics committees are often their most visible activities, the educational service of ethics committees represents their greatest contribution to institutions.

Policy Formulation and Review

Ethics committees and consultation services offer pivotal support in developing institutional procedures and policies. By outlining what the institution says it will do and specifying who is responsible for having it done, institutional procedures and policies offer accountability in the institution's care of patients. Examples of policies required by The Joint Commission that need the consultation (or origination) of the ethics committee include informed consent, advance directives, pain management, confidentiality, and treatment refusal. The committee can serve as a forum for—or orchestrate—the necessary debate on the understanding and wording of the policy. This process nearly always involves creating differing and alternative policies and selecting the best policy for the institution after involving leaders in the institution and community. Institutional culture evolves with the appearance of new therapies and clinicians; the ethics committee and its policies act as an institutional memory and ensure that institutional policies both make sense and reflect the culture of the institution. Also, policy development, which can be conducted effectively in subcommittee assignments, can offer a tremendous opportunity for education.

Case Consultation

Patient care ethics committees and consultation services work to help clinicians, patients, and their families make difficult moral, as well as clinically sound, decisions. Ethics consultation is what many ethics committee members consider to be their core task; they are being trained to help people make ethically correct and defensible clinical decisions within the institution. Patient care ethics consultation services differ from committees by following a more traditional medical model: a small team, typically led by a physician, offers guidance to the responsible medical care team regarding a specific patient's care. The guidance may be reviewed by a larger group, including sometimes a separate health care ethics committee, but the responsible medical care team can accept or decline the advice. A physician may lead health care ethics committees, but often other professionals, such as ethicists or attorneys, serve in this capacity.

Developing ethical clinical practices requires the conjunction of several elements: bioethics principles, ethics skills, and evidence-based clinical practice standards (Figure 16–1). Health care ethics committees and consultation services can help apply these basic elements as they assist clinicians, patients, and families. Although ethics committees and services are designed to be pragmatic and thus useful to the institutions they serve, ethics case consultations are nonetheless always confronted with novel situations. As such, their results remain rather variable, and they are not always appreciated—or even sought or permitted—by patients, families, or the health care team. As with other forms of clinical consultation, members of an ethics committee will ideally approach ethics consultation with respect for the complexity of the patient care situation, offering assistance and expert knowledge whenever possible, with an appreciation of the boundaries and scope of their role.

Discussion of cases is an ongoing educational goal and responsibility of ethics committees. Cases need to be explored in depth, and attempts to condense the reasoning loop (e.g., dismissing an issue of patient refusal of clearly beneficial treatment as "autonomy") may preclude appropriate assessment of the issues involved. Understanding novel ethics issues will require that individual members of multiple disciplines and backgrounds express the variety of values that each is depended on to contribute. Committees and consultative teams whose members have worked together for some time and encountered many kinds of patient care dilemmas can often reach the core of a case immediately. However, when members are less experienced and still learning, even simple cases require complex moral discussions that go beyond mere resolution of the case. Paradigmatic cases, cases from workbooks or case-study books, and foundational legal cases, as well as standard texts, all provide opportunities for exploring an ethical issue (for examples, see Dickenson and Fulford 2000; Horn 1998; Roberts and Hoop 2008; Roberts and Reicherter 2015).

It is very important to note that arriving at a clear consensus is not always the aim of an ethics consultation. Instead, identifying solutions that

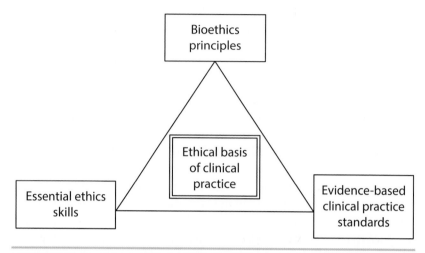

FIGURE 16–1.   The ethical basis of clinical practice: applying principles, skills, and evidence.

Source.   Reprinted from Roberts LW, Dyer AR: *Concise Guide to Ethics in Mental Health Care.* Washington, DC, American Psychiatric Publishing, 2004, p. 304. Copyright © 2004 American Psychiatric Publishing. Used with permission.

are acceptable—and defining solutions that are *not* acceptable—may be a more appropriate goal.

Ethics consultations are often called simply to shed light on ethical issues commonly witnessed in the institution, without necessarily referring to a particular case. For instance, a house officer unfamiliar with the health care law about advance directives might request assistance, which will not require a full consultation; or a staff member might initiate a discussion about a specific case or type of issue (e.g., a patient refusing what the health care team deems to be beneficial therapy). These types of cases are legitimately handled without the full consultation team or the committee. Indeed, consultations may occur through an ethics committee, a subset of that committee, or an individual consultant or consultation team.

It is critical that there be institutional support for the committee and/ or its consultation service, because consultation is a complex task with repercussions. A consultation service should be careful not to take on more than it can handle—that is, the complexity of the role should correspond to the level of sophistication of the service and the resources it has available. For this reason, some services may offer only information and education, others may provide a forum for discussion but not advice, still others might serve a mediation role, and some might even handle administrative or organizational ethics issues.

Institutional policies should be explicit about how the consultation service is to be approached, who can request a consultation, what the consultation service's role is, what types of cases can be addressed, whether recommendations will be offered, and when, if ever, such recommendations may be binding rather than advisory. Given the moral complexities in clinical care, most people believe that ethics consultations should be advisory only. There is always a possibility that any binding recommendation from the ethics committee will be perceived as coercive. Binding recommendations may be especially problematic when the health care team holds a different view from that of the ethics committee or the patient. Again, a psychiatrist or psychologist on a patient care ethics committee or consultation service can make an important contribution by observing and reflecting on the group process and fostering awareness of the boundaries and scope of the group's work together.

At most institutions, ethics committees may be approached for assistance by any stakeholder involved in a case, ranging from patients or family members to physicians or hospital administrators. Consultation services may be more restricted, with most (or all, by definition, in some institutions) requests deriving from the primary clinical care teams. Nevertheless, if an ethics consultation is to be done, notifying the attending physician is essential, regardless of whether that physician requested the consultation. It is just as important to notify and obtain the consent of the patient or surrogate, if possible.

Table 16–1 lists questions that may assist ethics discussions.

SELECTION OF MEMBERS

Ethics conversations require the representation of divergent viewpoints in order to be comprehensive and attuned to the complexity and diversity of situations encountered in health care. Ethics committees must include members from multiple disciplines, diverse cultures, and different social groups to serve their function well. It is helpful to have a professional ethicist on the committee. Attorneys likewise can provide a valuable perspective; however, participation of the lawyer representing the hospital would constitute a conflict of interest that should be disclosed and well understood among the committee members. Tolerating and being receptive to divergent viewpoints, which are important for cultural diversity and understanding, can help members to win the trust of various constituencies.

Many have recognized the critically important role of psychiatrists and other mental health professionals in health care committee discussions,

TABLE 16–1. Questions to help guide ethics committee discussions

1. What are the central medical considerations of this case?

2. What is the accepted standard of care for the patient? If not known, what are two or three possible courses of action that would meet current standards in this case?

3. What are the patient's preferences in this situation?

4. What is the patient's decision-making capacity? If the patient lacks capacity, what is understood about the patient's lifelong values? Are there advance directives? Is there an appropriate decision maker?

5. What are the significant human factors of the case? (Examples include patient's age, attitudes, occupation, religious beliefs, and values.)

6. Identify all of the related major value factors present for the patient, for the health care professionals, and for other relevant persons who are involved in the case. Which of these are health care values (e.g., comfort, benefit) and which are other kinds of considerations (e.g., economic, political)?

7. Identify and describe the major value conflict in the case.

8. Prioritize the ethical values that are in conflict in the case.

9. Has everyone who should be involved in the process been included?

Source. Reprinted from Roberts LW, Dyer AR: *Concise Guide to Ethics in Mental Health Care.* Washington, DC, American Psychiatric Publishing, 2004, p. 308. Copyright © 2004 American Psychiatric Publishing. Used with permission.

both to provide insight into key elements of the case and to track and facilitate the committee's process of reflection and deliberation. Attunement to the complexities of group process and collaborative decision making, combined with sophisticated knowledge of patient decisional capacity issues, may facilitate optimal committee processes. Moreover, poorly recognized psychiatric issues that exist in the case may precipitate ethics consultations. In many institutions, a high, and perhaps disproportionate, number of cases referred for consultation are triggered by issues that fall within the domain of psychiatry (e.g., delirium or cognitive distortions) or may benefit from the skill set of psychiatrists (e.g., family discord or grief).

Additionally, the personal qualities of committee members matter greatly. Committee members must possess integrity. They need to be interested in the work of the committee and the institution. They need to be respected, but that does not mean they need to be powerful. They need to be easy to talk with, willing to listen, and open to learning. They must have strength of character (rather than being merely oppositional) and must be communicative (not merely talkative). A health care ethics committee is known for its ability to shape ethical behavior in the institution and the community. Influence of committee members always depends on the respect they have earned among colleagues and seldom on any special skills they possess in a particular pedagogy.

PROFESSIONAL ASSOCIATION ETHICS COMMITTEES

Various professional organizations maintain ethics committees to review complaints from patients or clients, educate their members on matters of ethics, and sanction or discipline unethical members. Notably, those professions that engage in psychotherapeutic practices take these responsibilities particularly seriously. The American Psychiatric Association, the American Psychological Association, and the National Association of Social Workers maintain active ethics committees both nationally and locally. These associations have written codes of ethics or statements of ethics principles by which members agree to abide and against which complaints of unethical behavior may be judged. Professional codes and standards pertaining to ethical conduct serve both to delineate the profession's responsibility to the public and to offer guidance to its practitioners.

CONCLUSION

More than personal morality is involved in clinical ethics. The health care professions both require and rely on a larger code of professional conduct, an ethos for all practitioners that defines their social role and represents the integrity of the professions. When health care practitioners breach these standards, they jeopardize not only their personal identity but also any moral presence and contribution that the profession as a whole might have in society. Professionalism is neither fully formulated nor static; rather, it is constantly evolving as reflective clinicians and outside observers call for improvements or alterations in the practice of medicine to meet changing conditions. The many advances in technological capabilities in the past few decades have been accompanied by the appearance of new and dangerous diseases, economic and insurance instability, and increasing complexity in the delivery and receipt of health care. Patients trust their clinicians to do, or to advocate, what is understood to be clinically and socially best for the patient. At times, however, satisfactory clinical and ethical outcomes will naturally entail consultation with a committee or service specially constituted to help deliberate over choices and to represent diverse and complex views in the service of patients' interests and well-being.

CASE SCENARIOS

■ A 14-year-old boy with terminal glioblastoma has undergone innovative radiation treatments and multiple medication trials. He says that he is "done now" and wishes to die. "I tried to stay alive because it hurts my parents so much to think of me dying, but I am done." The staff calls for a psychiatry consult and refers the case to the ethics committee.

■ A second-year resident states that she will not "do shock therapy" on patients, even if the training program requires that she learn this clinical treatment procedure. She approaches her attending physician, who says that she must learn the procedure. She objects and requests an ethics consultation to discuss the situation.

■ A psychiatrist serving on the clinical ethics committee in an academic setting has set up his electronic mail account so that his executive assistant can read his messages without the senders knowing.

■ A physician at a mental health center collects unused medications from his patients. He takes them to his local church and distributes them to parishioners whom he thinks are "in need" but who lack adequate resources to get "their pills in the usual way from doctors." A parishioner who works at the medical center raises the issue for the patient care ethics committee to discuss.

■ A pharmaceutical representative brings coffee, doughnuts, and pens for distribution at a local continuing medical education event. The chief of the medical staff brings this question to the ethics consultation service to discuss.

17

Clinician Well-Being and Impairment

Mickey Trockel, M.D.

Merry N. Miller, M.D.

Laura Weiss Roberts, M.D., M.A.

Psychiatrists carry enormous personal burdens in their service to others—service as part of a profession that cannot be practiced impersonally. It is estimated that a psychotherapist has 10 productive years before burnout (Table 17–1) and disillusionment from working intensively with the psychological suffering of others overtake the idealism that motivated most people to enter a helping profession in the first place (Grosch and Olsen 1994). Moreover, psychiatrists experience the same threats to their health and well-being as other physicians, who commonly suffer from stress and stress-related disorders, substance abuse, depression, and personal and family problems. The probability of ever being divorced among physicians is 24.3%, a rate similar to that of other professionals such as dentists (25%), nurses (33%), and attorneys (27%), but the rate is dramatically higher among women physicians (Ly et al. 2015).

The overall annual physician suicide rate has been estimated to be more than twice that of the general population (American Foundation for Suicide Prevention 2016). In one study of nearly 8,000 U.S. surgeons, 15% reported

TABLE 17–1. Symptoms of burnout

Physical	Behavioral	Psychological	Spiritual	Clinical
Fatigue	Loss of enthusiasm	Depression	Loss of faith	Cynicism toward patients
Physical depletion	Coming late to work	Emptiness	Loss of meaning	Daydreaming during sessions
Irritability	Accomplishing little despite long hours	Negative self-concept	Loss of purpose	Hostility toward patients
Headaches	Quickness to frustration and anger	Pessimism	Feelings of alienation	Boredom toward patients
Gastrointestinal disturbances	Becoming increasingly rigid	Guilt	Feelings of estrangement	Quickness to diagnose
Back pain	Difficulty making decisions	Self-blame for not accomplishing more	Changes in religious beliefs	Blaming patients
Weight change	Closing out new input	Feelings of omnipotence	Changes in religious affiliation	
Change in sleep pattern	Increased dependence on/withdrawal from colleagues			
	Irritation with coworkers			

Source. Adapted from Grosch WN, Olsen DC: *When Helping Starts to Hurt: A New Look at Burnout Among Psychotherapists.* New York, WW Norton, 1994. Copyright © 1994 WW Norton. Used with permission.

having thoughts of ending their lives (7% in the prior year), and 39% were reluctant to seek psychiatric care due to fear of repercussions for their medical license (Shanafelt et al. 2011). Among female physicians the risk of suicide is especially high, with suicide completion rates that are as much as 4 times higher than those for females in the general population (Center et al. 2003; Council on Scientific Affairs 1987; Frank and Dingle 1999; Sargent 1987; Schernhammer and Colditz 2004).

Medical students and residents become exhausted; they have little time to establish patterns of preventive health; they are vulnerable to addiction, mental illness, and relationship problems; and they may fear academic repercussions if they acknowledge being ill or seeking personal health care (Roberts et al. 2001b). Physicians-in-training are at heightened risk for substance use disorders (Miller and McGowen 2000) and for suicide. In a six-school study with more than 2,000 medical student and resident participants, for instance, Goebert et al. (2009) found that 12% of respondents met criteria for probable major depression, worse among medical students and women in the study, and 6% reported recent suicidal ideation. The pattern of depression and suicidal ideation was heightened for underrepresented minority group members—especially among Alaska Native, Native American, Pacific Islander, and African American individuals. This pattern is of particular concern, given the number of new medical schools that are being introduced in the United States, a significant proportion of which are specifically seeking to train minority physicians as a core mission.

The mental distress and loss of life among health professionals is a tragedy of enormous personal, professional, and societal dimensions. The following ethical issues are relevant in this discussion:

- The ethical obligation to care for oneself—the ethical imperative as society's caretakers to remain healthy, both physically and emotionally
- Professional obligations to intervene when aware of an impaired professional, and personal obligations to help a distressed colleague
- Ethical dilemmas in caring for professional colleagues and their families
- The ethics of medicine's culture, which has traditionally rewarded self-denial and workaholism at the expense of healthy relationships and self-care
- The ethical failure of allowing residents-in-training to be obligated to work longer hours than optimal for their health by training programs in medical services delivery systems that benefit financially from doing so

Among these issues, the most consistently compelling ethical issues pertaining to physician wellness relate to the fact that physicians' wellness affects their performance as clinicians who provide medical care for others.

There is an emerging understanding of the ethical imperative for physicians, as society's caretakers, to keep physically and emotionally healthy. Indeed, the most refined, expensive, and important clinical "instrument" in the health system continues to be the physician, and from a purely mechanistic perspective, physician wellness is critical for optimal performance of the physician as a servant to patient well-being. Performance is optimized in part by self-care behaviors that improve cognitive functions in the short and long term. These behaviors include proper exercise, nutrition habits, and sleep. Physicians caring for their wellness will be more effective in caring for their patients. This observation alone places self-care for wellness among the set of responsibilities, also including adequate training and continuing education, that are ethically prescribed for practitioners of medicine to provide the best possible clinical care for their patients.

In addition to the ethical imperative for physician wellness for technical and cognitive performance, emotional wellness and social wellness are imperative for a physician's performance as a healer. The association between physician well-being and improved patient care outcomes was dramatically demonstrated by Halbesleben and Rathert (2008), whose study of physician–patient pairs indicated that patients had shorter recovery times following hospital discharge if their physicians were less emotionally exhausted and therefore experiencing fewer depersonalization symptoms of burnout. Close examination of the data in their report indicates that physician depersonalization at 1 standard deviation lower was associated with a 12-day shorter patient recovery time following discharge. One year earlier, Grepmair et al. (2007) published their findings of a randomized trial of mindfulness meditation training for psychotherapists. In comparison with patients treated by a control group of therapists, patients treated by therapists engaged in mindfulness meditation enjoyed far greater improvement in several mental health measures, including the Global Severity Index, depression, anxiety, obsessiveness, psychoticism, anger/hostility, and somatization.

In addition to enhanced performance in the science and art of medicine that optimal wellness affords, the relationship between physicians' personal health promotion practices and their effectiveness as advocates for positive health behavior is another ethical issue. A growing body of empirical evidence documents that physicians who actively engage in preventive health practices personally are more likely to support these practices for their patients. Physicians who engage in healthy lifestyle practices model this behavior for others, who look to them as experts in health. When physicians are engaged in healthy self-care behaviors, they are also more likely to advise their patients to do the same. Physicians "preach what they practice"

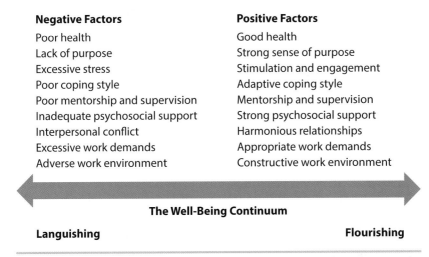

Negative Factors

Poor health
Lack of purpose
Excessive stress
Poor coping style
Poor mentorship and supervision
Inadequate psychosocial support
Interpersonal conflict
Excessive work demands
Adverse work environment

Positive Factors

Good health
Strong sense of purpose
Stimulation and engagement
Adaptive coping style
Mentorship and supervision
Strong psychosocial support
Harmonious relationships
Appropriate work demands
Constructive work environment

The Well-Being Continuum

Languishing   Flourishing

FIGURE 17–1. **Factors influencing the well-being of professionals.**
Source. Copyright © 2015 Laura Weiss Roberts, M.D., M.A. Used with permission.

(Lurie et al. 1987), which suggests that healthy doctors will generate greater health for their patients.

Thus, it is both ethical and rational to "prescribe" wellness for physicians—that is, those individuals who are entrusted with providing clinical care for others. Attention to wellness efforts, along with social support and mentorship, and other factors such as work demands and workplace milieu will allow physicians to flourish rather than languish (Figure 17–1). Attributes of physicians and the cultural context in which they practice may interact to prevent even the most professionally responsible doctors from attending to their own well-being. For these reasons, it is important to integrate wellness imperatives into the workplace, with strong leadership and role modeling at every level within an organization.

HEALERS AND SELF-CARE

The very qualities that attract people to the field of psychiatry, as well as to other areas of medicine and the health professions, and make them good at what they do also make them vulnerable to the demands of the work. Empathy, sympathy, intuition, thoroughness, a strong work ethic, perfectionism, and the ability to absorb, tolerate, and understand feelings are all qualities that are valuable in the helping professions. The willingness to take on the problems of others is seen as a mark of virtue. Yet there must be limits; the ability to help is not without bounds.

One important boundary is the clinician's need to care for himself or herself. The evolving evidence that burnout and fatigue relate to poor patient care practices and more frequent ethical transgressions and medical mistakes represents another ethically important concern. Stated more strongly, when physicians ignore their well-being, the consequences to their patients may be severe.

In a moving opinion piece published in *The New York Times* in 2014, Pranay Sinha wrote about the experience of being an intern as he reflected on the tragic suicides of two interns 2 weeks prior:

> [W]e must…ask if there are aspects of medical culture that might push troubled residents beyond their reserves of emotional resilience.… [The] drastic increase in responsibility can and does overwhelm most interns.… [M]y first two months were marked by severe fatigue, numerous clinical errors (that were promptly caught by my supervisors), a constant and haunting fear of hurting my patients and an inescapable sense of inadequacy. I kept up a charade of composure and humor to blend in with my talented colleagues.…
> Sick of feeling like a charlatan…I confessed [over dinner, to a more accomplished colleague] that I did not think I belonged in the program. He…then uttered the three most beautiful words I had ever heard: "Dude, me too!"
> We need to be able to voice these doubts and fears. We need to be able to talk about the sadness of that first death certificate we signed, the mortification at the first incorrect prescription we ordered, the embarrassment of not knowing an answer on rounds that a medical student knew. A medical culture that encourages us to share these vulnerabilities could help us realize that we are not alone and find comfort and increased connection with our peers. It could also make it easier for residents who are at risk to ask for help. And I believe it would make us all better doctors.… [A] tired and depressed doctor who is an island of self-doubt simply isn't as likely to improve the outcomes of his or her patients—or ever truly care for them. (Sinha 2014, p. A27)

This first-person narrative conveys the sense of fragility and exhaustion experienced by early physicians and shows the importance of support during this crucial period of professional development.

Ralph Waldo Emerson stated, "All the thoughts of a turtle are turtles." The argument that physician self-care is important could be viewed as a preoccupation with oneself. We gently suggest a different view. In a time in which health and economic disparities throughout the world may be addressed in new and transformative ways because of new technologies and greater resources, it is critical to think differently about physician self-care and wellness than in the past. The era of battle-worn, exhausted physicians and physicians-in-training has been replaced by a new model of professionalism in which physicians, including psychiatrists, can use their expertise and personal strengths to bring about greater health for individual patients and also to communities and entire populations. In light of the potential for amplified impact of individual physicians, the imperative is for them to remain healthy and to bring a commitment to prevention and optimal health practices—not merely chronic or late disease interventions. In the case of physicians working with patients who have mental disorders and co-occurring conditions, the imperative is heightened because of the lack of adequate numbers of specialists juxtaposed against the tremendous disease burden associated with these disorders and conditions throughout the world. Physicians should be viewed as a vital and scarce resource in this context, and systematic and unwavering support for advancing physician well-being is ever more critical as a result.

THE WOUNDED HEALER

Medical professionals are entrusted with self-governance and ethically obligated to intervene with a colleague when he or she is clearly distressed or impaired. In the context of professional ethics, *impairment* is defined as the inability to provide clinical care with reasonable skill and safety to patients by reason of physical or mental illness or substance dependence. Impairment reaches across a spectrum, ranging from mild forms to more severe. Worry and preoccupation with day-to-day problems may go largely unnoticed but yet may prevent a clinician from being optimally empathic. More severe impediments to effective practice include addictions and mental illness; such conditions are unlikely to resolve without appropriate treatment.

On the path to wellness, perfectionistic expectations probably represent the greatest resistance to treatment in patients and among professionals. For those conditioned to appear self-reliant, getting help seems an admission of weakness. Feelings of shame and thoughts of doubt accompany the recognition of the need for help and the first steps toward treatment.

In the past, addictions and mental illness were seen as moral shortcomings and were dealt with accordingly through punitive measures. Although such attitudes are often identified with remote periods of history, they sadly persist today. A therapeutic approach to impaired professionals is only gradually overcoming the older, more pejorative attitudes. Most states have now passed impaired-professional legislation, based on the model impaired-physician statute developed in the early 1970s by the American Medical Association (1973) Council on Mental Health. These legislative mandates provide a therapeutic alternative to loss of licensure for impaired professionals. Typically, an impaired professional voluntarily surrenders her or his license and agrees to enter a treatment program. Upon successful completion of the treatment, the license is restored with whatever monitoring may be deemed necessary.

Denial is also common among health professionals and clinicians-in-training, and the stigma many people associate with psychiatric illness prevents many individuals even within the field from getting help. In a study of 1,027 medical students at nine medical schools, Roberts et al. (2000, 2001b) found that although most medical students (90%) needed or wanted personal health care, nearly half had difficulty with access to care despite having insurance. A majority (57%) did not seek care at times, in part because of demands in the training situation, such as having no time to obtain care, and worries about confidentiality. Students acknowledged substantial fear of reprisal for having or seeking care for stigmatizing illnesses. Finally, this study revealed that when the participants were presented with scenarios depicting students with evidence of very serious illness (e.g., suicidal depression, severe substance dependence, uncontrolled diabetes), roughly one-third of them opted to protect the student/colleague's confidentiality rather than intervene to help him or her get care or report the student/colleague to the dean's office. In this study, the pattern of self-diagnosis and curbside consultation for medical treatment was documented to occur early in the clinical training years. In a follow-up study of residents, most (65%) reported a decline in their personal health, and many of these physicians-in-training did not seek necessary care or sought curbside consultations (Roberts and Kim 2015b). Hundreds of studies have documented the patterns of poor self-care among physicians and physicians-in-training, with psychiatric issues gaining in prominence. The repercussions of these untreated mental health problems among clinicians are widespread and include potential effects on patient care in addition to the obvious effects on individual clinicians and their families.

Responding to the mental health problems of professional colleagues brings with it a number of ethical dilemmas and personal challenges. Recognition that a colleague may need help raises questions about the level of intervention that is appropriate. It is easy for colleagues to collude with the "impaired" clinician in terms of denial and minimization. Overidentification may also result in an exaggerated concern about the impact of treatment on the impaired clinician's career. Aggressive interventions such as involuntary hospitalization for the seriously suicidal colleague may be less likely due to a perceived conflict between the ethical obligation to protect the colleague's career and reputation and the duty to protect the colleague's safety. Confidentiality issues can also become problematic in such situations, especially with widespread access to personal health information via the electronic medical record. It is accepted that the need for safety takes precedence over confidentiality concerns, but professionals may hesitate to apply this rule when the patient is also a colleague. Limit setting can also be more difficult when treating colleagues. The boundaries that are normally maintained between physician and patient may easily be blurred when the patient is a professional colleague. Such boundary crossings may lead to increased strain on the clinician and sometimes may result in inappropriate behaviors.

Even when clinicians do seek help, they are often treated differently from other patients (see Chapter 13, "Difficult Patients"). Colleagues may be treated as very important persons (VIPs) and may actually receive less-than-optimal care because exceptions are made for them, their denials are accepted, and confrontations are avoided. Being a VIP may also increase a clinician's sense of shame and resistance to treatment. Those who see themselves and who are seen by others as important and strong may have more difficulty admitting their problems and identifying themselves as in need of help. They also may be more likely to try to control and direct the treatment. In addition to the difficulties physicians face obtaining medical care in the institutional context where they work, other cultural factors also threaten their wellness and perpetuate barriers to wellness of the students and resident physicians they mentor.

NEGATIVE INFLUENCES IN THE CULTURE OF MEDICINE

Difficult training requirements, ongoing demands of patient care, and use of the electronic medical record, to name a few contributors, exert significant effects on physicians' well-being. Emotional exhaustion—what has been referred to more broadly as burnout (see Table 17–1)—among physicians and physicians-in-training has been tied to unprofessional behaviors and poor patient care practices. Although a comprehensive overview of this literature is beyond the scope of this chapter, some early studies have set the stage for thinking more deeply about the relationship of exhaustion, depersonalization, mistreatment, poor modeling, and abuse throughout the culture of medical training, as well as their ramifications.

Medicine has a culture in which self-denial and workaholism are rewarded at the expense of healthy relationships and self-care. The training process for clinicians in this culture raises many ethical dilemmas (see Chapter 20, "Clinical Training"). Training programs are known to be physically and emotionally stressful, often involving long working hours and even sleep deprivation. During medical school and residency training, physicians learn to distance themselves from patients, to take on more and more work without complaint, and to compartmentalize their feelings. In addition, many practice settings reward long hours and self-neglect. Perfectionism and workaholic standards are pervasive in medicine and may play a role in the increased rates of distress seen among clinicians. Obsessionality, which is not the same as thoroughness, is seen as a virtue rather than what may be a defense against unpleasant emotions. Physicians essentially are taught to ignore their needs if they want to be successful, and they may later have difficulty achieving balance in their lives.

The culture of medicine that has traditionally promoted an ideal of self-denial and workaholic standards is being challenged. The Accreditation Council for Graduate Medical Education (ACGME), for example, requires residency programs in every discipline to teach actively about self-care and to engage in practices that promote improved health, such as restructuring call schedules and expectations. As programs struggle to adapt to evolving standards, it is worthwhile to reflect on the higher ethical imperative to care for professionals as well as patients by setting more realistic limits. It is hoped that this change, once it is processed, will be the beginning of a shift away from the unhealthy traditions of the past toward a new era in which the health of health care professionals during and after training is more highly valued.

Dyrbye et al. (2008) performed a seven-school study of burnout with 2,248 medical student participants (52% response). The authors defined *burnout* as the triad of emotional exhaustion, depersonalization, and feelings of low personal accomplishment. In their study, 50% of students met criteria for burnout and 46% for depression; 11% had contemplated suicide in the prior year. Study participants overall had lower mental health quality-of-life scores than similar-age individuals in the general population. Importantly, when queried about a series of unprofessional behaviors, students who met criteria for burnout were far more likely to report more than one unprofessional behavior, such as taking credit for someone else's work or cheating on an examination. Moreover, students with burnout much more frequently reported worrisome behaviors affecting the care of patients, such as reporting that a lab test was pending when it was actually forgotten or reporting that it was normal without checking the actual result. In another study by Shanafelt et al. (2002), most residents met criteria for burnout, and these residents had 2–3 times increased probability of reporting that they had engaged in suboptimal care of patients at least monthly to weekly, such as failure to discuss treatment options or to answer patients' questions, treatment or medication errors, and less attentiveness to patient concerns. In yet another study of residents with depression or burnout, Fahrenkopf et al. (2008) found that depressed residents (20% of the sample) and residents with burnout (75% of the sample) had increased risk of medication errors in patient care.

These data should be placed in the context of the culture of medicine more broadly, which has dark aspects related to mistreatment and abuse of physicians-in-training. In 1990, Silver and Glicken published a landmark study on medical student abuse. Most medical students at the University of Colorado participated in the study ($n=431$; 83% response rate), and the authors reported that 17% had undergone abuse by the end of Year 1, 33% by the end of Year 2, 68% by the end of Year 3, and 81% by the end of Year 4 of medical school. The highest incidence occurred in the third year, with 20% of students reporting at least five episodes of abusive treatment that was of "major importance and very upsetting." Since 2000, in the now-annual survey conducted by the Association of American Medical Colleges, 13%–20% of graduating medical students have reported mistreatment in medical school. In 2013, approximately 23% of graduating students had witnessed significant mistreatment of a peer. On specific items in the 2013 questionnaire, students indicated occasionally or frequently being publicly belittled or humiliated (23%), being required to perform personal services (e.g., running personal errands) (9%), being subjected personally to offensive remarks (7%), receiving unwanted sexual advances (5%), being denied opportunities due to gender (6%), or receiving lower grades due to gender (6%) (Association of American Medical Colleges 2013).

In a large analytic project summarizing studies of harassment and discrimination in medical training, Fnais et al. (2014) assembled the existing evidence regarding harassment (51 studies; $n=38,353$ participants), verbal abuse (28 studies; $n=27,258$ participants), gender discrimination (13 studies; $n=6,237$ participants), sexual harassment (36 studies; $n=27,919$ participants), racial discrimination (10 studies; $n=19,455$ participants), and physical abuse (24 studies; $n=23,776$). In this remarkable collation of results, they found that verbal abuse was common (mean 63%, range 28%–94%) and more commonly reported as affecting medical students. Harassment (mean 60%, range 11%–100%), gender discrimination (mean 54%, range 19%–92%), and physical abuse (mean 15%, range 3%–100%) were common and more commonly reported as affecting residents. Sexual harassment (mean 33%, range 3%–93%) and racial discrimination (mean 24%, range 4%–58%) were common and affected medical students and residents equally.

These sobering data suggest that role modeling of professionalism is wanting in medical schools that train medical students and residents. Psychiatrists understand the impact of these distressing and even traumatizing experiences. Certainly, from an ethics perspective, physicians are not their best selves—able to be reflective and compassionate and objective—in the context of mistreatment and trauma. For these reasons, it is no surprise that such negative experiences in the culture of medicine may lead to diminished self-care and patient care practices.

Statistics indicating that many medical trainees suffer from depression and that the majority experience burnout (Dyrbye et al. 2014) underscore the effects of institutional factors such as obligated excessive work hours and other forms of mistreatment or abuse. Most physicians-in-training begin their careers with altruistic intentions to relieve suffering and enjoy connecting with people on a very personal level. They are prone to enjoy the practice of medicine. When trainees are forced to take on excessive clinical service duties requiring excessive work hours, however, they must choose between providing optimal care for their patients or cutting patient care corners to create time for self-care such as exercise and sleep and time for personal relationships outside of work. The resulting conflict between excessive patient care time demands and a need for self-care time in a context in which trainees have little power to alter their work schedules is likely to contribute to symptoms of burnout, including emotional exhaustion and depersonalization (Ishak et al. 2009). Financial incentives and service delivery needs may make adequate reductions in clinical duty hours for resident physicians difficult to achieve in some specialties.

Obligating resident physicians to assume excessive clinical duties renders obvious financial and service delivery benefits to clinical care delivery institutions where resident physicians work. Without institutional financial investment to hire providers to take on some of the excessive duties performed by resident physicians, attending physicians with already excessive work hours themselves will be likely to oppose resident duty-hour restrictions that add to the clinical burden they already struggle to carry (Wong and Imrie 2013). Creative restructuring of scheduling and work flow to force residents to do the same amount of work within duty-hour guidelines will grossly attenuate resident well-being benefits intended with work-hour restrictions (Auger et al. 2012). Absent financial support from their institutions to actually reduce some of the less educationally necessary duties residents perform, training program directors and other attending physicians who dictate resident workload may be unduly subject to bias stemming from their own well-being concerns when deciding ideal work-life balance for their trainees, which calls into question the validity of the clinical training faculty perspective (Reed et al. 2007) that reducing work hours attenuates the educational value of residency training. ACGME measures to limit resident work hours were met with resistance, even though the target limit was—and remains—80 hours per week averaged over 4 weeks, not including time for reading or study that optimal learning of new clinical competency also requires. Obligated excessive work hours and other institutional factors may explain mounting evidence that many current training programs are unhealthy experiences for aspiring healers-in-training.

Similar findings were reported in earlier studies of practicing physicians. Firth-Cozens and Greenhalgh (1997) found that 57% of physicians in their project believed that work-related stress, tiredness, exhaustion, or sleep deprivation negatively affected their patient care practices. These physicians commented on taking shortcuts or making procedural errors, with 7% leading to serious mistakes and 2%–4% leading to patient deaths. Williams and Skinner (2003), in their narrative review of outcomes of physician job dissatisfaction, reported that more dissatisfied physicians tend to have riskier prescribing profiles, less compliant patients, and less satisfied patients.

CONCLUSION

Inspiring new findings helping to establish the "healthy doctor=healthy patient" movement may lead to significant change in the culture of medicine. The Stanford Medicine (2015) WellMD program is one illustration of such change. Empirical studies have supported the connectedness of physician and patient well-being. For example, Dresner et al. (2010) performed a study of 429 physicians and 1,621 matched patient control subjects, revealing that health screening practices of physicians and their patients (e.g., evaluation for common cancers or health risk factors such as hypertension, elevated cholesterol, and tobacco use) were strongly correlated. Similarly, Duperly et al. (2009) performed a study of 661 medical students, revealing that personal health habits corresponded to preventive counseling behaviors in their care of patients. Early work on the compassion-preserving impact of experiences of medical students and residents as patients reinforces the idea that empathy, attention to communication, and investment in the therapeutic relationship may be salutary consequences of programs to support self-care. These findings, combined with the more worrisome findings about exhausted physicians and physicians-in-training being more prone to mistakes and ethical misjudgments, should motivate health systems to invest in the well-being of their physicians and to move their cultures in positive directions.

CASE SCENARIOS

- A 34-year-old resident becomes distressed after the suicide of one of her patients. She experiences persistent feelings of failure, has difficulty sleeping, and becomes afraid of being "fired" despite multiple evaluations documenting her excellent performance in the program. She increasingly uses alcohol to help her sleep.

- A 39-year-old psychiatrist becomes romantically involved with a patient seen on one occasion in the emergency department. "We were each getting over a divorce, and we had a lot in common," he told his supervisor. "She was never really my patient, because I was just a consultant on the case."

- A 42-year-old faculty attending physician at a psychiatric hospital is working 14-hour days and on weekends. He is irritable toward his patients, teammates, and family. He repeatedly fails to show up for his supervision sessions with the residents. He is having trouble sleeping, ignores his children, and has stopped exercising and pursuing his hobbies.

- A 26-year-old M.D.–Ph.D. student posts a note on his social media account stating that he is completely discouraged and doubts that he will be able to finish his program. He is observed to be losing weight, remaining in the laboratory until very late at night, and complaining of poor sleep. The student's advisor is on a 1-month sabbatical, and the lab manager decides to leave an anonymous tip on the campus "hotline."

- The 39-year-old associate training director of the psychiatry residency program asks one of the chief residents out on a date.

18

Psychiatric Research

Laura Weiss Roberts, M.D., M.A.

Psychiatric research is essential if new knowledge is to improve the understanding of mental disorders—their origins, prevention, treatment, and impact. Failure to conduct psychiatric research, particularly in light of the overwhelming burden of mental disorders across all world populations, is a social justice and health disparities issue that has been fueled by misunderstandings, stigma, and unfair resource distribution policies—not unlike the underdevelopment of clinical resources and systems for mental health care.

The strong imperative to conduct psychiatric research is, as with research involving other potentially vulnerable populations, balanced against ethical imperatives related to morally acceptable treatment of human beings. As I have written elsewhere, the following questions must be asked:

> Is human experimentation ever ethically permissible? Are human studies always and inevitably exploitative? Since the release of the Belmont Report…in 1979, the response to these difficult ethical questions has been that people may participate in scientific studies when the following two conditions have been met: the research must occur in a context of utmost trust and professionalism, and it must be conducted in a manner that wholly embodies the ethical principles of respect for persons, beneficence, and justice. When these conditions are fulfilled, the human being is not used as a "means to an end" by science. Rather, a well-informed and capable person

may engage with investigators, accepting freely the risks of research, in the shared pursuit of knowledge that may improve human health. (Roberts 2015a, p. 1506)

As noted in that quote, three ethics principles govern human research: 1) *respect for persons*, honoring the dignity and promoting the autonomy of research participants; 2) *beneficence*, the duty to seek maximal good and to do minimal harm through the conduct of research; and 3) *justice*, ensuring that the segment of the population bearing the greatest burden for research also benefits from it and ensuring that special groups are not exploited as a result of individual, interpersonal, or societal attributes or powerlessness. These bioethics principles were most elegantly and clearly articulated in the landmark Belmont Report (National Commission for the Protection of Human Subjects of Biomedical and Behavioral Research 1979) and are echoed throughout other historical research ethics documents. Federal regulations for human research are grounded in the Belmont principles and are referred to as the "Common Rule" (Table 18–1).

Modern views of ethically sound research embrace these three original principles of respect for persons, beneficence, and justice and add to them the notion of *integrity* (see Chapter 15, "Integrity and the Professional Roles of Psychiatrists"). These ideals are translated into practice through the design, methods, and safeguards of experimental protocols. Ethically sound research hinges on expertise and also on the integrity of investigators and the absence of significant conflicts of interest that might threaten objectivity, decisions, and/or actions. Moreover, ethically sound research seeks to advance the concerns and well-being of special groups and potentially vulnerable populations, including children.

DESIGN, METHODS, AND THE NEED FOR ETHICS SAFEGUARDS

Ethics and scientific design issues fit closely together in a few key respects:

1. It is widely accepted that a study's design should be based on a research question that is valuable, significant, timely, and justified and that the study's methods should test hypotheses in a manner that will produce meaningful, interpretable results. Concretely, the design and methods must be appropriate to prove or disprove the study's hypotheses. Otherwise, because of the principle of respect for persons and its underlying philosophical basis, it is not acceptable to include human beings as

TABLE 18–1. History of the Common Rule

Year	Title	Summary
1974	National Research Act	Codified U.S. Department of Health, Education, and Welfare (DHEW); issued moratorium on federally funded fetal research; mandated institutional review board (IRB) review of human research for DHEW funds.
1974–1978	National Commission for Protection of Human Subjects of Biomedical and Behavioral Research	Reported on research involving special populations; issued regulatory guidance for IRBs, informed consent. Developed the seminal Belmont Report, which was published in 1979, outlining ethical principles in protecting human subjects in research.
1978	Revised DHEW	Enacted regulations protecting pregnant women, fetuses, prisoners, and in vitro fertilization.
1978–1983	President's Commission for the Study of Ethical Problems in Medicine and Biomedical and Behavioral Research	Reviewed federal policies governing human research; recommended that all federal agencies adopt DHEW/U.S. Department of Health and Human Services (DHHS) regulations for the protection of subjects.
1981	Revision of DHHS	Mandated to provide oversight of IRB responsibilities and procedures. U.S. Food and Drug Administration (FDA) regulations were revised to correspond to DHHS.
1982	President's Science Advisor/Office of Science and Technology	Appointed to head interagency committee to develop a common policy for protection of human research subjects.
1983	DHHS regulation	Enacted protections governing children in research.

TABLE 18–1. History of the Common Rule *(continued)*

Year	Title	Summary
1991	Final common Federal Policy for the Protection of Human Research Subjects (i.e., the "Common Rule")	Issued by 15 federal agencies, provided regulations regarding human subject protection (combined via executive order) identical to basic DHHS policy for protection of research subjects; provided additional protections for pregnant women, fetuses, in vitro fertilization, prisoners, children. FDA informed consent and IRB regulations were changed to meet these standards.

Source. Adapted from Roberts LW, Dyer AR: *Concise Guide to Ethics in Mental Health Care.* Washington, DC, American Psychiatric Publishing, 2004, pp. 262–263. Copyright © 2004 American Psychiatric Publishing. Used with permission.

"objects" of study in research that lacks potential for a true scientific contribution and a greater social good.

2. An ethically sound study will employ a design and procedures that minimize risks to study participants. In essence, an experiment must not expose individuals to greater levels of risk than are necessary to ask its underlying scientific question. For this reason, an experiment should not use a relatively more risky design when a relatively less risky alternative design will suffice scientifically.

3. The scientific design and its interventions should not be so complex that they cannot be understood and their intent and ramifications appreciated by individuals who are considering participation in the study (Roberts 1998).

Various experimental designs have become the subject of controversy as scientific methods have evolved and awareness of ethical issues in research has increased. In the past, studies that entailed placebo trials, medication washout periods, or symptom challenge maneuvers raised difficult questions regarding their scientific necessity and true risks. Conceptual arguments have been developed both for and against these designs, yet few data are available on the personal and scientific impact of these approaches and their alternatives to help clarify the concerns surrounding them. For example, it is not known whether individuals who participate in placebo studies ultimately have worse outcomes than those who participate in other types of experiments or than patients who have never been in research protocols. Eventually, controversial or problematic designs may be discarded as they become scientifically obsolete. Meanwhile, special methodological approaches must arise around controversial or problematic designs to ensure that they are conducted ethically.

Special issues in the design of potentially higher-risk studies, such as deep brain stimulation trials, and in uncertain or psychosocial risk studies, such as psychiatric genetics research, pose a number of scientific design questions. In the absence of clear answers to these questions, investigators should work closely to design their studies with other experts, relevant stakeholders (e.g., institutional review boards [IRBs], local communities, and funding agencies), and representatives of the potential participant groups. The aim of the participatory process (Roberts 2013; Roberts et al. 2015) will be to develop scientific approaches that include more rigorous safeguards and yet take incremental steps that help bring valuable new knowledge but minimize potential for harm of study volunteers.

The process of building additional ethical safeguards has occurred with deception studies in the field of behavioral science. Deception studies, in general, are intended to explore phenomena in which awareness of the focus of the experiment will impair the ability to collect accurate data. Deception studies pose uncertain risk and have a history of leading to significant harm to unknowing volunteers. A deception study can meet current ethical standards if it explores nonstigmatizing phenomena, involves participants who have consented to the possibility of deception in the protocol, and provides an appropriate debriefing to participants at the conclusion of their involvement in the study. The issues are similar in biomedical research designs that use deception—that is, incomplete disclosure of the specific interventions that the participant will experience. For example, in a medication trial employing a double-blind design in which neither the investigator nor the participant knows which medication is being administered, it is possible to differentiate psychological (e.g., attitudinal) influences of the researchers and the participants from the "true" effects of the medications being studied.

Notorious, ethically disturbing psychological deception experiments have been conducted, however, such as studies of personal and sexual behaviors in which investigators did not appreciate the ethical ramifications of not informing or of deceiving participants outright. Such experiments have been experienced by participants and recognized by the scientific community as inordinately intrusive and exploitative. Consequently, special steps to ensure the ethical conduct of deception studies have been created and agreed upon within the fields of behavioral and biomedical science. These steps include an informed consent process that is broad enough to encompass the material actually being assessed within the study; recruitment of participants with sound decisional capabilities, given the object of the study; special sensitivity and efforts to minimize embarrassment or discomfort should these arise for participants; and appropriate debriefing at the end of each participant's study involvement. Similar ethically oriented methods may be employed to enhance the ethical protections around study participants in experiments whose designs pose special problems.

Certain experimental designs naturally will undergo careful scrutiny as scientific designs and methods advance. The fact that such questions arise should be viewed not as a failure of the science but rather as a scientific success in that investigators are openly accountable, self-observing, and thoughtful about the justification for their experimental methods. The key is to accurately assess the scientific necessity of and the alternatives to the design, determine the potential risks to participants, and collaborate with others to review these issues and develop additional ways of improving the ethical features of the design wherever possible.

ETHICS SAFEGUARDS

Several safeguards are built into the process of all biomedical experimentation to offer ethical protection to human participants. These safeguards are implemented at the level of the institution (e.g., medical center, source of funding) and the individual investigator, and they are codified and enforced through federal regulations (e.g., Office for Human Research Protection). The most critical of these safeguards include 1) IRBs; 2) informed consent; 3) advance, alternative, and collaborative decision making; 4) additional expert and peer review processes; and 5) confidentiality protections. In the following subsections, these safeguards are discussed in light of their theoretical bases and empirical support.

Institutional Review and Data and Safety Monitoring

IRBs prospectively review human research occurring in an institutional context. Their aim is threefold: to ensure that the science has merit, the study participants are treated ethically, and the "rights and welfare" of participants are protected. IRBs are empowered to approve research, to insist on modifications and revisions as a condition of approval, or to disapprove research before it is undertaken. Their decisions carry weight outside the institution as well, because most funding agencies will require IRB approval before supporting projects. Although the procedures of IRBs focus primarily on protocols prospectively (e.g., reviewing consent forms for their adequacy, examining the scientific rationale for the experiment), IRBs have responsibility for the ongoing monitoring of research within the institution. The IRB can stop research, even after it has been approved, if the research is found to be conducted incompetently, discovered to be performed significantly differently than originally described, or determined to pose inordinate risks to participants.

IRBs combine both expertise and representation. Members should be knowledgeable about both scientific issues and ethics protections, including the content of relevant regulations and literature. Membership should also allow for adequate representation of the viewpoints of potential research participants. For example, it has long been recognized that nonscientists, community representatives, and people of both genders should be included on IRBs. More recently, it has been proposed that people deriving from special groups, such as individuals with mental illness, should be included as voting members of IRBs. Greater diversity of perspectives and broader collaboration serve as the rationale for IRB membership constituted in this way.

The actual functioning of IRBs has been poorly understood, although a body of empirical work has developed around this topic. IRBs seldom receive sufficient attention and resources, given their critical role within biomedical and other research institutions. The cultures and actual procedures of individual IRBs may vary significantly according to the nature of the institution, the region of the country, and the kind of research most frequently reviewed. IRBs may delegate significant portions of their work to other elements of the institution—for example, by asking for the scientific review before IRB submission (e.g., through a departmental review process), which may result in less objective scrutiny of proposals. In addition, IRB members are not required to have formal preparation and commonly are volunteers who accept IRB duties in addition to their usual responsibilities. IRB members themselves may have role conflicts and conflicts of interest, including financial conflicts of interest—and the oversight of these factors, which may influence their judgments and decisional processes, is minimal. Finally, IRBs often may not receive adequate support (e.g., administrative staff, budget, space) to perform anything but the most basic prospective review and annual review activities. Some poorly implemented and some competent but overburdened IRBs have been faulted for inadequate review processes. Under more optimal circumstances, efforts to improve the education of IRB members and investigators, to conduct intermittent monitoring of certain protocols, to work more closely with communities and special groups, and to develop explicit policies and standards related to research might be possible.

Informed Consent

The doctrine of informed consent requires that all individuals truly understand and freely make choices about intrusions on their physical and psychological selves. As in informed consent for clinical care (see Chapter 4, "Informed Consent and Decisional Capacity"), informed consent for participation in research is a process, not a single event, and ideally occurs within the context of a professional relationship characterized by trust and integrity. Research consent, also like clinical consent, entails three elements: information sharing, decisional capacity, and voluntarism.

Information Sharing

Research consent involves accurate and complete information regarding the reason for and nature of the proposed intervention, its associated biological and psychosocial risks and benefits and their magnitude, the alternatives (including no intervention at all), who is responsible for the research, and other ramifications of participation, such as economic or social consequences. Sharing information reflects respect for the individual and the truth. Outside of the very specific situation of emergency research consent, this information should be imparted in a manner that is clear, that is not rushed, and that promotes the genuine understanding of the potential participant. For complex or risky protocols, it is important that disclosure associated with consent occur on at least two occasions and that supplementary materials (e.g., pamphlets or video recordings) be provided.

Decisional Capacity

An individual who is invited to enroll in a research project should be capable of making the decision to participate and of expressing his or her preferences. Decisional capacity has been described as having several components: the physical and cognitive ability to communicate effectively; the intellectual ability to take in new information and understand, work with, and apply ("rationally manipulate") it; and the integrated cognitive and emotional ability to make sense of the meaning and repercussions of the decision within the context of the participant's life ("appreciation"). Interventions to help support an individual's decisional capacity may include treatment for impairing symptoms; careful and open discussions with research staff; inclusion in the consent process of family members, spouses, and significant others whom the participant wishes to be present; and conversations with other research participants.

Voluntarism

Authentic voluntarism or autonomy is a third necessary element of informed consent. It may be understood as involving four domains: 1) developmental factors, 2) illness-related considerations, 3) psychological issues and cultural and religious values, and 4) contextual factors. Voluntarism is a difficult concept to operationalize, because there are so many subtle influences on an individual's true ability to make fully independent decisions and to act freely in certain situations or at specific points in time. For example, a man whose use of substances impairs his insight and motivation may not be able to fully understand his genuine internal wishes or to work toward enacting his personal choices. A parent who is immensely concerned about a seriously ill child may make decisions out of desperation. Similarly, an individual who is approached by his or her teacher, employer, nursing home director, longtime personal physician, military superior, or prison warden to participate in research may not feel able to refuse. A poor person may have such a need for the financial compensation associated with a study that the level of risk seems irrelevant. Finally, an elderly, ethnic minority person without health insurance may feel that he or she has few options when interacting with a clinical investigator who offers health care as part of a protocol. Under most circumstances, the criterion of voluntarism is superficially fulfilled by the absence of overt coercive influences (Roberts 2002). Such problems associated with autonomy provide further reason for the absolute integrity of investigators as a precondition for ethical human research.

The activities surrounding informed consent therefore should be designed to support information disclosure, enhance the participant's decisional abilities, and promote individual autonomy. The consent form represents only one concrete but important portion of the consent procedure. As such, the consent form should be clear and readable, contain relevant information, and clarify the voluntary nature of the participant's enrollment in the experiment.

Clinical observation and empirical studies indicate that a number of issues bear careful consideration in informed consent for participation in psychiatric investigations. Several studies suggest, for example, that people with psychiatric illnesses, when compared with control subjects without psychiatric illness or individuals with medical illness, have greater difficulty taking in, retaining, and recalling information presented at the time of consent disclosures for clinical care and research procedures. The landmark MacArthur Treatment Competence Study (Appelbaum and Grisso 1995; Grisso and Appelbaum 1995; Grisso et al. 1995) explored these cognitive elements inherent to clinical consent in 498 individuals from three groups: patients with schizophrenia or major depression, patients with ischemic heart disease, and nonpatient community volunteers. Cognitive measures showed that the psychiatric patients, when acutely ill, had significantly greater difficulty with decision making than did the patients with heart disease and the community volunteers. Similar findings, not unexpectedly, have been documented among people with dementia. Additionally, elements beyond cognitive factors also may greatly influence consent activities and adversely affect the decision-making capabilities of psychiatric patients—even those who appear cognitively intact. For example, any of the following may interfere with psychiatric patients' abilities to engage fully in a consent process: psychological distress; compromised insight; difficulties with interpersonal trust and communication; inaccurate beliefs; problems with motivation, initiative, and behavior; and relative powerlessness due to institutionalization or very severe symptomatology.

Advance, Alternative, and Collaborative Decision Making

Psychiatric research, like other areas of biomedical experimentation, at times may involve individuals with fluctuating or declining decisional abilities. For this reason, informed consent—the primary ethical safeguard for human research—may pose special problems in psychiatric experimentation. Advance, alternative, and collaborative decision making therefore can have a particularly important role in psychiatric research consent.

Advance decision making involves careful anticipatory planning by investigators with their study participants to examine situations that may arise in the course of experimentation and to clarify a participant's preferences in each possible situation. This process should be carefully documented (e.g., via a psychiatric advance directive) and can be enormously helpful if the participant becomes decisionally compromised or incapable. The participant may designate an alternative or surrogate decision maker to help implement the advance directives. Sometimes alternative decision makers may be identified or formally appointed in the absence of documented preferences of the participant, or if unexpected issues arise that were not identified in advance. In these contexts, it is critical that the decision makers seek to determine or perhaps extrapolate what the preferences of the participant would be and to make decisions accordingly. In other words, the alternative decision maker's task is to act faithfully and to adhere closely, to whatever extent possible, to the wishes of the participant. Collecting data on the participant's life values and past decisions, either directly from the individual or from family members, may facilitate this process. Only when the patient's preferences are unknowable should a best-interests standard for substitute decision making be employed.

All forms of decision making in the context of research participation should be viewed as collaborative. A collaboration takes place between participant and investigator, and in the difficult circumstances of decisional impairment, decision making may ultimately be shared by participants, spouses, family members, significant others, pastors or other individuals important to the participant, and members of the larger research team. This collaboration can be unwieldy, and confidentiality boundaries should be clarified in advance whenever possible to safeguard the participant's personal information. Such collaborative efforts, however, also help to build trust, to address problems and poor outcomes constructively, and to protect participants.

Additional Expert and Peer Review Processes

Additional expert and peer review processes may occur formally or informally. Within institutions, additional reviews may occur when seeking funding, space, or other resources or when requesting permission to perform research in certain settings. Guidelines for research involving special populations may suggest that protocol review be undertaken on a scale larger than individual institutions. In a highly controversial step, the National Bioethics Advisory Commission (1998) recommended the development of a national review panel for all proposed research that poses greater than minimal risk to participants who have limited decision-making abilities. Protocols may also undergo additional review and systematic monitoring through data and safety monitoring boards (DSMBs) to help ensure the safety of participants. Whereas IRBs were widely adopted in the late 1970s, DSMBs have been introduced more recently for safeguarding participants in clinical trials. They serve to evaluate trial procedures and data as they are gathered to determine whether participants are being exposed to inordinate or unexpected risks. Protections also exist after data have been gathered and analyzed. When manuscripts are submitted for publication or scientific presentations are given, the scientific and ethical rigor of the study often receives careful scrutiny. Because DSMBs allow for both prospective and retrospective evaluation and incorporate precise expert attention, these additional review activities are likely to become increasingly important in the repertoire of ethical safeguards.

Confidentiality Protections

Confidentiality is a privilege accorded to patients and to research participants that derives from the legal right of privacy and the ethical principle of respect for persons. In essence, the personal material gathered from and discovered about a research participant must be kept safe in all stages of data collection, analysis, and disclosure (e.g., publication, presentation). In many cases, this will mean that data will be confidentially recorded and encoded and perhaps analyzed in aggregate for scientific presentations and publications. Data should not be traceable to specific individuals unless they give special consent, such as for recorded personal interviews.

Researchers face many challenges, some traditional in nature and some astonishing and new. Posthumous publication of personal narratives, for example, is ethically very problematic. This topic has been considered in the field of psychiatry for many years, because many of the original teaching cases of Freud and others were not disguised. At this time, special efforts to obtain consent from the individual in advance—or perhaps from family members or advocates who act in accordance with the values and best interests of the individual—are undertaken to conform to ethics standards. New issues pertaining to confidentiality and privacy in research arise every day, however. Genetic research now poses almost infinite real-time and future ethical issues related to privacy, and many societal stakeholders are wholly engaged in developing boundaries. The unforeseeable nature of many of these issues and the problems associated with international genetics inquiry (e.g., the genetic code revision of human embryos in China in 2015) have made hard-and-fast rules for oversight impossible.

EXPERTISE, INTEGRITY, AND CONFLICTS OF INTEREST

Scientific *expertise* is critical to the ethical conduct of research. This idea is based on the notion that investigators should be knowledgeable and scientifically astute in order to justify the inclusion of human beings in an experiment as a "means to an end"—namely, the pursuit of scientific findings. In established areas of science, potential investigators should show mastery of their field of study. In newer areas of science, or when investigators newly enter their scientific careers, it is important that additional expertise be gathered from mentors and collaborators whose insights may help foster the scientific excellence of the work and help prevent mistakes that may place study participants at unnecessary risk. Moreover, by wide consensus, the proposed science must itself possess some fundamental, significant good for society. Science for the sake of science is not sufficient. To learn something solely for the purpose of knowing it, especially when the process of learning it may involve potential risk or overt cruelty such as occurred in some past experimentation, is not acceptable within current ethical and moral standards. In practical terms, the investigators must be capable of crafting a scientifically rigorous design, conducting the experiment carefully and skillfully, and interpreting the study's findings in a way that brings about direct benefit or greater knowledge that in turn may ultimately benefit others.

Scientific *integrity* is a necessary precondition for ethically sound scientific research. It is defined as the researcher's faithfulness, both in motivation and conduct, to the ethical duties associated with his or her professional role. For example, the scientist must intend—and act with—honesty in interactions with participants and colleagues. It is upon integrity that trust—the foundation of the profession of medicine and the field of science—is built. Without trust, informed consent, institutional review, and all other safeguards would be meaningless.

Significant threats to investigator integrity represent *conflicts of interest*, defined as motivations or situations in which health care professionals' "responsibilities to observe, judge, and act according to the moral requirements of their role are, or will be, compromised" (Shimm and Spece 1996, p. 1). Conflicts of interest may arise, for example, when investigators receive very large monetary incentives for enrolling individual participants in protocols or when investigators have large financial investment in the research enterprise itself or the entity sponsoring the protocol. Subtler, less concrete conflicts of interest may exist as well, such as the academic investigator's desire for institutional promotion and national recognition in conjunction with an experiment. Consequently, the investigator's faithfulness to his or her moral responsibilities within the clinician investigator role—that is, the capacity and commitment to serve with integrity—is important to the ethical conduct of human research (see Chapter 15, "Integrity and the Professional Roles of Psychiatrists").

Integrity is especially critical in human experimentation, in part because of the inherently conflicting "dual roles" of the clinician-investigator. For instance, the dual role of the clinical investigator may create conflicts when the good of the patient is subordinated to the needs of science. Arguably, this occurs every time a patient is placed on an experimental treatment or a placebo when a known effective treatment for the patient's disorder exists. The moral obligations of this dual role raise the problem of the therapeutic misconception with prospective study participants (Appelbaum et al. 1982). This problem, simply put, is that participants may believe that the clinical investigator will always act to promote the well-being of the individual participant. This beneficent aim is a fundamental expectation of other relationships with medical professionals but is not the exclusive aim of the clinical investigator, who must also serve the scientific goal of the experiment. This tension is perhaps most obvious in double-blind studies, in which clinical investigators themselves are not aware of the treatment received by individual study participants.

It is important to note that this potentially conflictual role of the clinical investigator does not represent an inherent conflict of interest, as has been suggested by some. To minimize ethical problems associated with the dual role, however, there should be no other elements that threaten the ability of the investigator to think and behave in accordance with the moral aspects of his or her role. The research participant should be truly aware of the dual demands faced by the clinical investigator. Finally, the research participant should consent in an informed and autonomous manner to collaborate with the investigator in the experiment.

SPECIAL GROUPS AND POTENTIALLY VULNERABLE POPULATIONS

Vulnerability is a concept related to the ideal of what makes a person fully human—that is, the capacities and freedoms that allow people to think, to love, to desire, to work, to experience, to use language, to act intentionally, to choose authentically, to nurture, to serve others, and the like. These capacities and freedoms reside within the self, integrated in the individual person through experience, self-reflection, thought, feeling, and behavior. From a theoretical perspective, the person who is truly vulnerable cannot or does not fulfill these capacities and freedoms, singly or in an integrated manner.

More concretely, special groups and potentially vulnerable populations can be conceptualized in relation to their members' potential capacities for informed consent. Individuals whose capacity for consent is more likely to be compromised because of problems with information processing, decisional abilities, capacity for effective communication, and/or other problems related to intrinsic or extrinsic susceptibility to coercion are considered to be potentially vulnerable. This potential vulnerability arises from these individuals' heightened risk of exploitation or, at least, diminished ability to advocate for themselves. This concept has been extended on theoretical grounds to highly diverse groups such as severely ill medical and psychiatric patients; children; women of childbearing age; very poor people; and institutionalized, captive, or dependent individuals (e.g., prisoners, nursing home residents, students, veterans). The concept of vulnerability also encompasses people who are severely developmentally disabled and have never been decisionally capable and elderly persons who have serious cognitive impairment and have lost their abilities to make independent decisions. Some theorists extend the concept of vulnerability to include human tissues deriving from fetuses, in vitro experiments, and cadavers (Advisory Committee on Human Radiation Experiments 1996).

In recent years, biomedical science and society at large have struggled with how to best protect potentially vulnerable individuals without being prejudicial or disrespectful of personhood, usurping personal autonomy, and denying access to potentially beneficial or otherwise highly valuable research endeavors. Significant efforts to develop ethically rigorous, genuinely respectful, and culturally sensitive participatory research guidelines have been undertaken (Roberts 2013; Roberts et al. 2015; Wallerstein 1999). Significant controversies have arisen in neuropsychiatric research regarding these issues, most notably in the research of schizophrenia, dementia, and childhood disorders. Advocates of psychiatric investigation describe the immense suffering associated with mental illnesses and the importance of their study to clinical medicine, science, and society. Those who oppose psychiatric research express concern about the adequacy of ethical safeguards and the past exploitation of this special group of individuals with multiple sources of vulnerability. Nearly all agree, however, that psychiatric research requires very special attention and safeguards to address the ethical complexities that will inevitably arise in such work (Dresser 1996). Table 18–2 lists questions to consider in relation to the ethical acceptability of psychiatric research protocols.

Research Involving Children

Individuals can participate in a research project if they provide informed consent and if multiple safeguards are in place. Legal precedent assumes that adults are competent to provide informed consent but that minors are not competent to provide their own consent. Significantly, the National Institutes of Health has a goal to increase the participation of children in research investigating the treatment of disorders that affect them. An important question to consider, then, is how researchers can include children in their studies, particularly when the focus of study is mental disorders or related phenomena.

Consent

The U.S. Department of Health and Human Services (DHHS; 2009) developed guidelines for conducting research with minors in its policy for the protection of human subjects (Subpart D: Additional Protections for Children Involved as Subjects in Research, 45 CFR §46.401–409). Children are identified as a vulnerable population that requires safeguards to protect their rights and to prevent the undue risk of harm. Scholars point out that the minors who are recruited for studies possess vulnerabilities beyond that of age. These youths are likely to have medical, psychiatric, or developmental disorders; to have school problems; or to be involved in juvenile justice or social service systems. Special rules, moreover, apply to children in research and individuals in the correctional system, adding greater layers of complexity in terms of ethics issues and regulatory compliance concerns.

Parents and guardians have the right to grant consent for their children. Although typically consent can be furnished only by the individual participating in the research, parents can provide permission for their children's participation. DHHS guidelines, however, require minors to assent to their own participation; this requirement translates to an affirmative agreement,

---

TABLE 18–2. Questions to consider regarding the ethical acceptability of psychiatric research protocols

---

1. **Scientific issues**

   Is the study scientifically valuable?

   Are the hypotheses adequately tested?

   Can the design and methods yield meaningful data?

   Does the protocol employ fully justifiable scientific techniques, either traditional or innovative?

2. **Research team and context issues**

   Does the investigative team have enough expertise and support to successfully complete the experiment?

   Is the institutional context sufficient to allow the research to progress smoothly?

   Are the researchers aware of research ethics issues and potential problems related to the protocol?

   Are the researchers in good standing within the scientific and professional communities?

   What conflicting roles and conflicts of interest exist in relation to this protocol? How will they be dealt with?

   Are the documentation features of the protocol adequate to monitor procedures and the professional accountability of the research team?

3. **Design issues related to *risk***

   Does the design minimize experimental risks to participants? Do alternative designs pose less risk?

   Does the protocol pose excessive risk to individual participants, the community, and/or larger society?

   If participants are likely to have emerging symptoms as a result of or during protocol involvement:
   - Has an appropriate mechanism for identifying and following symptom progression been built into the protocol?
   - Have criteria for disenrollment from the protocol been clarified?
   - Has an appropriate mechanism for providing alternative or traditional treatment been established?

4. **Design issues related to *benefit***

   What benefits exist for participants? Are benefits and their likelihood accurately described?

   Have benefits of the study been optimized for individuals and society without being coercive to potential participants?

   Is it expected that societal benefit derived from the protocol be specifically applicable to the population being studied?

TABLE 18–2. Questions to consider regarding the ethical acceptability of psychiatric research protocols *(continued)*

---

5. **Confidentiality**

    Is participant information carefully safeguarded during the collection, storage, and analysis stages of the study?

6. **Selection, exclusion, and recruitment issues**

    Does the process of selection, exclusion, and recruitment ensure that members of vulnerable populations, as currently defined, be included *only* if they are essential to the study's scientific hypotheses?

    Are understudied populations inappropriately excluded from participation? That is, are selection and recruitment practices potentially discriminatory?

    Is the recruitment process itself noncoercive?

7. **Informed consent and decisional capacity issues**

    Does the informed consent disclosure process include all relevant information, such as
    -   The study's purpose and the nature of the illness or the phenomenon being studied?
    -   Who is responsible for the scientific and ethical conduct of the study?
    -   Why the individual may be eligible for participation?
    -   The proposed intervention and its associated risks and benefits and their relative likelihood alternatives to participation?
    -   Key study design features (e.g., placebo use, randomization, medication-free intervals, frequency of visits, confidentiality, plans for use of data)?

    Is there reasonable assurance of adequate decisional capacity of participants with respect to their ability to understand, rationally analyze, and appreciate the meaning of the research decision?

    If participants have or are at risk for diminished decisional capacity at any time during protocol participation:
    -   Have efforts for enhancing or restoring the decisional capacity of a participant been undertaken?
    -   Is there an appropriate mechanism for identifying, following, and documenting a participant's level of diminished decisional capacity?
    -   Does the protocol include an appropriate mechanism for advance decision making by the participant or for identifying an alternative decision maker for the participant? Is it clear when the advance directive or alternative decision maker should be put into effect?

    Is the consent form concise, readable, accurate, and understandable?

    Is there reasonable assurance that individuals will not experience coercive pressure to participate in the project or continue in the project?

TABLE 18–2. Questions to consider regarding the ethical acceptability of psychiatric research protocols *(continued)*

8. **Compensation issues**

   Is compensation for participation sufficient, *without* being (or seeming to be) coercive to research participants?

   If health care is an opportunity that is highly valued and shapes the volunteer's decision to enroll, how will the patient's health care needs be met if disenrollment becomes necessary?

9. **Review issues**

   Has the protocol undergone appropriate scientific and ethical review?

   Should the protocol undergo any additional review steps (e.g., by community leaders)?

   Does the protocol have features (e.g., very high risk, very vulnerable participants) that merit ongoing external monitoring?

10. **Data presentation/authorship issues**

    Will the presentation of the data describe the ethical safeguards employed in the protocol?

    Will the presentation of the data meet current ethical standards with respect to authorship?

    Will the presentation of the data meet other current standards (e.g., accurate disclosure of conflicting roles and conflicts of interest)?

    Will participants' identities be adequately protected in data presentation?

Source. Adapted from Roberts LW, Geppert CM, Brody JL: "A Framework for Considering the Ethical Aspects of Psychiatric Research Protocols." *Comprehensive Psychiatry* 42(5):351–363, 2001. Used with permission from Elsevier.

with the absence of an objection representing an insufficient assent. Significantly, children can veto their participation. Information about the research must be presented to the minor at a level commensurate to the child's age and developmental level. Indeed, a child's capacity for assent is determined by his or her age, developmental maturity, and psychological state at the time of recruitment. Although children younger than age 7 years are typically not considered capable of providing assent, younger children still have the right to learn about the research and to assent to their own involvement. Some empirical work suggests age 9 years as a turning point in cognition and voluntarism, allowing for greater ability to provide consent (Ondrusek et al. 1998). Research on capacity for consent and assent also emphasizes the importance of noncognitive aspects of decision-making ability and of distinct coercive pressures that young people may experience (Roberts 2002).

Risk

DHHS demarcated the safeguards that serve to protect minors from the potential harm associated with research. Figure 18–1 presents a decision tree for this paradigm of weighing risks and benefits. Risk is ascertained by evaluating the risk to the participant, the benefit to the participant, the benefit to similar children or to children in general, and the minor's capacity to provide assent. If a study exposes the child to no more than minimal risk, the minor's participation is acceptable with one parent's permission and the child's assent, irrespective of the possible benefit to the participant. *Minimal risk* is defined as posing risks no greater than those experienced in children's daily lives, assuming that daily life represents a safe and caring environment. When the study presents more than minimal risk, minors can participate if the benefits are greater than the risks. The benefit to the participant must be at least equal to the potential benefit from the other treatments available to children with the same disorder. Participation can proceed if one parent grants permission and the child assents.

Research that exposes children to more than minimal risk and offers no direct benefit to the participant can advance only if the study is likely to generate knowledge that will benefit children who are being treated for the same disorder as the participant (Vitiello 2003). Furthermore, the minor must not endure any experiences that exceed in discomfort those sustained in a medical, dental, psychological, social, or educational situation (Rosato 2000). In these circumstances, permission of both parents, when applicable, and the assent of the minor are required. Past empirical work in this area emphasizes the importance of evaluating risk in relation to biological and psychosocial dimensions and from the perspective of the child, whose fears, physical discomfort, and expectations must be considered.

Emerging Issues

Current DHHS regulations do not recognize the concept of mature minors—that is, minors who are competent to provide consent. Competence is characterized by the ability to comprehend the relevant information, determine the risk-to-benefit ratio, and make a voluntary decision. A large body of research indicates that by age 14 years, most adolescents have developed the cognitive and social capacity to provide informed consent. Interestingly, many states allow adolescents to consent to certain medical and mental health interventions and adolescents with terminal illness to refuse life-sustaining care.

Many ethicists and scholars purport that the DHHS guidelines diminish the autonomy of mature minors (Melton 1999; Rosato 2000) and transitional age youth, more generally. Adolescents are regarded no differently

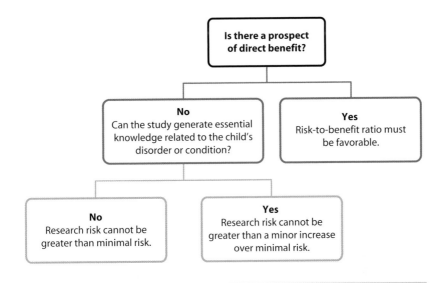

FIGURE 18–1. Federal requirements for more rigorous review regarding prospect of direct benefit in research with children.

Minimal risk is defined as posing risks no greater than those experienced in children's daily lives, assuming that daily life represents a safe and caring environment.

Source. Copyright © 2014 Laura Weiss Roberts, M.D., M.A. Used with permission.

from young children. Existing regulations do not allow an older adolescent to participate in a research protocol if the guardian refuses to grant permission. This regulation becomes an ethical dilemma when, in the absence of parental permission, an adolescent assents to participate in research because of its expected benefits either to the adolescent or to other adolescents with the same disorder. The Common Rule is currently in the process of revision, and new guidance regarding consent in research involving children may be more attuned to the issues faced by adolescent volunteers (Federal Register 2015).

Melton (1999) thoughtfully outlined mechanisms by which children and guardians can share the decision-making process. He proposed one model wherein children are afforded increased participation as they become more mature developmentally. He proposed another model in which guardians or other identified adults function as mentors or consultants for mature minors. In this model, the mature minor can provide consent.

An additional ethical consideration relates to a key societal justice issue that has been described as "scientific neglect" of vulnerable populations

(Roberts 1998). The vigorous self-advocacy of people with HIV and, to a lesser extent, of people with breast cancer has raised two important questions: First, does an individual have the right to access experimental research procedures, and second, do the health concerns of special populations, including elderly persons and children, receive adequate attention and resources? Within the field of psychiatry, the absence of adequate data on psychopharmacology in children results in providing health care that is not evidence based, potentially causing unmeasured and unstudied harm (Martin et al. 2000; Vitiello 2003). The off-label use of medications with children, which has significantly increased in recent years, represents even greater possibilities for harm (see Chapter 19, "Innovation in Psychiatry"). Rosato (2000) argued that children are essentially being used as research subjects, without the benefit of a supervised and controlled study, when they are administered psychopharmacological agents that have not been approved for their age cohort or clinical diagnosis. Similarly, the paucity of systematic outcome data on children's mental health has left judges, social workers, teachers, and clinicians without information on the true impact of major decisions affecting children's lives.

CONCLUSION

To be ethically sound, psychiatric research should remain faithful to the principles of respect for persons, beneficence, and justice; be conducted by investigators who possess expertise and integrity; have justifiable design and methods; and uphold safeguards shared throughout the field of biomedical research. A number of efforts can be made to assess and ensure the ethical conduct of research. Reviewing the list of questions in each of the domains provided in Table 18–2 may be helpful to prospective investigators, protocol reviewers, or concerned readers of scientific literature. The reader is referred to federal regulations that continue to evolve to include, for example, new guidelines related to special populations (e.g., prisoners) and parameters around conflict of interest (e.g., for IRB members and investigators). In addition, the Roberts Research Protocol Ethics Assessment Tool (RePEAT), an educational tool for reviewing and writing protocols, is presented in this chapter's Appendix. Finally, special efforts to address the attributes and circumstances of people with mental illness may further help mitigate against, and even reverse, their potential vulnerabilities with respect to participating in human research.

CASE SCENARIOS

■ A researcher struggles with the question of whether to enroll a homeless person diagnosed with schizophrenia in a medication protocol. She is concerned that the patient will feel coerced by the free medication and health care he will receive if he enrolls and that he will have few resources if he becomes seriously symptomatic and demands discharge during the medication-free run-in period.

■ A researcher who owns stock in a major pharmaceutical company becomes a primary investigator on a trial for a new medication.

■ An early-career researcher wants to test a new herbal medication in patients with panic disorder. The medication in question has undergone very few basic science studies of its safety or efficacy.

■ An IRB member serves as a principal investigator on a number of industry-based studies and approaches a fellow IRB member to become a coinvestigator.

■ A researcher is concerned that several of the patients in his neuroimaging study of dementia are not decisionally capable. Because the study poses minimal risks to participants, however, he allows them to remain in the study if they give assent and have a responsible surrogate decision maker.

Appendix: Roberts Research Protocol Ethics Assessment Tool (RePEAT)

Ethical domain	Acceptable		Unacceptable	
Scientific merit and design issues				
1. Do the study's hypotheses possess *scientific merit?*	Yes	Not applicable	Requires clarification	No
2. Does the *research design appropriately test* its hypotheses?	Yes	Not applicable	Requires clarification	No
Expertise, commitment, and integrity issues				
3. Does the research team have sufficient *expertise* to successfully conduct the study?	Yes	Not applicable	Requires clarification	No
4. Does the research team have sufficient *commitment, resources, and support* from the institution to successfully conduct the study?	Yes	Not applicable	Requires clarification	No
5. Are the members of the research team *knowledgeable* with respect to the ethics of human research and in *good standing* within the scientific and professional communities?	Yes	Not applicable	Requires clarification	No
6. Does evidence exist of *past misconduct* by members of the research team, individually or collectively?	No	Not applicable	Requires clarification	Yes
7. Do the financial, institutional, or other arrangements related to the protocol pose any *threat to the integrity* of members of the research team, individually or collectively (e.g., significant "conflicts of interest")?	No	Not applicable	Requires clarification	Yes

Appendix: Roberts Research Protocol Ethics Assessment Tool (RePEAT) *(continued)*

Ethical domain	Acceptable		Unacceptable	

Risks and benefits

Ethical domain	Acceptable		Unacceptable	
8. Are *experimental risks* to participants minimized by the research design?	Yes	Not applicable	Requires clarification	No
9. Does the protocol pose *excessive risk or other burdens* to individual participants, the community, and/or larger society?	No	Not applicable	Requires clarification	Yes
10. If participants are likely to have *emerging symptoms* (i.e., appearance of new symptoms or worsening of existing symptoms) as a result of or during protocol participation:				
a. Has an appropriate mechanism for *identifying and following symptom progression* been built into the protocol?	Yes	Not applicable	Requires clarification	No
b. Has an appropriate mechanism for *identifying when to discontinue protocol participation* in order to begin standard treatment for emerging symptoms that pose safety risks or involve enduring distress been built into the protocol?	Yes	Not applicable	Requires clarification	No
c. Has an appropriate mechanism for *referring or providing patients with standard treatment* for emerging symptoms that pose safety risks or enduring distress been built into protocol?	Yes	Not applicable	Requires clarification	No
11. Are *benefits* in association with research participation optimized by the research design for individuals and society?	Yes	Not applicable	Requires clarification	No

Appendix: Roberts Research Protocol Ethics Assessment Tool (RePEAT) *(continued)*

Ethical domain	Acceptable		Unacceptable	
Confidentiality				
12. Do the research design and plans for data use adequately protect participant *confidentiality?*	Yes	Not applicable	Requires clarification	No
Participant selection and recruitment				
13. Does the selection and recruitment process for the protocol ensure that members of *vulnerable populations* (e.g., children, institutionalized or decisionally impaired patients, women who are pregnant or may become pregnant) will be included only if essential to the study's scientific hypotheses?	Yes	Not applicable	Requires clarification	No
14. Are *understudied populations* inappropriately excluded from participation (i.e., are selection and recruitment practices potentially discriminatory)?	No	Not applicable	Requires clarification	Yes
15. Does the *selection and recruitment process* for the protocol ensure that potential participants may comfortably refuse protocol involvement (i.e., is the recruitment process itself noncoercive)?	Yes	Not applicable	Requires clarification	No
16. Will benefits derived from the protocol, if any, be conferred to the specific *population being studied* in the protocol?	Yes	Not applicable	Requires clarification	No

Appendix: Roberts Research Protocol Ethics Assessment Tool (RePEAT) *(continued)*

Ethical domain		Acceptable	Unacceptable

Informed consent and decisional capacity

17. Does the research design define an appropriate *informed consent process* including:

			Acceptable		Unacceptable
a.	*Disclosure of information* regarding:	Yes	Not applicable	Requires clarification	No
	—The study's purpose				
	—Who is responsible for the conduct of the study				
	—Why the individual may be eligible for participation				
	—The nature of the illness (or the phenomenon being studied)				
	—The proposed intervention				
	—The associated risks and benefits and their relative likelihood				
	—Alternatives to participation				
	—Key study design features (e.g., placebo use, randomization, medication-free intervals, frequency of visits, confidentiality, plans for use of data) and other issues?				
b.	Reasonable assurance of adequate *decisional capacity* of participants with respect to the ability to understand, rationally analyze, and appreciate the meaning of the research decision, OR reasonable assurance of adequately meeting all criteria listed under Item 18 below?	Yes	Not applicable	Requires clarification	No

Appendix: Roberts Research Protocol Ethics Assessment Tool (RePEAT) *(continued)*

Ethical domain	Acceptable		Unacceptable
c. Reasonable assurance that individuals will *not experience coercive pressure* to participate during the consent phase or during protocol involvement (e.g., timing of consent discussions so that individuals can think through the decision and seek advice from others; explicit acknowledgment that participation is voluntary and that individuals may refuse or withdraw from protocol involvement without adverse consequences; giving even decisionally incapable participants the right to refuse)?	Yes	Not applicable	Requires clarification No
d. A *concise, readable, accurate, and understandable* consent form, suited to the population under study?	Yes	Not applicable	Requires clarification No
18. If participants are likely to experience *diminished decisional capacity at any time* during protocol participation (including at the time of enrollment):			
a. Has an appropriate mechanism for *identifying, following, and documenting the level of diminished decisional capacity* of participants been built into the protocol?	Yes	Not applicable	Requires clarification No

Appendix: Roberts Research Protocol Ethics Assessment Tool (RePEAT) (continued)

Ethical domain	Acceptable		Unacceptable	
b. When possible, has an appropriate mechanism *for enhancing or restoring the decisional capacity* of the participant been built into the protocol?	Yes	Not applicable	Requires clarification	No
c. If a *period of diminished decisional capacity may be necessary* because of the scientific hypotheses of the study (e.g., a study of advanced dementia or of some life-threatening emergencies, or a psychopharmacology trial study involving a relatively brief medication-free interval), does the protocol include:				
(1) An appropriate mechanism *for advance decision making by the participant or for identifying an alternative decision maker* for the participant?	Yes	Not applicable	Requires clarification	No
(2) An appropriate mechanism *for implementing advance decisions or for preparing and utilizing the alternative decision maker* when necessary?	Yes	Not applicable	Requires clarification	No
Incentives				
19. Are *incentives for participation* sufficient and appropriately timed so that they compensate research participants *without* being coercive?	Yes	Not applicable	Requires clarification	No
Other issues				
20. Are the *documentation* practices adequate to monitor protocol procedures and the professional accountability of the research team?	Yes	Not applicable	Requires clarification	No

Appendix: Roberts Research Protocol Ethics Assessment Tool (RePEAT) (continued)

Ethical domain	Acceptable		Unacceptable	
21. Is an appropriate "debriefing" process built into the protocol so that participants may be informed of relevant study procedures and/or findings?	Yes	Not applicable	Requires clarification	No
22. Are *other ethical problems* apparent in this protocol? If "Yes," describe:	No	Not applicable	Requires clarification	Yes
23. Are there *other issues that interfere with protocol approval?* If "Yes," describe:	No	Not applicable	Requires clarification	Yes
24. Prior to its approval, does the protocol require *additional review* by others with more specialized expertise or by others with especially relevant interests and experience to assess its ethics or its science?	No	Not applicable	Requires clarification	Yes
Does the protocol, *in its present form,* meet minimal criteria for being ethically sound?*	Yes			No
Does the protocol, *in its present form,* require a more rigorous level of monitoring than is customary?	No	Yes**		
Comment:				

Note. This tool is intended for use in assessment of ethical aspects of research protocols involving human participants.

*All evaluative criteria (Items 1–24) must receive an acceptable response for the protocol to be *minimally acceptable* on ethical grounds. Problems, as indicated by responses in *either* of the second two columns, should be addressed formally and should undergo re-review prior to protocol approval.

** "Yes" is acceptable if specific protocols have been established.

Source. Copyright © 1999 Laura Weiss Roberts, M.D., M.A. Adapted with permission from Laura Weiss Roberts, M.D., M.A., 2015.

19

Innovation in Psychiatry

Laura Weiss Roberts, M.D., M.A.

Cynthia M.A. Geppert, M.D., M.A., M.P.H., M.S., D.P.S.

Necessity is the mother of invention, it is said. The tremendous need for knowledge and new ways to help people living with mental disorders and related conditions has inspired tremendous innovation in psychiatry. Every day psychiatrists improvise with off-label uses of medications and combinations of medications and other therapies to help patients in need. Leading-edge clinicians are engaged in "e-innovation," developing therapies that engage with technology and social media, such as asynchronous "text therapy." Psychiatric genetic studies, at times involving many thousands of individuals, are yielding new insights into the causes of and contributors to mental disorders. Master physicians are adapting approaches from other fields, such as deep brain stimulation and vagal nerve stimulation, to address the most severe symptoms of disabling mental disorders. Big data analytics are yielding new insights regarding prevention, early identification, and disease progression. Triangulation of biomarkers combining genetic, imaging, and clinical phenomenology, possible through remarkable advances in a number of fields, are helping to resolve some of the oldest questions in psychiatry, and to accelerate projects that align with the National Institute of Mental Health's Research Domain Criteria and the American Psychiatric Association's (2013a) *Diagnostic and Statistical Manual of Mental Disorders,* 5th Edition. Brilliant physician-scientists in psychiatry are applying optogenetic and stem cell techniques (Deisseroth et al. 2015) to study brain disorders and other conditions, such as chronic pain, making discoveries that will certainly change the future of human health.

This chapter focuses on the interface of clinical research and clinical innovation, genetics, and e-based therapies to illustrate ethical approaches to rapid advances in psychiatry. The principles and approaches may be adapted and generalized to innovations as they arise in psychiatry.

CLINICAL RESEARCH AND CLINICAL INNOVATION

Patients each day seek care for severe symptoms of mental disorders and co-occurring conditions for which there are no or too few treatments that have fulfilled U.S. Food and Drug Administration (FDA) approval. Some treatments have been approved by the FDA, but only for individuals who fall into other age groups or have conditions other than the disorder of the patient in need. Psychiatrists in practice commonly encounter these treatment challenges. Moreover, psychiatric care for potentially vulnerable populations, such as children and adolescents, pregnant women, and elders, has been especially limited by the lack of adequate clinical evidence.

In light of insufficient evidence that will clearly direct care practices and guidelines, how does the clinician think about protecting the rights and safety of individuals whose care may be directly or indirectly affected by innovation? Some innovations fall strictly under the purview of human research, and the ethics of these activities aligns with the principles and safeguards that have evolved in this area of biomedical science (see Chapter 18, "Psychiatric Research"). Because clinicians will be called on to design unique strategies—to improvise and innovate—to help their patients, it is imperative that every psychiatrist and trainee understand when he or she is doing something that meets criteria for human research. Human research, in a very basic and formal sense, is *research* that involves *human subjects,* as further described below according to federal guidelines for the protection of human subjects (U.S. Department of Health and Human Services 2009, 45 CFR §46.102, Definitions):

- *Research* is defined as "a systematic investigation, including research development, testing, and evaluation, designed to develop or contribute to generalizable knowledge."

- A *human subject* is defined as a "living individual about whom an investigator (whether professional or student) conducting research obtains (1) data through intervention or interaction with the individual, or (2) identifiable private information."

When activities with patients meet these definitions, the work is considered clinical research. Clinical research falls under human subjects regulations that require institutional review board approval and oversight and must fulfill many other safeguard conditions.

The nuances in these definitions of *research* and *human subject* are critically important. For example, the off-label use of a medication in the care of an individual patient does not qualify as clinical research and does not fall under the purview of an institutional review board, even if it is undertaken in a systematic fashion, because the primary intent is not to contribute to generalizable knowledge. Similarly, the use of data from an electronic medical record to improve quality practices on a hospital unit is not research, even if it is undertaken in a systematic fashion, because there is no intent to contribute to generalizable knowledge. When the psychiatrist decides to perform a case series in which off-label prescribing occurs in order to write up the series for a journal and when the quality assurance team decides to use its findings as preliminary data for a grant, poster, or publication, these professionals have stepped across the line separating innovation into research.

For novel efforts that remain on the clinical side of the line, clinicians should follow a disciplined thought process regarding whether the use of innovation is justified rather than remaining within traditional boundaries of care. Clinical activities represent clinical innovation (rather than clinical research) when the primary intention is to help the individual patient. Along with other clinicians, I have articulated that clinical innovation can be considered ethically justified if it occurs under specific circumstances (Figure 19–1; Hoop et al. 2009a). When choosing to implement innovation, the clinician should obtain the patient's consent with greater care, document the consent specially in the patient's medical record, and maintain careful documentation in the patient's medical record that addresses each of the four questions posed in Figure 19–1, and which are discussed further as follows:

1. There must be a substantial clinical need. Necessity drives innovation, ethically.
2. Standard treatment efforts must have been exhausted without success. Appropriate medications and other treatments that have been approved for the condition and would be appropriate for the individual must have

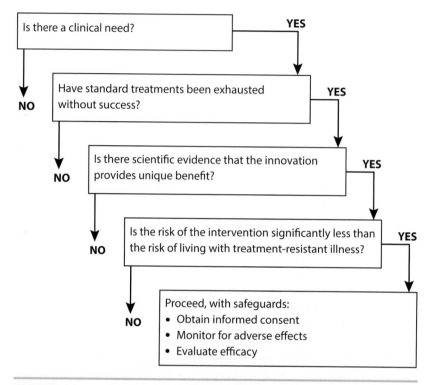

FIGURE 19–1. Decision tree for ethical use of clinical innovation.

Source. Reprinted from Hoop JG, Layde J, Roberts LW: "Ethical Considerations in Psychopharmacological Treatment and Research," in *Textbook of Psychopharmacology*, 4th Edition. Edited by Schatzberg AF, Nemeroff CB. Washington, DC, American Psychiatric Publishing, 2009, p. 1490. Copyright © 2009 American Psychiatric Publishing. Used with permission.

been given reasonable trials. When the proposed innovation is very low risk, it may be introduced before all possible traditional treatments have been exhausted. However, the possible opportunity cost of exposing an individual to risks, even small, and essentially depriving the patient of an approach that fits within usual standards of care should be considered very carefully.

3. Scientific evidence must support the innovation as potentially providing benefit. The amount of evidence required depends on the severity of the condition, the known risks and benefits of the treatment, and the patient's preferences. For example, relatively modest evidence of efficacy may be required to justify the use of an innovative agent that has excellent safety data if the patient prefers to try the new treatment and has severe treatment-resistant symptoms.

4. The anticipated likely risks of the intervention and the relatively rare but entirely possible risks must not be significantly greater than the risks associated with the underlying illness or condition. For example, the use of antipsychotics for transient mild anxiety would be inappropriate given the risks of significant side effects associated with this class of medication. In addition, appropriate safeguards to identify risks and side effects must be feasible and put in place.

Neuromodulation for different serious conditions using deep brain stimulation or repetitive transcranial magnetic stimulation techniques represents an emerging area of innovation. Using the criteria above, the clinician must consider whether there is clear and serious need for innovation, whether reasonable and formally approved alternatives have been attempted without sufficient success, whether evidence exists to suggest the potential for benefit, and whether the likely and rare-but-serious risks outweigh the potential for gain. Foremost is the question of whether the individual has sufficient decisional capacity to undertake the proposed treatment. Every effort to ensure optimal informed consent under these circumstances is essential. Careful attention should be given to the nature of the relationship with the patient; the decision at hand; the quality of information sharing; the capacity of the patient to communicate, comprehend, reason, and appreciate; and the authentic and free character of the decision. Other safeguards include safety in performing any procedure, clinical monitoring for adverse effects, efforts to evaluate the treatment's efficacy, and reevaluation of both the patient's need for the intervention and the scientific evidence supporting its use, if the intervention is ongoing.

PSYCHIATRIC GENETICS

Genetic advances are transforming the world and raising unprecedented ethical concerns. Genetic investigation has inspired the hopes of people living with mental disorders and their families. Although most psychiatric genetic work is now conducted in a research context, the coming years will see the translation of this science to the offices of clinical psychiatrists, neurologists, and some primary care clinicians. Psychiatric genetics may involve testing asymptomatic individuals with a predisposition to mental illness, persons who potentially carry susceptibility genes for psychiatric disorders, and mentally ill individuals with genetic variants or markers that might pertain to the efficacy and safety of medications (i.e., the new field of pharmacogenetics). One day in the not-too-distant future, gene therapy for mental disorders may be a part of psychiatric treatment. Therefore, it is important for practitioners to understand the fundamental ethics of informed consent and confidentiality as well as considerations of justice that surround innovation in psychiatric genetics.

Genetic information is of particular ethical significance for mental illness. Psychiatric genetic information is 1) complex, 2) probabilistic, 3) familial, and 4) existential. With few exceptions (e.g., Huntington's disease), every major neuropsychiatric disorder is thought to be a complex disorder. A complex genetic disorder is the result of not a single gene but of several genes interacting with each other and with the environment. A recent National Institute of Mental Health work group established a substantial complex genetic component for five major psychiatric disorders (Cross-Disorder Group of the Psychiatric Genomics Consortium 2013), but no single gene has yet been identified as a definitive cause of a major disorder such as bipolar disorder or schizophrenia.

Informed Consent, "Return of Results," and Confidentiality

The complex nature of psychiatric disorders means that even when genes are identified for their involvement in the development of psychiatric disorders, possession of these genes confers only a risk or probability, not a certainty, that an individual or a family member will develop a psychiatric condition. A person who has several family members diagnosed with schizophrenia clearly has a greater vulnerability than a member of the general population. Family history does not unalterably dictate the development of a disorder, however, or determine when the condition will emerge, how severe the course of illness will be, or whether treatment will be effective.

A detailed discussion of risks, benefits, and alternatives with attention to personal values is at the core of informed consent. Genetic information is statistical and probabilistic. Risks are expressed as statistical probabilities and as such are extremely abstract concepts that are difficult to interpret and explain. Studies suggest that it is problematic to adequately describe the risks and benefits of genetic research or interventions to healthy persons or to those with medical illnesses. Most medical treatments or studies involve physical risks that can be stated in concrete terms of expected pain and discomfort. Genetic testing involves nothing more invasive than a cotton swab scraped across a cheek or, at most, the drawing of a blood sample. The risks are not biological per se; instead, there are psychosocial dangers to family relationships and the ability to obtain or maintain employment and health insurance. Many individuals with serious mental illnesses have problems with attention, memory, and processing that impair their comprehension of this kind of abstract and complicated information.

Information about genetic testing and genetic interventions also challenges affective dimensions of decisional capacity in psychiatric patients confronted with choices regarding genetic testing. Genetics as a subject arouses powerful emotions. As one person stated recently, after learning about her genetic condition, "I feel like a bad seed—like I hurt my children with my genes." Guilt, fear, anxiety, confusion, self-doubt, anger, and shame may accompany individuals' experience of learning about their genetic makeup. These feelings are amplified in individuals with conditions such as schizophrenia, bipolar disorder, and substance abuse, which carry significant health repercussions and societal stigma.

The familial nature of genetic testing and treatment may negatively affect the capacity for voluntarism because individuals may feel unable to make a choice independent of other family stakeholders. Indeed, the consent decision of an individual affects an entire family. When a family is doing well, new information ("return of results") about the family's genetic susceptibilities may be difficult to handle. When a family is struggling, which is not uncommon in the context of mental illness, this new information can damage an already-fragile family system.

In terms of other aspects of informed consent and the return of results, no genetic interventions are available that can prevent, correct, or reverse the course of serious mental illnesses once they manifest. Researchers, patients, and clinicians must carefully weigh the psychological harm that may come from the knowledge of genetic status, given the absence of curative treatments and the uncertain benefits of early detection and treatment. Nevertheless, in the future, a test result suggesting greater vulnerability to developing schizophrenia or bipolar disorder may enable individuals and families to take preventive action, such as close monitoring of symptoms, avoidance of substance abuse and extreme stress that may trigger onset of a disorder, or even prophylactic or ameliorative pharmacology at the first signs of illness.

Learning the results of genetic tests can bring benefit, harm, or a little or a lot of both, depending on the individuals' personalities, the larger context, and the immediate circumstances. Some families will feel relief and a sense of control from being able to warn other family members and to make informed marital and reproductive decisions. Other individuals may feel discouraged or helpless when they learn of a susceptibility to mental illness. On the basis of this information, even though it is uncertain and probabilistic, family members may make significant life decisions, such as in relation to marrying or having children, according to empirical work in this arena.

   To illustrate, I discuss four very early studies of ethical issues related to schizophrenia and bipolar disorder genetics. Schulz et al. (1982) used the Family Attitudes Questionnaire to measure attitudes and perceptions toward the etiology, familial risk, and socioeconomic burden of schizophrenia, as well as childbearing plans and the acceptability of genetic counseling, in members of 17 families, each having a child with schizophrenia. They found that patients and well family members held radically different attitudes toward the disorder. For example, 92% of parents, compared with only 25% of ill individuals, identified schizophrenia as an extremely burdensome disorder. Only 29% of the parents, compared with 66% of ill persons, reported that they would have children based on their knowledge and experience of schizophrenia in their family. The same questionnaire was used in a study by Targum et al. (1981), this time focusing on bipolar disorder and yielding a similar result. A total of 19 individuals with bipolar disorder and their healthy spouses participated. In this study, 53% of well spouses, compared with only 5% of patients, reported that they would not have had children if they had known more about bipolar illness. In another study of bipolar disorder, Trippitelli et al. (1998) assessed the knowledge and attitudes of individuals with bipolar disorder and their spouses ($N=90$) regarding treatment response rates for bipolar disorder, probability of inheritance, genetic testing, disclosure of genetic information, abortion, marriage, and childbearing. The majority of the ill individuals and their spouses said that they would use genetic tests for bipolar disorder if they were available. Most patients and spouses believed that the benefits of knowledge of carrying a bipolar gene outweighed the risks. Smith et al. (1996) investigated attitudes toward bipolar disorder and genetic testing, including prenatal testing and possible pregnancy termination related to course and severity of illness. They surveyed members of a bipolar support group, medical students, and psychiatry residents ($n=113$), and nearly half reported that they would terminate a pregnancy if the child would definitely develop bipolar disorder in the future.

   Because genetic data are familial data, significant challenges arise in relation to protecting individual confidentiality. Most contemporary psychiatric genetic research depends on pedigrees and often blood or tissue samples from family members of the person enrolled in genetic testing or treatment—the proband. Diagnosing an individual with bipolar disorder reveals information about the presence or susceptibility of the index condition and often of related psychiatric disorders in parents, siblings, children, and even those who have died or are yet to be born. Hence, the disclosure of genetic information can have an impact—for good and ill—at three levels: the individual, the family, and the community. As part of the initial informed consent procedure in genetic research, the proband usually gives the investigators permission to contact his or her relatives to explain the study and to offer them participation. Researchers endeavor to protect the privacy and confidentially of all family members by revealing only the absolute minimum of information necessary to pursue the scientific goals of the study.

The issue of confidentiality is moot if, in fact, genetic information represents the true, unique biosignature of an individual. Stripping away a name, an address, a Social Security number, or other identifying data from the electronic health record means nothing if genetic data identify precisely one person—and, as previously described, reveal key insights about an entire family. All prior notions of privacy do not hold in such a circumstance. Current confidentiality safeguards and legislation are not sufficient to manage this astonishing development in human genetics.

Discrimination and Social Justice Issues

Too often, when genetic information is revealed at the social group and community level, the unfortunate result is stigma and discrimination. Because both persons with mental illness and persons with genetic disease have already been documented as objects of prejudice and injustice, persons with positive genetic findings for mental illness confront a double discrimination and overlapping vulnerabilities. An early court case from Hong Kong illustrates the enormous discriminative potential of psychiatric genetic information (Wong and Lieh-Mak 2001). Three young men had applied to serve in various branches of the protective forces (e.g., the fire and customs departments). They were refused employment on the basis of a family history of schizophrenia, which was held to indicate increased potential for violence. None of the applicants was symptomatic or had ever been diagnosed with a mental illness or received genetic testing, although a family history was substantiated in two of the cases. After testimony by numerous psychiatric genetic experts, the court ruled that it was unlawful for the civil service to discriminate in employment, for the sake of public safety, against people with a family history of mental illness. The court further ruled that an individualized assessment of specific risks, rather than the application of population-based lifetime risks, must be applied in determining fitness for work.

This case and reported examples of people with only a risk of inherited medical disorders who have lost their health insurance, employment, or other educational and occupational opportunities underscore the need to protect genetic information from unauthorized disclosure to third parties who might use it to exploit or harm the individuals and their families. Even false-positive results and incorrectly interpreted findings have led to persons being unable to obtain health insurance for their children or to be promoted at work (Lapham et al. 1996). Early studies with patients who have a high risk of developing breast cancer showed that fears of discrimination and stigmatization dissuade patients from participating in research and from seeking diagnosis and treatment until the disease has progressed (Armstrong et al. 2000).

The Genetic Information Nondiscrimination Act, or GINA, went into effect in 2009, motivated by cases and empirical evidence that demonstrated the need for better protections for people in the United States. The first part of the law prohibited genetic discrimination in health insurance. The second part made it illegal for employers to use a person's genetic information when making decisions about hiring, promotion, and other terms of employment. This law represents a landmark in U.S. history in protecting individuals from social harms of genetic information. Many other ethical questions have arisen related to ownership rights and genetic information and the broad application of genetic technologies never imagined or foreseen when GINA was enacted (Skloot 2011).

With colleagues, I performed a series of studies looking at how employees and employers regard the use of health and genetic information in the workplace (Geppert and Roberts 2005; Hoop et al. 2009b; Roberts et al. 2005a, 2005b, 2011a, 2012). In one project we administered an extensive online survey, with 570 participants who were employees at Sandia National Laboratories and the University of New Mexico. We found that respondents believed that genetic information was more sensitive than nongenetic health information and that they did not wish to share either type of information with employers due to fears of discrimination and stigma. This project also revealed a tension in that workers also believed that employers had fundamental responsibilities for protecting health and safety in the workplace, which could necessitate the need to know the health issues of workers.

Perhaps the most significant consideration related to discrimination and justice is that health benefits related to genetic innovation in psychiatry will be limited to a small segment of society for the near future. This observation fits within a larger set of concerns about health disparities and social inequities in global health. Because genetic information is existential and thus has import for the understanding of the nature of humanity, of where people have come from, and of what their destiny may be, this human inequity has special poignancy.

Ethically Sound Approaches

Interest in obtaining genetic services for psychiatric conditions is growing rapidly. Competent and compassionate psychiatric care that encompasses genetic counseling will be essential to maximize the therapeutic benefits of genetic research, testing, and therapy while minimizing the adverse consequences. Well-trained genetic counselors are in short supply. Clinical psychiatrists and neurologists, and possibly primary care clinicians, will be charged with counseling psychiatric patients and families about the promises and problems in genetics issues.

Clinicians can take the following steps to begin to develop the knowledge and skills needed for genetic counseling with psychiatric patients:

1. The decisional capacity and voluntarism of persons with mental illness to consent to genetic testing, research, and therapy must be prudently assessed, methodically respected, and patiently facilitated. Clinicians may need to have a series of discussions about genetic risks and benefits; utilize audiovisual materials, analogies, and problem-solving exercises to convey the valence of probabilities; and evaluate the need for a surrogate decision maker.

2. Clinicians need to invite and enhance family involvement from the initial stages of discussion and in an ongoing fashion, both to safeguard the autonomy, privacy, and confidentiality of all parties and to allow the "family patient" to receive the best care possible. It will be crucial to clarify personal, familial, and social values relevant to the decisions to be made.

3. Most practicing psychiatrists and neurologists will have received only rudimentary training in psychiatric genetics, and few psychologists, nurses, counselors, and social workers will have received even this level of preparation. Nevertheless, they can avail themselves of the growth in continuing medical education in genetics and the ethical, legal, religious, and social implications of genetic research offered through the Internet, conferences, books, and journals.

4. Clinicians can identify experts in ethics, religion, culture, and/or genetics at local university hospitals or research centers or ethics committees whom they may consult on an informal and formal basis.

Psychiatrists and other health professionals who follow these and other constructive suggestions will be well situated to apply the benefits of genetic research to the clinical care of patients with scientific rigor and ethical responsibility.

E-INNOVATION IN PSYCHIATRY

The engagement with technology and social media has transformed models of mental health care and the therapeutic relationship. The previously un-imagined is now here: video appointments conducted through the electronic medical record; patient advice telephone lines staffed by high school graduates who walk through protocols and direct care; psychotherapy performed exclusively via asynchronous texting between a clinician and patient who have never met face to face; and an entire array of issues such as psychiatrists being "Yelped" and "Googled" and "friended." Individuals have created Internet personae, with the cascade of issues that follow, as described by psychiatrist Elias Aboujaoude (2011, 2015) in his *New York Times* Best Sellers–listed book, *Virtually You: The Dangerous Powers of the E-Personality,* and his more recent book, *Mental Health in the Digital Age: Grave Dangers, Great Promise.* Cyberspace has become medicalized.

On one hand, e-innovations hold immense promise in that they may allow for real-time assistance to individuals throughout the world. Numerous Internet-supported interventions exist, including Web-based education interventions, self-directed therapeutic interventions, clinician-supported therapeutic interventions, online counseling, Internet-operated software, and blogs, podcasts, online support groups, and online assessments (Barak et al. 2009). Empirical studies have shown tremendous benefits to some of these new interventions (Jones et al. 2014; Trockel et al. 2014). A recent study examining the feasibility and acceptability of using text messages for mental health promotion in poor areas of India suggests the potential for bringing culturally accepted, inexpensive, and helpful interventions to vulnerable populations in very underserved areas (Chandra et al. 2014). E-innovations may represent the first genuine opportunity to reduce global mental health disparities, particularly with psychosocial treatment modalities.

On the other hand, these new models and approaches present new challenges. The practice of a psychiatrist who is judicious about prescribing substances with addictive potential can be damaged by anonymous criticisms posted on unregulated Web sites. Recent research exploring the early experiences with telehealth and other e-innovation has documented a number of concerns of both mental health service users and mental health professionals, such as how to manage issues that come up in discussion forums, e-mail, and video-based care and where additional education is needed before e-health methods (e.g., unsupported computerized assessment tools or therapies) can be used more broadly (Jones and Ashurst 2013).

More than a decade ago, a joint committee of the International Society for Mental Health Online and the Psychiatric Society for Informatics suggested principles of professional ethics for the online provision of mental health services (Hsiung 2001). The principles encompass informed consent, operating procedures, and emergency responses. The principles touch on important issues such as addressing possible misunderstandings in e-based care; managing expectations related to turn-around time, privacy, and boundaries; ensuring competence of the e-care service provider; addressing legal issues; and ensuring that there is sufficient local backup if patients become distressed. Many of these same principles have been advanced in more recent recommendations, such as in the context of marriage and family therapy (Jordan et al. 2014). Recommended principles for incorporating social media into treatment include guidelines for informed consent, multiple relationships, confidentiality, professional competence and integrity, responsibility to supervisees and trainees, and responsibility to research participants. Guidelines for each area have been articulated for their ethical importance and impact, with the hope that these ideals will better inform professional guidelines.

Indeed, updated and newer recommendations are evolving and are being introduced by professional societies in real time. The American Psychiatric Association (2009) has encouraged that practicing psychiatrists think carefully about how traditional principles of ethics, such as respect for persons and beneficence, may inform novel e-health and related practices. The inclusion of mobile technology into therapeutic work with a patient, as an adjuvant care strategy, may be ethically appropriate. However, advising patients to use mobile technology for mental health care independent of the doctor–patient relationship is not yet ethically acceptable, because most mobile technologies do not have a sound evidence base evaluating their value and impact (Darcy et al. 2016; Hsin et al. 2016). In psychiatry, a question has arisen about the ethics of inquiring about the background or activities of new or ongoing patients via the Internet. Simple curiosity is not a sufficient reason to query a patient's history or circumstances, according to the American Psychiatric Association (2016). However, use of the Internet or social media, if motivated solely by concern for the well-being of the patient, such as looking for contextual cues in an adolescent who is at risk for suicide, may be ethically acceptable. If informed consent is explicitly obtained, engagement of social media in treatment is ethically acceptable, but again other safeguards (e.g., confidentiality) are still necessary.

CONCLUSION

With each passing day, innovation is under way, and applications to enhance overall well-being and mental health are in evidence. Much of this innovation should and will be embraced by psychiatry across diverse settings because it means that life may get better for people with mental disorders throughout the world. Simply stated, for things to get better, many factors must change. Creativity and innovation should therefore be supported by ethical guidelines. Elsewhere I have written,

> [W]e are entrusted with finding a path to a better future for all whose lives are touched by mental disorders, neurodevelopmental conditions, addictions, and co-occurring disorders. These conditions represent the greatest health burdens experienced by millions of people throughout the world today. Even if we could provide access to current treatment for all people in need, the efforts still would not be adequate. How will we find this path forward to this better future, if not through creativity? I suggest that our responsibilities in fulfilling productivity expectations, delivering on performance metrics, and assuring compliance standards are important to real-time institutional and public accountability, but that these duties pale in comparison with our larger responsibility to build and sustain an environment in which creative ideas—novel connections with meaningful outcomes—may emerge. (Roberts 2015c, p. 471)

In this chapter I have articulated these ethical principles and a decisional tool (see Figure 19–1) to help analyze whether innovation is ethically defensible, and I have provided examples to illustrate nuances that arise in psychiatric innovation. For good to come from change and creativity, the work itself must be grounded in principles that have sustained discovery, whether in clinical innovation or in human research, in our society.

CASE SCENARIOS

- ■ A 16-year-old student-athlete with attention difficulties and post-concussive syndrome asks his psychiatrist if they can begin texting daily rather than meeting for individual therapy sessions every week.

- ■ A psychiatrist who cares for very difficult patients with personality disorders finds that she has had many Internet postings criticizing her clinical care practices. She attempts to have the postings removed, but the sites will only do so if she pays (significant) fees.

- ■ A 46-year-old mother of two grown children whose own mother died of early-onset Alzheimer's requests genetic testing for the disease. When discussing the possibility of a positive test with the counselor, she states that she would kill herself before becoming seriously "demented."

- A person with obsessive-compulsive disorder seeks treatment for his condition, requesting deep brain stimulation. He is young, has severe disease, is decisionally capable, and states, "I don't want to go through years of failed treatment. I want this fixed and in my control."

- A 27-year-old computer engineer is offered a job with a high-security technology firm. He briefly received treatment for depression as a graduate student and had a grandmother who committed suicide. When the company physician reviews his mental health history, the previous offer of employment is withdrawn.

20

Clinical Training

Laura Weiss Roberts, M.D., M.A.

Physicians-in-training, both medical students and residents, face unique ethical challenges as they acquire the knowledge and skills that will allow them to care competently and compassionately for human beings who may be suffering under the heavy burdens of life. Each stage of training represents different ethical tasks and dilemmas, which, if successfully mastered, lead to the attainment of a higher level of ethical sensitivity and professional responsibility. It is essential that supervisors and educators be attuned and attentive to these developmental stages of ethical growth so that they may intentionally create opportunities to foster self-awareness, habits of self-care, and humanistic and empathic patient–physician relationships. This awareness is indeed necessary if clinical education is to be more than on-the-job training at best and exhausting, traumatic, and cynicism-engendering labor at worst. In psychiatric training, appropriate didactic and experiential teaching, mentoring, and support can assist in preserving the moral foundation of the profession of psychiatry and in building optimal ethical knowledge, skills, and attitudes of these physicians who dedicate their careers to the care of individuals with mental illness.

Education leaders increasingly are making explicit their commitment to the moral foundation of clinical medicine. The Association of American Medical Colleges in 1998 developed a formal set of recommendations regarding the learning objectives for medical student education centered on the following premises: 1) physicians must be altruistic, 2) physicians must be knowledgeable, 3) physicians must be skillful, and 4) physicians must be dutiful. The American Psychiatric Association has recommended that ethics training for psychiatry residents encompass several key content, skill, and attitude domains (Table 20–1). The Accreditation Council for Graduate Medical Education (2011) continues to implement clearer and more rigorous standards for residency programs regarding the evaluation of resident competency, including the related areas of ethics, professionalism, and communication skills.

SPECIAL ETHICAL CHALLENGES

Clinical trainees inhabit three ethically important roles: as students, as trainees within the profession of medicine, and as early-career clinicians-in-training within a specialty area. These roles have much in common in terms of their goals and ethical imperatives. For example, they all value truth telling, promise keeping, and honest dealings with others. They all value respect, effort, and diligence. The three roles are nevertheless distinct, and their differences may create conflicts from time to time for clinicians-in-training. For instance, the student's responsibility is to learn, whereas the clinician's responsibility is to provide an optimal—or at least appropriate—standard of care to patients. When the student is learning to be a clinical professional, it is inevitable that mistakes, or the potential for mistakes, will occur. People with mental illness may be vulnerable and unable to advocate for themselves in clinical situations in which mistakes take place. These considerations are very important, especially in the context of caring for individuals with diminished interpersonal power (e.g., institutionalized persons; ill children or elderly persons; adults with serious mental illness; individuals with diminished societal power and roles, such as undocumented immigrants who have mental illness). In essence, the roles of early-career professionals learning to care for people with mental illness carry ethical imperatives and tensions, some of which are unique to the developmental situation of training and many of which will accompany trainees throughout their professional lives.

Clinical training thus presents predictable and developmentally necessary ethical challenges. Here I will highlight four.

1. Clinical trainees carry enormous patient care responsibilities during a period in which they are not yet fully clinically competent. On inpatient rotations, medical students and residents perform psychiatric evaluations and physical examinations for large numbers of patients. In emergency

TABLE 20–1. Model curriculum for psychiatric training recommended by the American Psychiatric Association

Knowledge

Existence of overlaps and differences between legal and ethical issues and how to access relevant laws

Importance and history of ethical codes to the profession of medicine and how the principles continue to apply to evolving situations

Basic philosophical principles, such as paternalism, autonomy, beneficence, nonmaleficence, and justice, which can be used to analyze ethical conflicts

The content of *The Principles of Medical Ethics With Annotations Especially Applicable to Psychiatry* and the practical meaning and application of each section

    Competent and respectful treatment

    Honest dealing and disclosure

    Respect for the law

    Respect for confidences and colleagues

    Commitment to study and obtain consultation

    Practice environment and terminating treatment

    Improving the community and relationships with government

Skills

Provide competent psychiatry evaluation and treatment

Avoid boundary violations with patients and colleagues

Avoid sexual exploitation of patients and colleagues

Preserve patient confidentiality

Evaluate and manage suicidal patients

Evaluate and manage homicidal patients

Obtain and use proxy decisions from patients

Institute involuntary commitment

Manage patient treatment refusal

Relate professionally and ethically with colleagues, faculty, and supervisors

Recognize and resolve competing ethical interests

Recognize legal obligations

Recognize the limits of one's own abilities and seek consultation when necessary

Recognize and intervene with impaired or unethical colleagues

---

TABLE 20–1. Model curriculum for psychiatric training recommended by the American Psychiatric Association *(continued)*

Skills *(continued)*

Apply ethical principles to consultation for medical colleagues or the courts

Admit and discharge patients

Participate in utilization review and peer review

Bill for psychiatric services

Attitudes

Compassion and honest dealing with patients and colleagues

Respect for human dignity

Respect for the law

Respect for the rights and confidences of patients, colleagues, and other health professionals

Commitment to providing competent medical service to patients

Commitment to one's own continued professional development

Commitment to improving the profession and the community

Source.   Reprinted from Roberts LW, Dyer AR: *Concise Guide to Ethics in Mental Health Care.* Washington, DC, American Psychiatric Publishing, 2004, pp. 244–245. Copyright © 2004 American Psychiatric Publishing. Used with permission.

departments, interns and residents are often the ones making decisions about a number of challenging dilemmas—for example, whether an intoxicated patient who is threatening suicide but refuses hospitalization is allowed to leave the facility, how grave "grave passive neglect" needs to be for a person with psychosis and poor self-care to be admitted involuntarily to a psychiatric unit, whether an elderly patient with early dementia needs a treatment guardian to make medication decisions, and whether a report should be filed with child protective services when an adolescent offhandedly mentions that his mom is "on drugs" and "never around." In some settings, the clinical trainee may be the only person with any advanced mental health training to actually see the patient. Although the trainee receives supervision from an attending physician or a more senior team member on such cases, these decisions often ride solely on the trainee's history taking, mental status examination, and assessment, as well as on his or her hunches, which may or may not be well attuned to the complexities of the patient's clinical presentation.

2. Clinical education inherently involves an ethical conflict. Being in training means learning on actual people, which is not a comfortable thought for individuals who are sensitive to the ethical meaning of the training experience. In surgery or medicine, this necessary learning process may mean performing procedures on ill individuals without much preparation ("see one, do one, teach one"). There must always be a first time for a physician-student to set a fractured bone, gather an arterial blood sample, suture a wound, or detect (or not) a serious pathological murmur. In psychiatric training, a fledgling clinician can potentially make any of dozens of judgment errors, big or small and involving omission or commission. Errors may occur as a trainee learns psychotherapy skills by conducting psychotherapy with a patient who is depressed or traumatized, or as a resident learns appropriate medication dosing by treating a frail elderly patient who has mental illness. Trainees who are not yet prepared for the complicated, nuanced clinical and ethical aspects of decisional capacity assessments are nonetheless confronted with the necessity to perform such assessments from the first week of residency, when they may be required to appear in court for a patient's involuntary commitment hearing. Often, the greater risk of error is balanced by the extra thoroughness and care that trainees give to their patients and to their work, but the consequences of errors can be serious, ranging from medication side effects to unanticipated suicide attempts.

3. Clinical trainees often must do things that they find alien, uncomfortable, or culturally "wrong" in caring for people with mental illness. The range of possibilities is broad—from asking a patient about the intimate details of her sexual history and behaviors to taking away a patient's personal liberty by involuntarily committing him to psychiatric treatment, from turning away a patient with mental health needs because of lack of insurance to caring for a patient who exhibits beliefs and violent behaviors that are disquieting, from giving a medication because it is on the formulary to withholding valuable treatment because of legal imperatives. The frequency with which such hard situations are encountered is a difficult aspect of the newly acquired clinical role. Interestingly, learning to provide mental health care means paying attention to one's inner sense of things. When an individual is learning to become a psychiatrist or other mental health professional, his or her principal instrument is the self. The clinical trainee is thus encouraged to shut off certain insights while attending to others. For these reasons, the educational experience involves moments that feel, at best, uneasy and confusing and, at worst, coercive and painful.

4. Another ethical challenge in preparing trainees to care for people with mental illness pertains to stress and self-care during the training process (Feeley and Ross 2015; Williams et al. 2015; Zuardi et al. 2011). More than other clinical specialty areas, the mental health professions clearly recognize the importance of clinicians themselves being psychologically sound and emotionally resilient and engaging in appropriate self-care as necessary to be able to provide mental health care to others. The irony, of course, is that the training process is exhausting and demanding, leaving little time or energy for the clinical trainee to pursue healthy and emotionally sustaining activities. The combination of heavy workload, sleep deprivation, and academic, clinical, and personal obligations can render even the most psychologically healthy resident vulnerable to stress.

In psychiatry, as in psychology but not in many of the disciplines of medicine, trainees are involved in supervision that touches on personal issues and they are often engaged in personal psychotherapy. In a recent study (Kovach et al. 2015), of the 133 psychiatry residents who participated in an e-mail-based anonymous study (40% response rate), one-quarter indicated that they were in psychotherapy themselves. Most were seen weekly in psychodynamically oriented treatment, not associated with their academic program. Nearly half identified personal stress, substance-related issues, or mood and anxiety issues, and overall those in treatment saw this experience as highly important to their development as psychiatrists.

As described in some detail in Chapter 17, "Clinician Well-Being and Impairment," trainees are at significant risk for mental health, addiction, and some physical health issues by virtue of the rigors of their educational preparation. Simply witnessing the suffering of people with mental illness generates pain within a mental health trainee; beyond this fact of professional work, some programs within mental health care are experienced as unkind or overtly abusive toward their trainees. Even in the most humane programs, faculty supervisors may become stressed and overwhelmed, providing poor role models for their early-career colleagues. The message of training is thus an ambiguous, conflicted one, conveying superhuman, or perhaps inhuman, expectations. From an ethical perspective, these conditions are critically important, because, as described in Chapter 1, "Ethics Principles and Professionalism," being self-reflective and nondefensive is essential to the process of sound ethical decision making. Furthermore, decades of conceptual and empirical work suggest that the clinical training process too often inculcates cynicism and diminishment of the self rather than imparting ideals of the profession and affirming the self in preparing trainees to help alleviate the suffering of others.

EMPIRICAL STUDIES

Many empirical studies have been performed on ethics and ethics instruction in clinical education (Jain et al. 2010, 2011a, 2011b; Lapid et al. 2009; Marrero et al. 2013). A uniform finding has been that clinical trainees have a strong interest in patient care ethics and the desire for more substantive preparation for the ethical aspects of clinical care responsibilities. For example, in an early postgraduate education study, Jacobson et al. (1989) surveyed 202 internal medicine residents at three training programs and found that a majority wanted more training on ethics-related topics. In an analogous study, Roberts et al. (1996) surveyed 181 psychiatry residents in 10 training programs in the United States. Seventy-six percent reported that they had encountered an ethical dilemma for which they felt unprepared, and 92% reported that ethics training had been useful in helping them respond to ethical dilemmas arising with patients. One-third reported receiving no ethics preparation during medical school, and 46% reported receiving none in residency. A majority of the residents expressed the belief that more curricular attention should be given to many ethics-related topics and topics related to legal and financial issues in patient care. Coverdale et al. (1992) found similar results in their study of 121 psychiatry chief residents and program directors, which revealed that although 40% of the programs had no formal ethics curriculum, the trainees expressed enthusiasm for additional ethics teaching.

Some colleagues and I performed a more recent ethics education study with 336 medical students and residents at the University of New Mexico (Roberts et al. 2004). The participants strongly endorsed the importance of professionalism among physicians, the prevalence of ethical conflicts in everyday practice, and the perception that ethics training is helpful in resolving ethical conflicts. They also identified the goals of ethics preparation as improving patient care and clinical decision making, gaining a better recognition of ethics issues, developing interpersonal skills useful in resolving ethics conflicts, learning strategies for clarifying values-laden choices, and acquiring a working knowledge of social science, philosophy, religion, and the law as they apply to clinical care. Similar to findings of other studies, clinically oriented learning approaches overall were perceived as far superior to more isolated or less relevant approaches, and formal assessment of ethics skills was seen as acceptable and appropriate.

All of these studies have revealed the beneficial impact of positive role models and direct involvement of clinicians in patient care and the importance of teaching methods that are integrated into clinical and supervisory routines of training. Empirical and observation-based literature also suggests that there is a strong commitment by learners and teachers regarding topics related to ethics such as, for example, instilling empathy and compassion (Aggarwal and Guanci 2014; Roberts et al. 2011b). The literature also suggests differential interest and commitment to ethics education by students of different backgrounds and attributes. Female trainees have consistently shown greater interest and more diverse learning preferences than their male counterparts, and interest in specific topics appears to be driven largely by the unique demands and nature of clinical specialty areas.

In a best-evidence medicine review, Birden et al. (2013) conducted a rigorous search to identify 3,522 references on medical professionalism in multiple electronic databases. This large number of papers was carefully whittled down to 218 published manuscripts on teaching professionalism, including 17 qualitative and 6 quantitative studies with best-quality evidence, and 3 qualitative and 4 quantitative studies with second-tier evidence. They also identified viewpoint pieces, case reports, systematic reviews, and books, and of these, the most publications were second-tier evidence viewpoint pieces ($n=95$), conveying perspectives on the topic.

From this comprehensive review, Birden et al. (2013) noted, "There is still no unifying theoretical or practical model to use as a format to integrate the teaching of professionalism in the medical curriculum that has gained wide acceptance" (p. e1263). This statement affirmed the claim made in a commentary by Bloch and Green (2009, p. 89):

> Based on time allocated and the nature of programs offered in the four countries [Australia, Canada, United Kingdom, United States]…we can summarize our own assessment of teaching developments in four main points:
>
> 1. Educational initiatives have been episodic, precluding sustained progress.
> 2. Only a small number of teaching programs stand out as potential models.
> 3. Psychiatric training bodies have generated only embryonic programs.
> 4. Reporting on specific teaching projects has been scanty and limited in its impact.

Birden et al. (2013), on the basis of their systematic review, suggested that role modeling and mentoring are crucial approaches in imparting professionalism, as reflected in the highest-quality teaching programs. Efforts to integrate professionalism education in clinical settings are perhaps the best received and may have special importance. The institutional milieu, which harbors both the formal and the informal, or "hidden," curriculum, greatly influences professionalism education as it is currently practiced and experienced.

The failure of the educational system to provide sufficient ethics training and the overall problem of lack of a coherent curricular approach to this area are nevertheless worrisome in light of empirical evidence suggesting that clinical education has a detrimental effect on the humanistic values, attitudes, and behaviors of clinical trainees. Recent literature has further highlighted an association between emotional exhaustion and breaches in ethics and professionalism in medical training (Dyrbye et al. 2010a, 2012). Much more encouraging is the early body of literature documenting the positive impact of ethics-related educational interventions in clinical training. Clinically relevant educational activities appear to improve the sensitivity and competence exhibited and the confidence felt by trainees as they respond to ethical problems (Baldwin et al. 1998; Bebeau and Thoma 1994; Bellini et al. 2002; Carter and Roberts 1997; Ende et al. 1986; Feudtner et al. 1994; Firth-Cozens 1987; Gann et al. 1991; Green et al. 1995; Hughes et al. 1991; Junek et al. 1979; Lo and Schroeder 1981; Scheidt et al. 1986; Self et al. 1998; Siegler et al. 1982; Sulmasy et al. 1990, 1994).

A number of resources for ethics and professionalism education in psychiatry have been developed and published (Gabbard et al. 2012; Roberts and Hoop 2008; Roberts and Reicherter 2015; Schwartz et al. 2009), and their lessons echo and embellish beyond these mixed observations and conclusions. The American Psychiatric Association specifically recommends topics to be covered in resident ethics curricula (see Table 20–1). Topics of emerging interest in psychiatric ethics for trainees relate to empathy and patient-centered care, conflict of interest and relationships with the pharmaceutical industry, professional boundaries in the era of the Internet, lapses in professionalism, and health systems–related and equity issues. Table 20–2 outlines other recommendations for ethics teaching in clinical training.

Still, the question of the goal of ethics training begs broad engagement and resolution. Bloch and Green (2009) have persuasively outlined the goal of ethics education for psychiatry residents as achieving three key outcomes:

1. The trainee should be able to appreciate "the relevance of ethical aspects of clinical practice" (p. 90) and to give them equal weight with scientific aspects of the case.
2. The trainee should be able to identify ethical issues accurately and in context.
3. Ethics training should assure that the trainee has attained the skills needed to handle the ethical issues encountered.

Table 20–3 lists goals and objectives of ethics training. Table 20–4 outlines strategies for teaching ethics and achieving these goals through psychiatric supervision.

TABLE 20–2. Recommendations for clinical ethics teaching in clinical training

Design curricula that address clinically relevant issues in mental health ethics, including confidentiality, informed consent, decisional capacity, and commitment.

Develop special events that highlight the importance and value of ethics (e.g., grand rounds, invited visiting professors, evidence-based ethics research presentations).

Create diverse contexts for learning and self-reflection and draw out the ethical meaning within routine clinical situations.

Find ways to provide additional educational opportunities for trainees who have a greater interest in ethics topics and skills.

Respectfully and sensitively guide trainees in identifying their responses and defenses to clinical ethical issues.

Provide access to ethics resources and encourage the engagement of colleagues, supervisors, and expert consultants in addressing ethically complex situations.

Encourage faculty mentors with an interest in ethics to obtain formal training and provide time and resources to support ethics teaching for trainees.

Include ethics knowledge, skill, and professional attitudes in the formal evaluation of trainees.

Help trainees as they deal constructively with their limitations and errors; without losing sight of clinical competence standards, work with trainees to perceive mistakes and bad-outcome situations as unfortunate but as offering formative lessons.

Seek opportunities for trainees to discuss the stresses of training and their impact on patient care activities, including ethically important decision making.

Source.   Adapted from Roberts LW, Dyer AR: *Concise Guide to Ethics in Mental Health Care.* Washington, DC, American Psychiatric Publishing, 2004, p. 254. Copyright © 2004 American Psychiatric Publishing. Used with permission.

CONCLUSION

Effective preparation for the ethical and professional aspects of caring for individuals with mental illness will have several characteristics: It should be developmentally attuned and ecologically sound, naturally evolving from the structure and realities of psychiatric training. It should not be treated as an add-on topic. Experience in ethics teaching and empirical evidence suggest the important contribution of role models, consultants, and innovative and integrated methods. Finally, ethics education in clinical training should be explicitly evaluated, not only in the sense of how well the trainees enjoyed the curriculum but also in regard to how well it imparted clinically important ethics skills.

TABLE 20–3. Goals and objectives for ethics education

Early in clinical training, achieve the ability to:

- Define and use ethics terms accurately.
- Identify values-laden aspects and ethical considerations present in a clinical care situation.
- Apply ethics principles to understand and select among different ethically sound approaches to clinical care situations.
- Perform literature searches on ethics topics related to issues present in clinical care situations.
- Recognize the limits of one's knowledge and role in a clinical care situation.
- Use clinical information, ethics guidelines, and empirical evidence to clarify ethical questions.
- Observe and characterize a clinical interaction and then identify how factors in the interaction may affect the ethical dimensions of the patient's care.
- Describe and reflect upon one's professional training experiences within the context of professional attitudes, values, and ethics.

Later in clinical training, demonstrate mastery of the above, plus ability to:

- Assess more sophisticated, complex clinical care situations in light of clinical, ethical, psychosocial, and legal issues.
- Identify, assess, and anticipate sequelae for different approaches to more sophisticated, complex clinical care situations in light of clinical, ethical, psychosocial, and legal issues.
- Demonstrate appropriate self-directed learning and growth in ethics and professionalism.
- Apply formal ethical decision-making models to ethically complex situations.

In preparation for the transition to independent clinical practice, demonstrate mastery of the above, plus ability to:

- Identify and respond to subtle clinical, ethical, psychosocial, and legal issues present in a clinical care situation.
- Perform key ethically important clinical tasks (e.g., obtaining informed consent or refusal for care, safeguarding confidentiality, addressing stigmatizing health issues) in a manner that reflects sensitivity, demonstrates awareness of ethical complexities present in the situation, and fulfills accepted standards of care.

TABLE 20–3. Goals and objectives for ethics education *(continued)*

- Identify a course of action that employs advanced clinical ethics problem–resolution techniques (e.g., recognizing the limits of one's knowledge, pursuing additional data gathering, seeking collaboration and consultation with individuals with cross-disciplinary expertise, such as law or medical subspecialties).

- Reflect upon one's professional training experiences, to characterize how one's value system may influence one's clinical practices, and to safeguard against one's personal biases.

Source. Adapted from Roberts LW, Dyer AR: *Concise Guide to Ethics in Mental Health Care.* Washington, DC, American Psychiatric Publishing, 2004, pp. 255–256. Copyright © 2004 American Psychiatric Publishing. Used with permission.

TABLE 20–4. Strategies for implementing ethics in clinical supervision

Help the resident define the clinical aspects of the patient's case.

Guide the resident to identify ethical issues and conflicts in the clinical situation, while giving the resident an opportunity to describe personal thoughts and concerns relating to the case.

Collaborate with the resident in gathering information and necessary clinical and ethical expertise.

Explore possible responses to the clinical and ethical problems with the resident, deciding what acceptable choices exist and anticipating the outcomes of these possible decisions.

Provide guidance and support as the resident implements the decision.

Create a context for reflection and review.

Source. Adapted from Roberts LW, Dyer AR: *Concise Guide to Ethics in Mental Health Care.* Washington, DC, American Psychiatric Publishing, 2004, p. 256. Copyright © 2004 American Psychiatric Publishing. Used with permission.

CASE SCENARIOS

- ■ The medical director of a community health center tells a second-year resident that a patient she evaluated in the emergency department 8 months ago has committed suicide.

- ■ A first-year resident becomes upset during inpatient rounds when she is chastised by teammates for admitting a patient the night before and immediately "being manipulated into" giving the patient the privilege of visiting his home. The patient was diagnosed with a personality disorder.

- A third-year resident with anorexia nervosa seeks psychiatric care for a relapse precipitated by the stresses of training. She learns that the only eating disorder specialist is her residency program director.

- A patient asks a resident to write a prescription for a medication at twice the recommended dose, so that he will be able to stretch the pills over a longer period of time and pay less money out of pocket at the pharmacy.

- A resident at an intake clinic is encouraged to record a different diagnosis on the billing sheet so insurance will pay more.

21

Population Health and Evolving Systems of Care

Laura Weiss Roberts, M.D., M.A.

Systems of health care in the United States are rapidly evolving, and perceptions of what constitutes ethically sound care within these systems are changing as well. Beyond ethics principles governing the care of individual patients, there is a newer emphasis on principles of ethics that relate to resource distribution and social justice issues across patient populations. Meeting the needs of individual patients while wisely shepherding scarce resources has been identified as a component of the profession of medicine's "social contract" (ABIM Foundation et al. 2002; McCurdy et al. 1997).

Balancing the health care needs of populations with the health care needs of individuals, however, has created often unforeseen ethical binds for clinicians, including psychiatrists, in both the private and the public sectors. Managed care organizations in particular have been identified as disrupting the clinician–patient relationship, which traditionally has been based on the patient's ability to choose a clinician by considering clinician competence, communication and compassion in the clinical relationship, continuity of care, and the absence of conflicts of interest (Hall 1997). Initiatives such as the medical home, the ambulatory intensive care unit, and a range of patient-centered managed care programs for chronically ill individuals have attempted to bring a therapeutic team-based care model, often with great success and high levels of patient satisfaction. Nevertheless, these programs are underdeveloped with respect to mental health and addiction treatment and service to people with mental illness and co-occurring disorders.

As resource priorities have been made within society and within new systems of care, stigma and poor recognition of the importance of mental illness have sometimes in the past acted together to diminish resources for people with psychiatric and comorbid disease. With the introduction of the Affordable Care Act in 2010, admissions to psychiatric inpatient units have increased (Golberstein et al. 2015), with accompanying bed shortages and longer stays in emergency departments. Ironically, although many more individuals have insurance in the United States in 2015 than in 2013, about 16% of people in the United States remain uninsured as a consequence of improved employment rates and the coverage associated with the Affordable Care Act (Carman et al. 2015). Individuals with mental health needs continue to have little access to services, particularly individuals who have few financial resources, derive from underrepresented minority backgrounds, and live in rural areas.

The lack of adequate resources for mental health services is a topic that has been elevated in the national dialogue on health care reform. The tragic suicide death of the son of Virginia legislator Creigh Deeds in 2009 serves as one example in which media attention helped bring greater awareness to the disparities in care given to people in mental health crises in comparison with physical health crises. The media have also highlighted the fact that the criminal justice system has become a new, and disheartening, mental health system in the United States (Steinberg et al. 2015).

People living with mental disorders have always posed special challenges in the provision of clinical services and continue to encounter heightened obstacles to adequate treatment in these new systems of care. With greater understanding of the prevalence of mental illness, the role of behavioral issues in physical disorders, and the impact of addictions on all aspects of health, there is an increased interest in developing integrated health services to help foster the goals of population health. The interest is particularly keen in helping to improve health outcomes in chronically ill adults who are high utilizers of health care services (Melek et al. 2014) and in children, who have a lifetime of health—or chronic disease—ahead of them (Boat 2015). In this chapter, I define specific ethical principles and values that should guide the development of mental health service systems, outline ethically important features of mental health services, and discuss strategies for addressing ethical conflicts in evolving systems of care.

ETHICAL PRINCIPLES IN EVOLVING SYSTEMS OF CARE

A number of critically important ethical principles should guide the development and implementation of mental health services (Table 21–1). *Respect for persons* is the principle that ensures that the dignity and the basic rights of individual patients will be recognized and upheld in interactions and procedures within a system of care. Closely related to this concept is the notion of *autonomy*—supporting the ability of the individual patient to make informed, independent decisions regarding his or her physical body and emotional self. The professional duty to respect the individual's right to self-governance does not mean that clinicians must provide everything that patients desire or request. Nevertheless, in some health care settings, the concept of patient autonomy in mental health care is moot because there is no access to mental health services. Moreover, in other settings where services do exist, some patients may receive marked pressure to accept certain kinds of treatments that are convenient or less expensive (e.g., medication) rather than treatments that are more in keeping with the patient's beliefs and values (e.g., psychotherapy or combined psychosocial and biological interventions).

Integrity refers to the consistent fulfillment by the clinician, both in word and in behavior, of the ideals of the profession of medicine, as discussed in several ways throughout this book. In practice, integrity means, for example, that the patient's well-being and best interests should be the clinician's primary concern (i.e., *beneficence*). Moreover, with rare exceptions, as noted in the section "Resolving Conflicts Between the Needs of Individuals and Populations" later in this chapter, the system should support the clinician's ability to help each patient according to current standards of care, faithfully seeking to ameliorate and alleviate suffering and to provide curative treatments wherever possible (i.e., *fidelity*). Financial conflicts of interest, such as economic incentives to clinicians for providing minimal services and substandard treatment, represent significant threats to the integrity and fidelity of clinicians. Such incentives have been highly contested and criticized, yet they persist in many systems in which physicians are employed. Clinicians should be very wary of managed care organizations that proffer contracts that contain provisions specifying, for example, that the reimbursement plan is contingent on withholding care (e.g., limiting tests ordered or numbers or kinds of prescriptions written). Furthermore, clinicians should consider potential implicit threats to fidelity, such as extreme, sustained productivity requirements that indirectly affect their ability to provide quality care to existing patients.

TABLE 21–1. Ethical principles in systems of care

Ethical principle	Application to systems of care
Respect for persons: Ensures that the dignity and rights of the individual are recognized and upheld	In its interactions and procedures, the system should recognize the dignity and uphold the rights of the patient.
Autonomy: Supports the ability of the individual to make informed, independent decisions about his or her body and self	The system should sufficiently support patient autonomy so that patients are not pressured to accept treatments contrary to their values because of expense or expedience. This does not mean that clinicians must provide what patients desire or request.
Integrity: Consistent adherence to the ideals of the medical profession	The system should support the principle that the patient's best interests are the clinician's primary goal.
Beneficence: The patient's well-being is the physician's central concern	The system should support the clinician's ability to • Adhere to high standards of care. • Alleviate suffering. • Provide cure where possible.
Fidelity: Faithfulness to the ideals of medicine and the good of the patient	Clinicians need to be wary of conflicts of interest, such as where the system proffers • Economic incentives to provide minimal services or substandard treatment. • Contracts specifying that reimbursement is contingent upon withholding of care.
Veracity: Truthfulness in the physician–patient relationship	Clinicians need to be wary of system contracts that threaten honesty (e.g., nondisclosure clauses that require physicians not to inform patients of superior treatment available outside the system).

Population Health and Evolving Systems of Care

TABLE 21–1. Ethical principles in systems of care (*continued*)

Ethical principle	Application to systems of care
Confidentiality: The positive duty to protect personal information in the absence of patient consent or legal exceptions	The issues are highly complex and overlapping in managed care systems, and employers or insurers may be informed of personal health information.
Fairness: The ideal of social justice in which goods, harms, and burdens are equitably distributed	The enormous income of for-profit systems may be obtained at the cost of providing substandard care, especially to ill individuals without alternatives.

Source. Adapted from Roberts LW, Dyer AR: *Concise Guide to Ethics in Mental Health Care.* Washington, DC, American Psychiatric Publishing, 2004, pp. 221–222. Copyright © 2004 American Psychiatric Publishing. Used with permission.

Veracity, or truthfulness, is a fundamental value within medicine, and it also can be threatened by practices within some systems of care. For instance, contracts that include nondisclosure clauses requiring that clinicians not inform patients of standard or superior treatments that are available outside of their system violate the professional duty to deal with patients honestly.

Confidentiality has been a significant ethical challenge in evolving systems of care that rely on team-based care, integrated care settings, and the electronic medical record. Patients often may not be aware of the providers involved in their treatment behind the scenes and may not be informed of the extent to which their health care documentation is shared, or can be breached, when the electronic record is accessed.

Fairness in resource allocation is the ethics principle that poses the greatest challenge in many of the newly emerging health care systems. Fairness derives from the ideal of social justice, which states that benefits and burdens of society should be shared by individuals within different segments of society in an equitable manner. Systems of health care are often assessed in relation to fairness. For example, universal health insurance is one policy initiative that has been advanced on the basis of a social justice rationale. The very striking financial gains attained by some for-profit managed care systems that provide substandard clinical care have been criticized on the grounds that they are fundamentally unfair to those ill individuals within their systems who may not have other viable alternatives for care.

Although it is apparent that current systems of care and resource distribution in the United States are not fair, it is unclear how health disparities can be fully addressed. The Affordable Care Act sought, among other goals, to decrease the number of uninsured individuals in the United States by expanding public and private coverage options, and by ensuring "universal insurability" of individuals regardless of preexisting health conditions (Hall and Lord 2014). It does not, however, achieve true universal or equitable coverage of all individuals, so equitable access to care and quality of care continue to remain subjects of wide debate. Current pressures on providers, hospitals, and insurers to provide high-quality care while increasing access and cutting costs are immense. Fortunately, this necessity has spurred some interesting new developments in care delivery and reimbursement, such as team-based medical care and value-based (rather than volume-based) payment programs (Hall and Lord 2014). Further studies are needed on the clinical effectiveness of these developments. Regardless of practice setting, all physicians have a stake in the natural evolution of health care systems within their national boundaries, and certainly within the United States, significant growth pains at the systems level are likely to permeate individual patient care interactions. In this context, it becomes all the more pertinent to realize that achieving greater fairness and broadly improved health care outcomes are vital goals of any ethically acceptable system of health care, as well as of all clinicians practicing within that system.

EVOLVING SYSTEMS OF CARE FOR MENTAL ILLNESS

To be clinically effective and ethically sound, health services optimally will be adapted to address the specific nature and core attributes of the health issues of the people served. Ideally, mental health services will be structured to respond to the high prevalence of mental disorders and the frequency of comorbidity with medical and substance-related disorders.

Using data summarized from several sources, the Centers for Disease Control and Prevention (2013) describes the burden of mental illness across various categories. For example, depression is the leading cause of disability in middle- and high-income countries but the eighth-place cause in low-income countries. Worldwide prevalence of schizophrenia ranges between 0.5% and 1%. In the United States, frequent mental distress affects 9.4% of adults. In addition, anxiety disorders are common in the United States, with an estimated lifetime prevalence of any anxiety disorder over 15%. Also in the United States, nearly 7% of adults reported experiencing an episode of major depression in the prior year, with women more commonly affected, and 4% of U.S. adults had bipolar disorder, with men and women equally affected. Alzheimer's disease now affects more than 5 million individuals in the United States, and it has become the fifth-leading cause of death for adults age 65 and older and the sixth-leading cause of death overall (Tejada-Vera 2013). By 2050, more than 10 million U.S. adults will have Alzheimer's disease, by current estimates.

Almost 50% of adult Americans will suffer from a significant mental disorder at one time or another in their lives (Centers for Disease Control and Prevention 2011) and a large proportion of people with mental illness are homeless (Nieto et al. 2008). As noted in Chapter 14, "People Living With Addictions," addiction to tobacco, alcohol, and illicit drugs produces untold suffering and more than $700 billion in direct and indirect costs in the United States each year (National Institute on Drug Abuse 2015). These conditions greatly affect physical health as well as mental health.

Symptoms of mental illness are highly prominent in general clinic settings, as was shown in early studies by Regier et al. (1993), Spitzer et al.

(1995), Johnson et al. (1995), and Olfson et al. (1997), which found that between 30% and 45% of primary care patients had diagnosable mental disorders. More than 50% of patients with any mental illness are treated exclusively within a primary care setting (Kamerow 1986). Interestingly, as mental health treatment access has decreased, costs have shifted to the medical health care side of many systems of care. Tanielian et al. (1997), for instance, found that the number of general hospital discharges with a documented primary mental disorder rose from 1.41 million in 1988 to 1.67 million in 1993; this increase of 18.3% is dramatically higher than the 0.1% rise of discharges with a primary diagnosis of a general medical disorder during the same time period. According to a recent study commissioned by the American Psychiatric Association (Melek et al. 2014), an estimated $26–$48 billion could be saved each year in the United States by integrating physical and mental health services.

Beyond simply recognizing the burden of need for mental health care, evolving systems ideally will be responsive to the psychosocial and societal impact of mental illness. It is well documented that individuals with mental illness have diminished overall quality of life and, by definition, some compromise in interpersonal and social roles. Moreover, the symptoms of some mental illnesses, such as amotivation, apathy, mistrust, impaired insight, and poor relatedness, may serve as barriers to pursuit of care. This problem of symptoms interfering with care-seeking is especially salient in systems in which patients must navigate a series of gatekeeping steps before being seen by a mental health specialist.

In addition to the level of individual suffering, the societal effects of mental illness are substantial. The Global Burden of Disease study by the World Health Organization (WHO; 2008) found that mental illness, including suicide, ranks highly as a cause of disability and premature mortality in economically robust nations. The WHO study discovered that research that examined only deaths vastly underestimated the negative impact of mental illness on quality of life. The WHO therefore used a method of comparing disease burden known as disability-adjusted life years (DALYs), which assigns a value to premature death and to severity and length of disability. When DALYs were used, major depression ranked second only to ischemic heart disease in magnitude of disease burden. Schizophrenia, bipolar disorder, obsessive-compulsive disorder, panic disorder, and posttraumatic stress disorder also contributed significantly to the burden represented by mental illness (Murray and Lopez 1996). These disturbing data highlight the immediacy and significance of mental health as a public health problem and strongly argue for increases in the resources allocated for diagnosis and treatment of mental illness.

Ethically sound systems of mental health services will be adapted to the need for scientific study and educational training related to these poorly understood, devastating disorders. Remaining attentive to the imperatives for scientific discovery and creative innovations and to the mission of training the next generation of scientists and physicians is essential. Moreover, the evolution of systems that are committed to continuously enhancing and learning new and beneficial approaches is crucial if gains are to be made in improving patient and population health outcomes. Academic medical centers, which traditionally have provided care for large segments of the chronically ill population in the United States, are struggling to survive. With the financial restructuring of academic departments, research and training programs have been severely and negatively affected, a situation that bodes especially poorly for academic departments of psychiatry and the future care of mentally ill individuals.

One example of an evolving system that has been shaped by these considerations is integrated care—a model in which behavioral health is incorporated into a primary care setting, with a mental health clinician serving in a consultative role to the primary care provider (Runyan et al. 2013). The clinician's goal within this context is to improve patient functioning in collaboration with a medical team, including providing access to mental health treatment for those in need of it. The integrated care model seeks to address the broad mental health burden of a primary care patient population, while also aiming to decrease barriers to mental health care and synergistically improve medical and mental health outcomes for patients. Understandably, this system of practice has already raised several important ethical considerations, including how best to manage informed consent, confidentiality, and conflicting provider roles in a team-based arrangement (Hodgson et al. 2013). Additional ethical discussions and safeguards specific to the integrated care setting are becoming increasingly important (Runyan et al. 2013). As mental health systems evolve to meet population needs, therefore, the ethical practice of individual patient care may need to be reevaluated and protected, as highlighted in the next section.

RESOLVING CONFLICTS BETWEEN THE NEEDS OF INDIVIDUALS AND POPULATIONS

Within the currently evolving systems of care in the United States, legitimate ethical conflicts may arise between the clinical needs of the individual patient and the shared clinical resource needs of a larger set of individuals. In such situations, key principles such as respect for persons, truth telling, fairness, and confidentiality should not be compromised. The physician's commitment is to improve quality of care and access to care, to foster just distribution of finite resources, and to maintain trust by managing conflicts of interest. Additional efforts to enhance the process of clinical care and to clarify the values underlying resource distribution decisions are essential to ethically sound care in these systems.

Some managed care organizations have been criticized for their practices, which interfere with informed consent in such "rationing" situations. For example, the quality of communication and information exchange between clinician and patient may be compromised by time constraints, inaccessibility of a consistent care provider, perceived double agency, and, historically, gag rules. On a broader level, ideally there will be a community assent process for any large resource decisions affecting patient care, and alternative avenues for care will be identified and communicated. In light of the potential for ethical conflicts primarily related to resource distribution, Hall (1997) years ago proposed several prerequisites for an optimal health delivery system. These prerequisites aim to prevent and resolve problems that emerge when individuals are competing for resources within the managed system. Hall indicated that the system must be responsive to patients, provide adequate and compassionate care, encourage physician excellence, be accessible, reduce bureaucracy to a minimum, provide humane treatment based on scientific merit, and be accountable to the patient. Many leading thinkers have urged that optimal and ethical systems should place significant emphasis on prevention and early illness interventions, which are relatively cost-effective at the population level and yet greatly benefit individual patients as well as large groups of people (Adelsheim 2014).

An argument can be made for ensuring the high-quality care of the few who have severe mental illness and have consequently been afforded less care by society, even if this may be cost-ineffective; the hope is that cost savings from prevention efforts aimed at other individuals may help offset this burden. Care systems that support scientific inquiry and foster continuous learning are increasingly recognized as important ethically, especially given the negative impact of managed care systems on scientific activities at U.S. academic medical centers.

Sabin (1996) proposed four ethical premises for clinicians serving in mental health care systems, commenting on strategies for resolving resource conflicts:

1. Ethical clinicians should dedicate themselves to caring for their patients in a relationship of fidelity and at the same time act as stewards of society's resources.

2. Ethical clinicians should recommend the least costly treatment alternative unless they have substantial evidence that a more costly intervention is likely to yield a superior outcome.
3. In their stewardship role, ethical clinicians need to advocate for justice in the health care system, just as in their clinical role they need to advocate for the welfare of their patients.
4. Ethical clinicians insist that potentially beneficial interventions should be withheld only on the basis of explicit standards that have been established with the participation of the affected populations and that are acknowledged by the individual patient.

Sabin further suggested that these ethical premises place special responsibilities on clinicians and the public to insist that managed health systems truly improve the effectiveness of care (i.e., improve outcomes in relation to resources spent), echoing the concepts that underlie "learning health care systems." A committee report by the Institute of Medicine (2012) defines a *learning health care system* as one that is effective and constantly improving and innovating to ensure optimal patient care practices and outcomes. Moreover, Sabin stated that clinicians and the public must insist that a genuine informed consent process occur at both national and regional levels, in communities, and with patients. Finally, Sabin argued that clinicians and the public should insist that all people in the United States have access to an adequate standard of health care. Failure to pursue these steps will ultimately lead to unethical conduct by clinicians, because they will have participated in a system of care that is not beneficent, honest, or just. Now, two decades later, this exhortation for the ethical clinician still rings true.

CONCLUSION

In the United States, newly emerging managed systems of health care, including mental health care, are not inherently unethical, but they do pose special ethical problems as the needs of individuals come into conflict with the needs of populations. Indeed, many leaders and stakeholders believe that the prudent shepherding of health care resources congruent with ethical principles such as respect for persons, autonomy, beneficence, and social justice is itself a new moral imperative. Nevertheless, focused attention on practices, policies, and conflict-resolution strategies is essential to ethically sound care for individuals with mental illness within evolving systems of care.

CASE SCENARIOS

- A patient is no longer suicidal but requires several more days to stabilize in the hospital after a mixed bipolar episode. The health maintenance organization refuses to pay for a longer stay. The psychiatrist writes in the notes, "Patient continues to be at high risk of suicide."

- Clinicians at an academic medical center are told that patients with newly diagnosed depression can only be treated with a single medication unless they fail a trial or have severe side effects from the first-line medication on the formulary, because offering alternative medications is too expensive.

- A child psychiatrist must decide whether to send an 8-year-old boy with psychotic symptoms out of state, because there are no beds in his region. The parents cannot afford to accompany the child.

- A partial hospital program is told by the administration that it will be closed if it cannot demonstrate improved outcomes and shortened stays for the dually diagnosed patients in its program.

- An insurance company denies a claim for psychotherapy from a psychiatrist treating a woman for severe social phobia but tells the patient it will pay for six sessions with a social worker.

References

Abide MM, Richards HC, Ramsay SG: Moral reasoning and consistency of belief and behavior: decisions about substance abuse. J Drug Educ 31(4):367–384, 2001 11957392

ABIM Foundation. American Board of Internal Medicine; ACP-ASIM Foundation. American College of Physicians-American Society of Internal Medicine; European Federation of Internal Medicine: Medical professionalism in the new millennium: a physician charter. Ann Intern Med 136(3):243–246, 2002 11827500

Aboujaoude E: Virtually You: The Dangerous Powers of the E-Personality. New York, WW Norton, 2011

Aboujaoude E, Starcevic V: Mental Health in the Digital Age: Grave Dangers, Great Promise. New York, Oxford University Press, 2015

Accreditation Council for Graduate Medical Education: The Common Program Requirements. July 1, 2011. Available at http://www.acgme.org/acgmeweb/Portals/0/PDFs/Common_Program_Requirements_07012011%5B2%5D.pdf. Accessed December 17, 2015.

Accreditation Council for Graduate Medical Education: Program Requirements for Graduate Medical Education in Psychiatry. February 3, 2014. Available at https://www.acgme.org/acgmeweb/portals/0/pfassets/programrequirements/400_psychiatry_07012014.pdf. Accessed December 14, 2015.

Adelsheim S: From school health to integrated health: expanding our children's public mental health system. Acad Psychiatry 38(4):405–408, 2014 24912970

Ad Hoc Committee of the Harvard Medical School to Examine the Definition of Brain Death: A definition of irreversible coma. Report of the Ad Hoc Committee of the Harvard Medical School to Examine the Definition of Brain Death. JAMA 205(6):337–340, 1968 5694976

Advisory Committee on Human Radiation Experiments: The Human Radiation Experiments: Final Report of the Advisory Committee on Human Radiation Experiments. New York, Oxford University Press, 1996

Aggarwal R, Guanci N: Teaching empathy during clerkship and residency. Acad Psychiatry 38(4):506–508, 2014 24687373

Aging with Dignity: Five Wishes Online. Tallahassee, FL, 2011. Available at: https://www.agingwithdignity.org/five-wishes.php. Accessed August 26, 2015

Allen LB, Glicken AD, Beach RK, et al: Adolescent health care experience of gay, lesbian, and bisexual young adults. J Adolesc Health 23(4):212–220, 1998 9763157

Altman LK: Two doctors cited for work developing artificial kidney. The New York Times, September 22, 2002

American Academy of Child and Adolescent Psychiatry: Code of Ethics. Washington, DC, American Academy of Child and Adolescent Psychiatry, 2014

American Foundation for Suicide Prevention: Facts About Physician Depression and Suicide. Available at: http://afsp.org/our-work/education/physician-medical-student-depression-suicide-prevention. Accessed January 4, 2016.

American Medical Association: The sick physician: impairment by psychiatric disorders, including alcoholism and drug dependence. JAMA 223(6): 684–687, 1973 4739202

American Medical Association: Principles of medical ethics. Chicago, IL, American Medical Association, 2001. Available at: http://www.ama-assn.org/ama/pub/physician-resources/medical-ethics/code-medical-ethics/principles-medical-ethics.page. Accessed September 29, 2015.

American Psychiatric Association: Diagnostic and Statistical Manual of Mental Disorders, 4th Edition, Text Revision. Washington, DC, American Psychiatric Association, 2000

American Psychiatric Association: The Internet in Clinical Psychiatry. Arlington, VA, American Psychiatric Association, October 2009. Available at: http://www.psychiatry.org/File%20Library/Psychiatrists/Directories/Library-and-Archive/resource_documents/rd2009_Internet.pdf. Accessed January 6, 2016.

American Psychiatric Association: Diagnostic and Statistical Manual of Mental Disorders, 5th Edition. Arlington, VA, American Psychiatric Association, 2013a

American Psychiatric Association: The Principles of Medical Ethics With Annotations Especially Applicable to Psychiatry, 2013 Edition. Arlington, VA, American Psychiatric Association, 2013b. Available at: http://www.psychiatry.org/psychiatrists/practice/ethics. Accessed September 27, 2015.

American Psychiatric Association: Opinions of the Ethics Committee on The Principles of Medical Ethics With Annotations Especially Applicable to Psychiatry, 2016 edition. Arlington, VA, American Psychiatric Association, 2016. Available at: http://www.psychiatry.org/File%20Library/Psychiatrists/Practice/Ethics/Opinions-of-the-Ethics-Committee.pdf. Accessed January 6, 2016.

Anfang SA, Appelbaum PS: Twenty years after Tarasoff: reviewing the duty to protect. Harv Rev Psychiatry 4(2):67–76, 1996 9384976

Annie E. Casey Foundation: Kids Count Data Book. Baltimore, MD, Annie E. Casey Foundation, 2000

Appelbaum PS, Grisso T: Assessing patients' capacities to consent to treatment. N Engl J Med 319(25):1635–1638, 1988 3200278

Appelbaum PS, Grisso T: The MacArthur Treatment Competence Study I. Law Hum Behav 19:105–174, 1995 11660290

Appelbaum PS, Gutheil TG: Drug refusal: a study of psychiatric inpatients. Am J Psychiatry 137(3):340–346, 1980 7356063

Appelbaum PS, Roth LH, Lidz C: The therapeutic misconception: informed consent in psychiatric research. Int J Law Psychiatry 5(3–4):319–329, 1982 6135666

Armstrong K, Calzone K, Stopfer J, et al: Factors associated with decisions about clinical BRCA1/2 testing. Cancer Epidemiol Biomarkers Prev 9(11):1251–1254, 2000 11097234

Association of American Medical Colleges: Medical School Objectives Project. Washington, DC, American Association of Medical Colleges, 1998

Association of American Medical Colleges: Diversity in Medical Education: Facts and Figures. Washington, DC, Association of American Medical Colleges, 2012. Available at: https://members.aamc.org/eweb/upload/Diversity%20in%20Medical%20Education_Facts%20and%20Figures%202012.pdf. Accessed February 15, 2015.

Association of American Medical Colleges: Medical School Graduation Questionnaire: All Schools Summary Report. Washington, DC, Association of American Medical Colleges, 2013. Available at: https://www.aamc.org/download/350998/data/2013gqallschoolssummaryreport.pdf. Accessed August 13, 2015.

Auger KA, Landrigan CP, Gonzalez del Rey JA, et al: Better rested, but more stressed? Evidence of the effects of resident work hour restrictions. Acad Pediatr 12(4):335–343, 2012 22626586

Baldwin DC Jr, Daugherty SR, Rowley BD: Unethical and unprofessional conduct observed by residents during their first year of training. Acad Med 73(11):1195–1200, 1998 9834704

Balon R, Beresin EV, Coverdale JH, et al: College mental health: a vulnerable population in an environment with systemic deficiencies. Acad Psychiatry 2015 26327172 [Epub ahead of print]

Barak A, Klein B, Proudfoot JG: Defining Internet-supported therapeutic interventions. Ann Behav Med 38(1):4–17, 2009 19787305

Baylis P: Medical negligence. Trans Med Soc Lond 89:75–80, 1973 4805632

Beauchamp TL, Childress JF: Principles of Biomedical Ethics, 7th Edition. New York, Oxford University Press, 2012

Bebeau MJ, Thoma SJ: The impact of a dental ethics curriculum on moral reasoning. J Dent Educ 58(9):684–692, 1994 7962920

Beecher HK: Ethics and clinical research. N Engl J Med 274(24):1354–1360, 1966 5327352

Bellini LM, Baime M, Shea JA: Variation of mood and empathy during internship. JAMA 287(23):3143–3146, 2002 12069680

Birden H, Glass N, Wilson I, et al: Teaching professionalism in medical education: a Best Evidence Medical Education (BEME) systematic review. BEME Guide No. 25. Med Teach 35(7):e1252–e1266, 2013 23829342

Blackhall LJ, Frank G, Murphy S, et al: Bioethics in a different tongue: the case of truth-telling. J Urban Health 78(1):59–71, 2001 11368203

Bloch S, Green SA: Promoting the teaching of psychiatric ethics. Acad Psychiatry 33(2):89–92, 2009 19398616

Blow FC, Bohnert ASB, Ilgen MA, et al: Suicide mortality among patients treated by the Veterans Health Administration from 2000 to 2007. Am J Public Health 102(suppl 1):S98–S104, 2012 22390612

Boat TF: Improving lifetime health by promoting behavioral health in children. JAMA 313(15):1509–1510, 2015 25898042

Bonham C, Salvador M, Altschul D, et al: Training psychiatrists for rural practice: a 20-year follow-up. Acad Psychiatry 38(5):623–626, 2014 24705826

Boonstra H, Nash E: Minors and the right to consent to health care. The Guttmacher Report on Public Policy 3(4):4–8, 2000. Available at: http://www.guttmacher.org/pubs/tgr/03/4/gr030404.pdf. Accessed October 16, 2015.

Boyd KM, Higgs R, Pinching AJ: The New Dictionary of Medical Ethics. London, BMJ Publishing, 1997

Bradley EH, Peiris V, Wetle T: Discussions about end-of-life care in nursing homes. J Am Geriatr Soc 46(10):1235–1241, 1998 9777905

Brandeis LD: Business: A Profession. Charleston, SC, BiblioLife, 2009

Branson BM, Handsfield HH, Lampe MA, et al: Revised recommendations for HIV testing of adults, adolescents, and pregnant women in health-care settings. MMWR Recomm Rep 55(RR-14):1–17, 2006 16988643 Available at: http://www.cdc.gov/mmwr/preview/mmwrhtml/rr5514a1.htm. Accessed February 5, 2016

Breitbart W, Rosenfeld BD, Passik SD: Interest in physician-assisted suicide among ambulatory HIV-infected patients. Am J Psychiatry 153(2):238–242, 1996 8561205

Brennan TA, Horwitz RI, Duffy FD, et al: The role of physician specialty board certification status in the quality movement. JAMA 292(9):1038–1043, 2004 15339894

Buchanan D, Khoshnood K, Stopka T, et al: Ethical dilemmas created by the criminalization of status behaviors: case examples from ethnographic field research with injection drug users. Health Educ Behav 29(1):30–42, 2002 11822551

Bush NE, Reger MA, Luxton DD, et al: Suicides and suicide attempts in the U.S. military, 2008–2010. Suicide Life Threat Behav 43(3):262–273, 2013 23330611

Cabrera DE, Benedek DM: Combat stress reactions and psychiatric disorders after deployment, in Care of Military Service Members, Veterans, and Their Families. Edited by Cozza SJ, Goldenberg MN, Ursano RJ. Washington, DC, American Psychiatric Publishing, 2014, pp 91–118

Carlsson JM, Mortensen EL, Kastrup M: Predictors of mental health and quality of life in male tortured refugees. Nord J Psychiatry 60(1):51–57, 2006 16500800

Carman KG, Eibner C, Paddock SM: Trends in health insurance enrollment, 2013–15. Health Aff (Millwood) 34(6):1044–1048, 2015 25947173

Carpenter WTJr, Gold JM, Lahti AC, et al: Decisional capacity for informed consent in schizophrenia research. Arch Gen Psychiatry 57(6):533–538, 2000 10839330

Carter D, Roberts LW: Medical students' attitudes toward patients with HIV infection. A comparison study of 169 first-year students at the University of Chicago and the University of New Mexico. J Gay Lesbian Med Assoc 1:209–226, 1997

Cassileth BR, Lusk EJ, Guerry D, et al: Survival and quality of life among patients receiving unproven as compared with conventional cancer therapy. N Engl J Med 324(17):1180–1185, 1991 2011162

Cedfeldt AS, English C, El Youssef R, et al: Institute of Medicine committee report on resident duty hours: a view from a trench. J Grad Med Educ 1(2):178–180, 2009 21975974

Center C, Davis M, Detre T, et al: Confronting depression and suicide in physicians: a consensus statement. JAMA 289(23):3161–3166, 2003 12813122

Center for Behavioral Health Statistics and Quality: Behavioral health trends in the United States: Results from the 2014 National Survey on Drug Use and Health. HHS Publication No. SMA 15-4927, NSDUH Series H-50. September 2015. Available at: http://www.samhsa.gov/data/sites/default/files/NSDUH-FRR1-2014/NSDUH-FRR1-2014.pdf. Accessed January 20, 2016.

Centers for Disease Control and Prevention: Recommendations for Preventing Transmission of Human Immunodeficiency Virus and Hepatitis B Virus to Patients During Exposure-Prone Invasive Procedures. Morbidity and Mortality Weekly Report. July 12, 1991 / 40(RR08);1–9. Available at http://www.cdc.gov/mmwr/preview/mmwrhtml/00014845.htm. Accessed December 17, 2015.

Centers for Disease Control and Prevention: HIV, Hepatitis, STD and TB Partners: Partner Services Factsheet. May 27, 2009. Available at http://www.cdc.gov/nchhstp/partners/Partner-Services-FS.html. Accessed December 17, 2015.

Centers for Disease Control and Prevention: CDC Report: Mental Illness Surveillance Among Adults in the United States. December 2, 2011. Available at: http://www.cdc.gov/mentalhealthsurveillance/fact_sheet.html. Accessed February 1, 2016.

Centers for Disease Control and Prevention: Burden of mental illness. October 4, 2013. Available at: http://www.cdc.gov/mentalhealth/basics/burden.htm. Accessed August 24, 2015.

Centers for Disease Control and Prevention: HIV/AIDS: State Laboratory Reporting Laws: Viral Load and CD4 Requirements. March 18, 2015. Available at: http://www.cdc.gov/hiv/policies/law/states/reporting.html. Accessed December 17, 2015.

Chandra PS, Sowmya HR, Mehrotra S, et al: 'SMS' for mental health—feasibility and acceptability of using text messages for mental health promotion among young women from urban low income settings in India. Asian J Psychiatr 11:59–64, 2014 25453699

Cheng TL, Savageau JA, Sattler AL, et al: Confidentiality in health care. A survey of knowledge, perceptions, and attitudes among high school students. JAMA 269(11):1404–1407, 1993 8441216

Chipp C, Dewane S, Brems C, et al: "If only someone had told me…": lessons from rural providers. J Rural Health 27(1):122–130, 2011 21204979

Clouser KD: What is medical ethics? Ann Intern Med 80(5):657–660, 1974 4823818

Cogswell BE: Cultivating the trust of adolescent patients. Fam Med 17(6):254–258, 1985 3870794

Comas-Díaz L, Jacobsen FM: Ethnocultural transference and countertransference in the therapeutic dyad. Am J Orthopsychiatry 61(3):392–402, 1991 1951646

Cornette MM, deRoon-Cassini TA, Fosco GM, et al: Application of an interpersonal-psychological model of suicidal behavior to physicians and medical trainees. Arch Suicide Res 13(1):1–14, 2009 19123105

Council on Ethical and Judicial Affairs: Code of Medical Ethics of the American Medical Association, 2014–2015. Chicago, IL, American Medical Association, 2014

Council on Scientific Affairs: Results and implications of the AMA-APA Physician Mortality Project. Stage II. JAMA 257(21):2949–2953, 1987 3573294

Coverdale JH, Bayer T, Isbell P, et al: Are we teaching psychiatrists to be ethical? Acad Psychiatry 16(4):199–205, 1992 24435428

Cross-Disorder Group of the Psychiatric Genomics Consortium: Identification of risk loci with shared effects on five major psychiatric disorders: a genome-wide analysis. Lancet 381(9875):1371–1379, 2013 23453885

Dao J, Lehren AW: Baffling rise in suicides plagues the U.S. military. The New York Times, May 15, 2013. Available at: http://www.nytimes.com/2013/05/16/us/baffling-rise-in-suicides-plagues-us-military.html. Accessed January 21, 2015.

Darcy AM, Louie AK, Roberts LW: Machine learning and the profession of medicine. JAMA 315(6):551–552, 2016 26864406

Davidoff F: Changing the subject: ethical principles for everyone in health care. Ann Intern Med 133(5):386–389, 2000 10979885

Davis JH: Hacking of Government Computers Exposed 21.5 Million People. The New York Times. July 15, 2015. Available at: http://www.nytimes.com/2015/07/10/us/office-of-personnel-management-hackers-got-data-of-millions.html?_r=0. Accessed January 13, 2016.

DeAngelis CD: Medical professionalism. JAMA 313(18):1837–1838, 2015 25965231

Deisseroth K, Etkin A, Malenka RC: Optogenetics and the circuit dynamics of psychiatric disease. JAMA 313(20):2019–2020, 2015 25974025

Dickenson D, Fulford B: In Two Minds: A Casebook of Psychiatric Ethics. New York, Oxford University Press, 2000

Drane JF: Competency to give an informed consent: a model for making clinical assessments. JAMA 252(7):925–927, 1984 6748193

Dresner Y, Frank E, Baevsky T, et al: Screening practices of Israeli doctors' and their patients. Prev Med 50(5–6):300–303, 2010 20167233

Dresser R: Mentally disabled research subjects: the enduring policy issues. JAMA 276(1):67–72, 1996 8667543

Drossman DA: The problem patient: evaluation and care of medical patients with psychosocial disturbances. Ann Intern Med 88(3):366–372, 1978 629502

Duperly J, Lobelo F, Segura C, et al: The association between Colombian medical students' healthy personal habits and a positive attitude toward preventive counseling: cross-sectional analyses. BMC Public Health 9:218, 2009 19575806

Dyer AR: Ethics and Psychiatry: Toward Professional Definition. Washington, DC, American Psychiatric Press, 1988

Dyrbye LN, Thomas MR, Massie FS, et al: Burnout and suicidal ideation among U.S. medical students. Ann Intern Med 149(5):334–341, 2008 18765703

Dyrbye LN, Massie FS Jr, Eacker A, et al: Relationship between burnout and professional conduct and attitudes among U.S. medical students. JAMA 304(11):1173–1180, 2010a 20841530

Dyrbye LN, Thomas MR, Power DV, et al: Burnout and serious thoughts of dropping out of medical school: a multi-institutional study. Acad Med 85(1):94–102, 2010b 20042833

Dyrbye LN, Harper W, Moutier C, et al: A multi-institutional study exploring the impact of positive mental health on medical students' professionalism in an era of high burnout. Acad Med 87(8):1024–1031, 2012 22722352

Dyrbye LN, West CP, Satele D, et al: Burnout among U.S. medical students, residents, and early career physicians relative to the general U.S. population. Acad Med 89(3):443–451, 2014 24448053

Emanuel EJ, Fairclough DL, Daniels ER, et al: Euthanasia and physician-assisted suicide: attitudes and experiences of oncology patients, oncologists, and the public. Lancet 347(9018):1805–1810, 1996 8667927

Ende J, Pozen JT, Levinsky NG: Enhancing learning during a clinical clerkship: the value of a structured curriculum. J Gen Intern Med 1(4):232–237, 1986 3772597

Epstein RS, Simon RI: The Exploitation Index: an early warning indicator of boundary violations in psychotherapy. Bull Menninger Clin 54(4):450–465, 1990 2268752

Epstein RS, Simon RI, Kay GG: Assessing boundary violations in psychotherapy: survey results with the Exploitation Index. Bull Menninger Clin 56(2):150–166, 1992 1617326

Eva KW, Reiter HI, Rosenfeld J, Norman GR: The ability of the multiple mini-interview to predict preclerkship performance in medical school. Acad Med 79(10 Suppl):S40–S42, 2004a 15383385

Eva KW, Reiter HI, Rosenfeld J, et al: The relationship between interviewers' characteristics and ratings assigned during a Multiple Mini-Interview. Acad Med 79(6):602–609, 2004b 15165983

Eva KW, Rosenfeld J, Reiter HI, et al: An admissions OSCE: the Multiple Mini-Interview. Med Educ 38(3):314–326, 2004c 14996341

Fahrenkopf AM, Sectish TC, Barger LK, et al: Rates of medication errors among depressed and burnt out residents: prospective cohort study. BMJ 336(7642):488–491, 2008 18258931

Fawcett J: Treating impulsivity and anxiety in the suicidal patient. Ann N Y Acad Sci 932:94–102, discussion 102–105, 2001 11411193

Fazel M, Wheeler J, Danesh J: Prevalence of serious mental disorder in 7000 refugees resettled in Western countries: a systematic review. Lancet 365(9467):1309–1314, 2005 15823380

Federal Register: Proposed Rule: Federal Policy for the Protection of Human Subjects. September 8, 2015. Available at: https://www.federalregister.gov/articles/2015/09/08/2015-21756/federal-policy-for-the-protection-of-human-subjects. Accessed January 4, 2016.

Feeley RJ, Ross DA: The creation and implementation of a wellness initiative in a large adult psychiatry residency program. Acad Psychiatry 2015 25778669 [Epub ahead of print]

Feudtner C, Christakis DA, Christakis NA: Do clinical clerks suffer ethical erosion? Students' perceptions of their ethical environment and personal development. Acad Med 69(8):670–679, 1994 8054117

Finkelstein L: The impostor: aspects of his development. Psychoanal Q 43(1):85–114, 1974 4814473

Firth-Cozens J: Emotional distress in junior house officers. Br Med J (Clin Res Ed) 295(6597):533–536, 1987 3117213

Firth-Cozens J, Greenhalgh J: Doctors' perceptions of the links between stress and lowered clinical care. Soc Sci Med 44(7):1017–1022, 1997 9089922

Fisher CB: Addiction research ethics and the Belmont principles: do drug users have a different moral voice? Subst Use Misuse 46(6):728–741, 2011 21073412

Fletcher JC, Lombardo PA, Marshall MF, et al: Introduction to Clinical Ethics, 2nd Edition. Hagerstown, MD, University Publishing Group, 1997

Flory J, Emanuel E: Interventions to improve research participants' understanding in informed consent for research: a systematic review. JAMA 292(13):1593–1601, 2004 15467062

Fnais N, Soobiah C, Chen MH, et al: Harassment and discrimination in medical training: a systematic review and meta-analysis. Acad Med 89(5):817–827, 2014 24667512

Foglia MB, Pearlman RA, Bottrell M, et al: Ethical challenges within Veterans Administration healthcare facilities: perspectives of managers, clinicians, patients, and ethics committee chairpersons. Am J Bioeth 9(4):28–36, 2009 19326309

François G, Hambach R, van Sprundel M, et al: Inspecting asylum seekers upon entry—a medico-ethical complex. Eur J Public Health 18(6):552–553, 2008 19028711

Frank E, Dingle AD: Self-reported depression and suicide attempts among U.S. women physicians. Am J Psychiatry 156(12):1887–1894, 1999 10588401

Fuller Torrey E, Kennard AD, Eslinger D, et al: More Mentally Ill Persons Are in Jails and Prisons Than Hospitals: A Survey of the States. Arlington, VA, Treatment Advocacy Center, 2010

Gabbard GO, Roberts LW, Crisp-Han H, et al: Professionalism in Psychiatry. Washington, DC, American Psychiatric Publishing, 2012

Galvin J, Crooks R: Medico-legal aspects of sexually transmitted infections. Medicine 42(7):390–393, 2014

Gann PH, Anderson S, Regan MB: Shifts in medical student beliefs about AIDS after a comprehensive training experience. Am J Prev Med 7(3):172–177, 1991 1931147

Ganzini L, Lee MA, Heintz RT, et al: The effect of depression treatment on elderly patients' preferences for life-sustaining medical therapy. Am J Psychiatry 151(11):1631–1636, 1994 7943452

Ganzini L, Volicer L, Nelson WA, et al: Ten myths about decision-making capacity. J Am Med Dir Assoc 5(4):263–267, 2004 15228638

Garcia HA, McGeary CA, Finley EP, et al: The influence of trauma and patient characteristics on provider burnout in VA post-traumatic stress disorder specialty programmes. Psychol Psychother 2015 25643839 [Epub ahead of print]

Gardner EM, McLees MP, Steiner JF, et al: The spectrum of engagement in HIV care and its relevance to test-and-treat strategies for prevention of HIV infection. Clin Infect Dis 52(6):793–800, 2011 21367734

Geppert CM, Roberts LW: Ethical issues in the use of genetic information in the workplace: a review of recent developments. Curr Opin Psychiatry 18(5):518–524, 2005 16639111

Geppert CMA, Roberts LW: The Book of Ethics: Expert Guidance for Professionals Who Treat Addiction. Center City, MN, Hazelden Foundation, 2008

Gerstein DR, Johnson RA, Larison CL, et al: Alcohol and Other Drug Treatment Outcomes for Parents and Welfare Recipients: Outcomes, Costs, and Benefits, Final Report. Washington, DC, U.S. Department of Health and Human Services, Office of the Assistant Secretary for Planning and Evaluation, 1997

Gilligan C: In a Different Voice: Psychological Theory and Women's Development. Boston, MA, Harvard University Press, 1993

Givelber DJ, Bowers WJ, Blitch CL: Tarasoff, myth and reality: an empirical study of private law in action. Wis L Rev 1984(2):443–497, 1984 11653756

Goebert D, Thompson D, Takeshita J, et al: Depressive symptoms in medical students and residents: a multischool study. Acad Med 84(2):236–241, 2009 19174678

Golberstein E, Busch SH, Zaha R, et al: Effect of the Affordable Care Act's young adult insurance expansions on hospital-based mental health care. Am J Psychiatry 172(2):182–189, 2015 25263817

Gopal AA: Physician-assisted suicide: considering the evidence, existential distress, and an emerging role for psychiatry. J Am Acad Psychiatry Law 43(2):183–190, 2015 26071508

Government Accountability Office: Anthrax Vaccine: GAO's Survey of Guard and Reserve Pilots and Aircrew (GAO Publ No 02-445). Washington, DC, U.S. Government Printing Office, 2002

Government Accountability Office: VA Mental Health: Number of Veterans Receiving Care, Barriers Faced, and Efforts to Increase Access (GAO Publ No 12-12). Washington, DC, U.S. Government Printing Office, 2011

Grant BF, Saha TD, Ruan WJ, et al: Epidemiology of DSM-5 Drug Use Disorder: Results From the National Epidemiologic Survey on Alcohol and Related Conditions-III. JAMA Psychiatry 73(1):39–47, 2016 26580136

Green B, Miller PD, Routh CP: Teaching ethics in psychiatry: a one-day workshop for clinical students. J Med Ethics 21(4):234–238, 1995 7473644

Grepmair L, Mitterlehner F, Loew T, et al: Promoting mindfulness in psychotherapists in training influences the treatment results of their patients: a randomized, double-blind, controlled study. Psychother Psychosom 76(6):332–338, 2007 17917468

Grisso T, Appelbaum PS: The MacArthur Treatment Competence Study, III: Abilities of patients to consent to psychiatric and medical treatments. Law Hum Behav 19(2):149–174, 1995 11660292

Grisso T, Appelbaum PS, Mulvey EP, et al: The MacArthur Treatment Competence Study, II: Measures of abilities related to competence to consent to treatment. Law Hum Behav 19(2):127–148, 1995 11660291

Grosch WN, Olsen DC: When Helping Starts to Hurt: A New Look at Burnout Among Psychotherapists. New York, WW Norton, 1994

Gross R, Olfson M, Gameroff M, et al: Borderline personality disorder in primary care. Arch Intern Med 162(1):53–60, 2002 11784220

Hahn SR, Thompson KS, Wills TA, et al: The difficult doctor-patient relationship: somatization, personality and psychopathology. J Clin Epidemiol 47(6):647–657, 1994 7722577

Haider AH, Sexton J, Sriram N, et al: Association of unconscious race and social class bias with vignette-based clinical assessments by medical students. JAMA 306(9):942–951, 2011 21900134

Haire B, Kaldor JM: Ethics of ARV based prevention: treatment-as-prevention and PrEP. Developing World Bioeth 13(2):63–69, 2013 23594312

Halbesleben JR, Rathert C: Linking physician burnout and patient outcomes: exploring the dyadic relationship between physicians and patients. Health Care Manage Rev 33(1):29–39, 2008 18091442

Hall MA, Lord R: Obamacare: what the Affordable Care Act means for patients and physicians. BMJ 349:g5376, 2014 25338761

Hall RC: Ethical and legal implications of managed care. Gen Hosp Psychiatry 19(3):200–208, 1997 9218988

Hall RC, Platt DE, Hall RC: Suicide risk assessment: a review of risk factors for suicide in 100 patients who made severe suicide attempts. Evaluation of suicide risk in a time of managed care. Psychosomatics 40(1):18–27, 1999 9989117

Hamaoka D, Bates MJ, McCarroll JE, et al: An introduction to military service, in Care of Military Service Members, Veterans, and Their Families. Edited by Cozza SJ, Goldenberg MN, Ursano RJ. Washington, DC, American Psychiatric Publishing, 2014

Hannah SD, Carpenter-Song E: Patrolling your blind spots: introspection and public catharsis in a medical school faculty development course to reduce unconscious bias in medicine. Cult Med Psychiatry 37(2):314–339, 2013 23681466

Hanssens C: Legal and ethical implications of opt-out HIV testing. Clin Infect Dis 45(suppl 4):S232–S239, 2007 18190292

Harris EC, Barraclough B: Excess mortality of mental disorder. Br J Psychiatry 173:11–53, 1998 9850203

Harris GT, Rice ME: Risk appraisal and management of violent behavior. Psychiatr Serv 48(9):1168–1176, 1997 9285978

Hasin DS, Stinson FS, Ogburn E, Grant BF: Prevalence, correlates, disability, and comorbidity of DSM-IV alcohol abuse and dependence in the United States: results from the National Epidemiologic Survey on Alcohol and Related Conditions. Arch Gen Psychiatry 64(7):830–842, 2007 17606817

Heaton RK, Clifford DB, Franklin DR Jr, et al; CHARTER Group: HIV-associated neurocognitive disorders persist in the era of potent antiretroviral therapy: CHARTER Study. Neurology 75(23):2087–2096, 2010 21135382

Hem MH, Molewijk B, Pedersen R: Ethical challenges in connection with the use of coercion: a focus group study of health care personnel in mental health care. BMC Med Ethics 15:82, 2014 25475895

Henderson G, King NMP, Strauss RP, et al: The Social Medicine Reader. Durham, NC, Duke University Press, 1997

Henderson GE, Wolf SM, Kuczynski KJ, et al: The challenge of informed consent and return of results in translational genomics: empirical analysis and recommendations. J Law Med Ethics 42(3):344–355, 2014 25264092

Hickson GB, Federspiel CF, Pichert JW, et al: Patient complaints and malpractice risk. JAMA 287(22):2951–2957, 2002 12052124

Hiday VA, Swartz MS, Swanson JW, et al: Criminal victimization of persons with severe mental illness. Psychiatr Serv 50(1):62–68, 1999 9890581

Hiday VA, Swartz MS, Swanson JW, et al: Impact of outpatient commitment on victimization of people with severe mental illness. Am J Psychiatry 159(8):1403–1411, 2002 12153835

High DM: Who will make health care decisions for me when I can't? J Aging Health 2(3):291–309, 1990 10105399

High DM: Surrogate decision making. Who will make decisions for me when I can't? Clin Geriatr Med 10(3):445–462, 1994 7982161

Hill RM, Pettit JW: Perceived burdensomeness and suicide-related behaviors in clinical samples: current evidence and future directions. J Clin Psychol 70(7):631–643, 2014 24421035

Hiroeh U, Appleby L, Mortensen PB, et al: Death by homicide, suicide, and other unnatural causes in people with mental illness: a population-based study. Lancet 358(9299):2110–2112, 2001 11784624

Hodgson J, Mendenhall T, Lamson A: Patient and provider relationships: consent, confidentiality, and managing mistakes in integrated primary care settings. Fam Syst Health 31(1):28–40, 2013 23566125

Hoop JG, DiPasquale T, Hernandez JM, et al: Ethics and culture in mental health care. Ethics Behav 18(4):353–372, 2008

Hoop JG, Layde J, Roberts LW: Ethical Considerations in Psychopharmacological Treatment and Research, in Textbook of Psychopharmacology, 4th Edition. Edited by Schatzberg AF, Nemeroff CB. Washington, DC, American Psychiatric Publishing, 2009a, pp 1477–1495

Hoop JG, Roberts LW, Hammond KA: Genetic testing of stored biological samples: views of 570 U.S. workers. Genet Test Mol Biomarkers 13(3):331–337, 2009b 19405873

Horn P: Clinical Ethics Casebook. Belmont, CA, Wadsworth Publishing Company, 1998

Hsin H, Torous J, Roberts L: An adjuvant role for mobile health in psychiatry. JAMA Psychiatry 73(2):103–104, 2016 26747695

Hsiung RC: Suggested principles of professional ethics for the online provision of mental health services. Stud Health Technol Inform 84(Pt 2):1296–1300, 2001 11604937

Hughes PH, Conard SE, Baldwin DC Jr, et al: Resident physician substance use in the United States. JAMA 265(16):2069–2073, 1991 2013925

Hundert EM: A model for ethical problem solving in medicine, with practical applications. Am J Psychiatry 144(7):839–846, 1987 3605395

Institute of Medicine: Committee on Quality of Health Care in America. To Err Is Human: Building a Safer Health System. Edited by Kohn LT, Corrigan JM, Donaldson MS. Washington, DC, National Academy Press, 2000

Institute of Medicine: Best Care at Lower Cost: The Path to Continuously Learning Health Care in America. September 2, 2012. Washington, DC, The National Academies Press, 2013. Available at: http://iom.nationalacademies.org/Reports/2012/Best-Care-at-Lower-Cost-The-Path-to-Continuously-Learning-Health-Care-in-America.aspx. Accessed February 1, 2016.

Ishak WW, Lederer S, Mandili C, et al: Burnout during residency training: a literature review. J Grad Med Educ 1(2):236–242, 2009 21975985

Jackson D, Hickman LD, Hutchinson M, et al: Whistleblowing: an integrative literature review of data-based studies involving nurses. Contemp Nurse 48(2):240–252, 2014 25549718

Jackson JL, Kroenke K: Difficult patient encounters in the ambulatory clinic: clinical predictors and outcomes. Arch Intern Med 159(10):1069–1075, 1999 10335683

Jacobson JA, Tolle SW, Stocking C, et al: Internal medicine residents' preferences regarding medical ethics education. Acad Med 64(12):760–764, 1989 2590359

Jain S, Hoop JG, Dunn LB, et al: Psychiatry residents' attitudes on ethics and professionalism: multisite survey results. Ethics Behav 20(1):10–20, 2010

Jain S, Dunn LB, Warner CH, et al: Results of a multisite survey of U.S. psychiatry residents on education in professionalism and ethics. Acad Psychiatry 35(3):175–183, 2011a 21602439

Jain S, Lapid MI, Dunn LB, et al: Psychiatric residents' needs for education about informed consent, principles of ethics and professionalism, and caring for vulnerable populations: results of a multisite survey. Acad Psychiatry 35(3):184–190, 2011b 21602440

Järvinen M, Miller G: Selections of reality: applying Burke's dramatism to a harm reduction program. Int J Drug Policy 25(5):879–887, 2014 24702965

Jibson MD, Cobourn LA, Seibert JK: The impact of financial disclosure on attendee assessment of objectivity in continuing medical education programs in psychiatry: a randomized, controlled trial. Acad Psychiatry 2015 26017619 [Epub ahead of print]

Johnson JG, Spitzer RL, Williams JB, et al: Psychiatric comorbidity, health status, and functional impairment associated with alcohol abuse and dependence in primary care patients: findings of the PRIME MD-1000 study. J Consult Clin Psychol 63(1):133–140, 1995 7896978

Jones M, Kass AE, Trockel M, et al: A population-wide screening and tailored intervention platform for eating disorders on college campuses: the Healthy Body Image program. J Am Coll Health 62(5):351–356, 2014 24621000

Jones RB, Ashurst EJ: Online anonymous discussion between service users and health professionals to ascertain stakeholder concerns in using e-health services in mental health. Health Informatics J 19(4):281–299, 2013 24255052

Jonsen AR, Siegler M, Winslade WJ: Clinical Ethics: A Practical Approach to Ethical Decisions in Clinical Medicine, 4th Edition. New York, McGraw-Hill, 1998

Jonsen AR, Siegler M, Winslade WJ: Clinical Ethics: A Practical Approach to Ethical Decisions in Clinical Medicine, 8th Edition. New York, McGraw-Hill Education, 2015

Jordan NA, Russell L, Afousi E, et al: The ethical use of social media in marriage and family therapy: recommendations and future directions. Fam J (Alex Va) 22(1):105–112, 2014

Junek W, Burra P, Leichner P: Teaching interviewing skills by encountering patients. J Med Educ 54(5):402–407, 1979 439126

Kaldjian LC, Jones EW, Rosenthal GE: Facilitating and impeding factors for physicians' error disclosure: a structured literature review. Jt Comm J Qual Patient Saf 32(4):188–198, 2006 16649649

Kamerow DB: Research on mental disorders in primary care settings: rationale, topics, and support. Fam Pract Res J 6(1):5–11, 1986 3455110

Kass LR: Professing ethically: on the place of ethics in defining medicine. JAMA 249(10):1305–1310, 1983 6827708

Katz J: Experimentation With Human Beings. New York, Russell Sage Foundation, 1972

Katz J: The Nuremberg Code and the Nuremberg Trial: a reappraisal. JAMA 276(20):1662–1666, 1996 8922453

Kemp J, Bossarte R: Suicide data report, 2012. Available at: http://www.va.gov/opa/docs/Suicide-Data-Report-2012-final.pdf. Accessed January 18, 2015.

Kessler RC, McGonagle KA, Zhao S, et al: Lifetime and 12-month prevalence of DSM-III-R psychiatric disorders in the United States. Results from the National Comorbidity Survey. Arch Gen Psychiatry 51(1):8–19, 1994 8279933

Kessler RC, Heeringa SG, Stein MB, et al: Thirty-day prevalence of DSM-IV mental disorders among nondeployed soldiers in the U.S. Army: results from the Army Study to Assess Risk and Resilience in Servicemembers (Army STARRS). JAMA Psychiatry 71(5):504–513, 2014 24590120

Khazan O: Why are there so few doctors in rural America? The Atlantic, Aug 28, 2014. Available at: http://www.theatlantic.com/health/archive/2014/08/why-wont-doctors-move-to-rural-america/379291/. Accessed August 21, 2015.

Kitson A, Marshall A, Bassett K, et al: What are the core elements of patient-centred care? A narrative review and synthesis of the literature from health policy, medicine and nursing. J Adv Nurs 69(1):4–15, 2013 22709336

Kitto S, Bell M, Peller J, et al: Positioning continuing education: boundaries and intersections between the domains continuing education, knowledge translation, patient safety and quality improvement. Adv Health Sci Educ Theory Pract 18(1):141–156, 2013 22167577

Kondo KK, Johnson ME, Ironside EF, et al: HIV/AIDS research in correctional settings: perspectives on training needs from researchers and IRB members. AIDS Educ Prev 26(6):565–576, 2014 25490736

Kovach JG, Dubin WR, Combs CJ: Use and characterization of personal psychotherapy by psychiatry residents. Acad Psychiatry 39(1):99–103, 2015 25424637

Kuhn L, Susser I, Stein Z: Can further placebo-controlled trials of antiretroviral drugs to prevent sexual transmission of HIV be justified? Lancet 378(9787):285–287, 2011 21763941

Lapham EV, Kozma C, Weiss JO: Genetic discrimination: perspectives of consumers. Science 274(5287):621–624, 1996 8849455

Lapid M, Moutier C, Dunn L, et al: Professionalism and ethics education on relationships and boundaries: psychiatric residents' training preferences. Acad Psychiatry 33(6):461–469, 2009 19933889

Layde JB: The legal framework of medical ethics in the United States, in Professionalism and Ethics in Medicine: A Study Guide for Physicians and Physicians-in-Training. Edited by Roberts LW, Reicherter D. New York, Springer Science+Business Media, 2015, pp 27–38

Levy J, Jones A: Nothing small about microaggression. Posit Aware 25(6):32–35, 2013 24847586

Lidz CW, Meisel A, Osterweis M, et al: Barriers to informed consent. Ann Intern Med 99(4):539–543, 1983 6625386

Lidz CW, Hoge SK, Gardner W, et al: Perceived coercion in mental hospital admission: pressures and process. Arch Gen Psychiatry 52(12):1034–1039, 1995 7492255

Lindenthal JJ, Thomas CS: Psychiatrists, the public, and confidentiality. J Nerv Ment Dis 170(6):319–323, 1982 7077307

Link BG, Phelan JC, Bresnahan M, et al: Public conceptions of mental illness: labels, causes, dangerousness, and social distance. Am J Public Health 89(9):1328–1333, 1999 10474548

Lo B, Schroeder SA: Frequency of ethical dilemmas in a medical inpatient service. Arch Intern Med 141(8):1062–1064, 1981 7247591

Lorem GF, Hem MH, Molewijk B: Good coercion: patients' moral evaluation of coercion in mental health care. Int J Ment Health Nurs 24(3):231–240, 2015 25394674

Loue S: Ethical issues in a study of bipolar disorder and HIV risk among African-American men who have sex with men: case study in the ethics of mental health research. J Nerv Ment Dis 200(3):236–241, 2012 22373761

Loue S, Pike EC: The informed consent process, in Case Studies in Ethics and HIV Research. Edited by Loue S, Pike EC. New York, Springer, 2007, pp 23–35

Ludmerer KM: Redesigning residency education—moving beyond work hours. N Engl J Med 362(14):1337–1338, 2010 20375412

Ludwig AS, Peters RH: Medication-assisted treatment for opioid use disorders in correctional settings: an ethics review. Int J Drug Policy 25(6):1041–1046, 2014 25249444

Lurie N, Manning WG, Peterson C, et al: Preventive care: do we practice what we preach? Am J Public Health 77(7):801–804, 1987 3592032

Ly DP, Seabury SA, Jena AB: Divorce among physicians and other healthcare professionals in the United States: analysis of census survey data. BMJ 350:h706, 2015 25694110

Malebranche DJ, Peterson JL, Fullilove RE, et al: Race and sexual identity: perceptions about medical culture and healthcare among black men who have sex with men. J Natl Med Assoc 96(1):97–107, 2004 14746359

Maniglio R: Severe mental illness and criminal victimization: a systematic review. Acta Psychiatr Scand 119(3):180–191, 2009 19016668

Mannheim CI, Sancilio M, Phipps-Yonas S, et al: Ethical ambiguities in the practice of child clinical psychology. Prof Psychol Res Pr 33(1):24–29, 2002

Marder SR, Mebane A, Chien CP, et al: A comparison of patients who refuse and consent to neuroleptic treatment. Am J Psychiatry 140(4):470–472, 1983 6132559

Marlowe DB, Kirby KC, Bonieskie LM, et al: Assessment of coercive and noncoercive pressures to enter drug abuse treatment. Drug Alcohol Depend 42(2):77–84, 1996 8889406

Marrero I, Bell M, Dunn LB, Roberts LW: Assessing professionalism and ethics knowledge and skills: preferences of psychiatry residents. Acad Psychiatry 37(6):392–397, 2013 23771251

Marson DC, Ingram KK, Cody HA, et al: Assessing the competency of patients with Alzheimer's disease under different legal standards: a prototype instrument. Arch Neurol 52(10):949–954, 1995 7575221

Martin A, Kaufman J, Charney D: Pharmacotherapy of early onset depression. Update and new directions. Child Adolesc Psychiatr Clin N Am 9(1):135–157, 2000 10674194

Mathews SC, Pronovost PJ: Commentary: establishing safety and quality as core values: a hospital road map. Am J Med Qual 27(4):348–349, 2012 22205770

Mazor KM, Simon SR, Gurwitz JH: Communicating with patients about medical errors: a review of the literature. Arch Intern Med 164(15):1690–1697, 2004 15302641

McCarty T, Roberts LW: The difficult patient, in Medicine: A Primary Care Approach. Edited by Rubin RH, Voss C, Derksen DJ, et al. Philadelphia, PA, WB Saunders, 1996, pp 395–399

McCrady BS, Bux DA Jr: Ethical issues in informed consent with substance abusers. J Consult Clin Psychol 67(2):186–193, 1999 10224728

McCurdy L, Goode LD, Inui TS, et al: Fulfilling the social contract between medical schools and the public. Acad Med 72(12):1063–1070, 1997 9435712

McDonald KM, Bryce CL, Graber ML: The patient is in: patient involvement strategies for diagnostic error mitigation. BMJ Qual Saf 22(suppl 2):ii33–ii39, 2013 23893394

McGinnis JM, Foege WH: Mortality and morbidity attributable to use of addictive substances in the United States. Proc Assoc Am Physicians 111(2):109–118, 1999 10220805

McLoyd VC: Socioeconomic disadvantage and child development. Am Psychol 53(2):185–204, 1998 9491747

McManus M, White P, Barbour A, et al: Pediatric to adult transition: a quality improvement model for primary care. J Adolesc Health 56(1):73–78, 2015 25287984

Melek SP, Norris DT, Paulus J: Economic Impact of Integrated Medical-Behavioral Healthcare: Implications for Psychiatry. Denver, CO, Milliman, 2014

Melrose RJ, Tinaz S, Castelo JMB, et al: Compromised fronto-striatal functioning in HIV: an fMRI investigation of semantic event sequencing. Behav Brain Res 188(2):337–347, 2008 18242723

Melton GB: Parents and children: legal reform to facilitate children's participation. Am Psychol 54(11):935–944, 1999

Merikangas KR, He JP, Burstein M, et al: Service utilization for lifetime mental disorders in U.S. adolescents: results of the National Comorbidity Survey–Adolescent Supplement (NCS-A). J Am Acad Child Adolesc Psychiatry 50(1):32–45, 2011 21156268

Metz ME, Seifert MH: Women's expectations of physicians in sexual health concerns. Fam Pract Res J 7(3):141–152, 1988 3274682

Meyer EG: The importance of understanding military culture. Acad Psychiatry 39(4):416–418, 2015 25690349

Miller NM, McGowen RK: The painful truth: physicians are not invincible. South Med J 93(10):966–973, 2000 11147478

Miller-Keane, O'Toole MT: Encyclopedia and Dictionary of Medicine, Nursing, and Allied Health, 7th Edition. St. Louis, MO, WB Saunders, 2003

Miyaji NT: The power of compassion: truth-telling among American doctors in the care of dying patients. Soc Sci Med 36(3):249–264, 1993 8426968

Molodynski A, Turnpenny L, Rugkåsa J, et al: Coercion and compulsion in mental healthcare: an international perspective. Asian J Psychiatr 8:2–6, 2014 24655618

Moser DJ, Schultz SK, Arndt S, et al: Capacity to provide informed consent for participation in schizophrenia and HIV research. Am J Psychiatry 159(7):1201–1207, 2002 12091200

Mouton C, Teno JM, Mor V, et al: Communication of preferences for care among human immunodeficiency virus-infected patients: barriers to informed decisions? Arch Fam Med 6(4):342–347, 1997 9225705

Murdoch I: Metaphysics as a Guide to Morals: Philosophical Reflections. New York, Viking, 1992

Murray JL, Lopez AD: The Global Burden of Disease: A Comprehensive Assessment of Mortality and Disability From Diseases, Injuries, and Risk Factors in 1990 and Projected to 2020. Cambridge, MA, Harvard School of Public Health, 1996

Myers JS, Nash DB: Graduate medical education's new focus on resident engagement in quality and safety: will it transform the culture of teaching hospitals? Acad Med 89(10):1328–1330, 2014 25054414

National Bioethics Advisory Commission: Research Involving Subjects With Mental Disorders That May Affect Decision Making Capacity. Rockville, MD, National Bioethics Advisory Commission, 1998

National Commission for the Protection of Human Subjects of Biomedical and Behavioral Research: The Belmont Report: Ethical Principles and Guidelines for the Protection of Human Subjects of Research. Washington, DC, U.S. Government Printing Office, 1979. Available at: http://www.hhs.gov/ohrp/humansubjects/guidance/belmont.html. Accessed October 22, 2015.

National Institute on Drug Abuse: Trends & Statistics: Costs of Substance Abuse. August 2015. Available at http://www.drugabuse.gov/related-topics/trends-statistics. Accessed December 17, 2015.

National Institute on Drug Abuse: National Survey on Drug Use and Health: Trends in Prevalence of Various Drugs for Ages 12 or Older, Ages 12 to 17, Ages 18 to 25, and Ages 26 or Older; 2012–2014. National Institute on Drug Abuse, Bethesda, MD. Available at: http://www.drugabuse.gov/national-survey-drug-use-health. Accessed January 4, 2016.

National Institute of Mental Health: Any Disorder Among Children. Available at: http://www.nimh.nih.gov/health/statistics/prevalence/any-disorder-among-children.shtml. Accessed January 4, 2016a.

National Institute of Mental Health: Use of Mental Health Services and Treatment Among Children. Available at: http://www.nimh.nih.gov/health/statistics/prevalence/use-of-mental-health-services-and-treatment-among-children.shtml. Accessed January 4, 2016b.

Newman SJ: Prevention, not prejudice: the role of federal guidelines in HIV-criminalization reform. Northwest Univ Law Rev 107(3):1403, 2012

Nie JB: The fallacy and dangers of dichotomizing cultural differences: the truth about medical truth telling in China. Virtual Mentor 14(4):338–343, 2012 23352071. Available at: http://journalofethics.ama-assn.org/2012/04/msoc1-1204.html. Accessed October 22, 2015.

Nieto G, Gittelman M, Abad A: Homeless mentally ill persons: a bibliography review. International Journal of Psychosocial Rehabilitation 12(1):1, 2008. Available at: http://www.psychosocial.com/IJPR_12/Homeless_Mentally_Ill_Nieto.html. Accessed February 1, 2016.

Nock MK, Deming CA, Fullerton CS, et al: Suicide among soldiers: a review of psychosocial risk and protective factors. Psychiatry 76(2):97–125, 2013 23631542

Nock MK, Stein MB, Heeringa SG, et al: Prevalence and correlates of suicidal behavior among soldiers: results from the Army Study to Assess Risk and Resilience in Servicemembers (Army STARRS). JAMA Psychiatry 71(5):514–522, 2014 24590178

Novack DH, Detering BJ, Arnold R, et al: Physicians' attitudes toward using deception to resolve difficult ethical problems. JAMA 261(20):2980–2985, 1989 2716130

O'Donoghue B, Roche E, Shannon S, et al: Perceived coercion in voluntary hospital admission. Psychiatry Res 215(1):120–126, 2014 24210740

Olfson M, Fireman B, Weissman MM, et al: Mental disorders and disability among patients in a primary care group practice. Am J Psychiatry 154(12):1734–1740, 1997 9396954

Ondrusek N, Abramovitch R, Pencharz P, et al: Empirical examination of the ability of children to consent to clinical research. J Med Ethics 24(3):158–165, 1998 9650109

Owen GS, David AS, Hayward P, et al: Retrospective views of psychiatric in-patients regaining mental capacity. Br J Psychiatry 195(5):403–407, 2009 19880929

Paasche-Orlow M: The ethics of cultural competence. Acad Med 79(4):347–350, 2004 15044168

Perez B, Knych SA, Weaver SJ, et al: Understanding the barriers to physician error reporting and disclosure: a systemic approach to a systemic problem. J Patient Saf 10(1):45–51, 2014 24553443

Posternak MA, Mueller TI: Assessing the risks and benefits of benzodiazepines for anxiety disorders in patients with a history of substance abuse or dependence. Am J Addict 10(1):48–68, 2001 11268828

President's Commission for the Study of Ethical Problems in Medicine and Biomedical and Biobehavioral Research: Deciding to Forgo Life-Sustaining Treatment: A Report on the Ethical, Medical and Legal Issues in Treatment Decisions. Washington, DC, U.S. Government Printing Office, 1983

Price AR: Anonymity and pseudonymity in whistleblowing to the U.S. Office of Research Integrity. Acad Med 73(5):467–472, 1998 9609854

Prine C: Privacy breaches in VA health records wound veterans. Pittsburgh Tribune-Review, October 12, 2013. Available at: http://triblive.com/news/allegheny/4656034-74/privacy-health-veterans#axzz3lAzmMWEP. Accessed August 5, 2015.

Puchalski C, Romer AL: Taking a spiritual history allows clinicians to understand patients more fully. J Palliat Med 3(1):129–137, 2000 15859737

Reed DA, Levine RB, Miller RG, et al: Effect of residency duty-hour limits: views of key clinical faculty. Arch Intern Med 167(14):1487–1492, 2007 17646602

Regier DA, Narrow WE, Rae DS, et al: The de facto U.S. mental and addictive disorders service system. Epidemiologic Catchment Area prospective 1-year prevalence rates of disorders and services. Arch Gen Psychiatry 50(2):85–94, 1993 8427558

Reuben DB: Miracles, choices, and justice: tragedy of the future commons. JAMA 304(4):467–468, 2010 20664050

Rhoades LJ: Office of Research Integrity: New Institutional Research Misconduct Activity, 1992–2001. Washington, DC, Office of Research Integrity, Office of Public Health and Science, U.S. Department of Health and Human Services, 2004

Rice DP, Kelman S, Miller LS: Estimates of economic costs of alcohol and drug abuse and mental illness, 1985 and 1988. Public Health Rep 106(3):280–292, 1991 1905049

Rich JD, Wohl DA, Beckwith CG, et al: HIV-related research in correctional populations: now is the time. Curr HIV/AIDS Rep 8(4):288–296, 2011 21904902

Rid A, Wendler D: Treatment decision making for incapacitated patients: is development and use of a patient preference predictor feasible? J Med Philos 39(2):130–152, 2014 24556152

Riecken HW, Ravich R: Informed consent to biomedical research in Veterans Administration Hospitals. JAMA 248(3):344–348, 1982 7045434

Robbins JM, Beck PR, Mueller DP, et al: Therapists' perceptions of difficult psychiatric patients. J Nerv Ment Dis 176(8):490–497, 1988 3404141

Roberts LW: The ethical basis of psychiatric research: conceptual issues and empirical findings. Compr Psychiatry 39(3):99–110, 1998 9606575

Roberts LW: Informed consent and the capacity for voluntarism. Am J Psychiatry 159(5):705–712, 2002 11986120

Roberts LW: Community-Based Participatory Research for Improved Mental Healthcare: A Manual for Clinicians and Researchers. New York, Springer Science+Business Media, 2013

Roberts LW: Advancing science in the service of humanity: professionalism and ethical safeguards. JAMA Intern Med 175(9):1506–1508, 2015a 26167792]

Roberts LW: Sacrifice and service, protectors and teachers: the role of military and veteran patients in training early-career psychiatrists. Acad Psychiatry 39(4):349–350, 2015b 26077009

Roberts LW: Water pie: creativity and leadership in academic psychiatry. Acad Psychiatry 39(4):470–471, 2015c 25977099

Roberts LW, Dyer AR: Concise Guide to Ethics in Mental Health Care. Washington, DC, American Psychiatric Publishing, 2004

Roberts LW, Hoop JG: Professionalism and Ethics: Q and A Self-Study Guide for Mental Health Professionals. Washington, DC, American Psychiatric Publishing, 2008

Roberts LW, Kim JP: Attunement and alignment of people with schizophrenia and their preferred alternative decision-makers: an exploratory pilot study comparing treatment and research decisions. J Psychiatr Res 71:70–77, 2015a 26453915

Roberts LW, Kim JP: Informal health care practices of residents: "curbside" consultation and self-diagnosis and treatment. Acad Psychiatry 39(1):22–30, 2015b 24923781

Roberts LW, Reicherter D (eds): Professionalism and Ethics in Medicine: A Study Guide for Physicians and Physicians-in-Training. New York, Springer Science+Business Media, 2015

Roberts LW, McCarty T, Lyketsos C, et al: What and how psychiatry residents at ten training programs wish to learn about ethics. Acad Psychiatry 20(3):131–143, 1996 24442690

Roberts LW, Muskin PR, Warner TD, et al: Attitudes of consultation-liaison psychiatrists toward physician-assisted death practices. Psychosomatics 38(5):459–471, 1997 9314715

Roberts LW, Battaglia J, Smithpeter M, et al: An office on Main Street: health care dilemmas in small communities. Hastings Cent Rep 29(4):28–37, 1999a 10451837

Roberts LW, Mines J, Voss C, et al: Assessing medical students' competence in obtaining informed consent. Am J Surg 178(4):351–355, 1999b 10587199

Roberts LW, Warner TD, Carter D, et al: Caring for medical students as patients: access to services and care-seeking practices of 1,027 students at nine medical schools. Acad Med 75(3):272–277, 2000 10724317

Roberts LW, Geppert CMA, Brody JL: A framework for considering the ethical aspects of psychiatric research protocols. Compr Psychiatry 42(5):351–363, 2001a 11559861

Roberts LW, Warner TD, Lyketsos C, et al: Perceptions of academic vulnerability associated with personal illness: a study of 1,027 students at nine medical schools. Compr Psychiatry 42(1):1–15, 2001b 11154710

Roberts LW, Geppert CM, Bailey R: Ethics in psychiatric practice: essential ethics skills, informed consent, the therapeutic relationship, and confidentiality. J Psychiatr Pract 8(5):290–305, 2002 15985891

Roberts LW, Geppert C, McCarty T, et al: Evaluating medical students' skills in obtaining informed consent for HIV testing. J Gen Intern Med 18(2):112–119, 2003a 12542585

Roberts LW, Monaghan-Geernaert P, Battaglia J, et al: Personal health care attitudes of rural clinicians: a preliminary study of 127 multidisciplinary health care providers in Alaska and New Mexico. Rural Ment Health 28:29–39, 2003b

Roberts LW, Green Hammond KA, Geppert CM, et al: The positive role of professionalism and ethics training in medical education: a comparison of medical student and resident perspectives. Acad Psychiatry 28(3):170–182, 2004 15507551

Roberts LW, Geppert CM, Warner TD, et al: Perspectives on use and protection of genetic information in work settings: results of a preliminary study. Soc Sci Med 60(8):1855–1858, 2005a 15686815

Roberts LW, Warner TD, Geppert CM, et al: Employees' perspectives on ethically important aspects of genetic research participation: a pilot study. Compr Psychiatry 46(1):27–33, 2005b 15714191

Roberts LW, Warner TD, Hammond KG: Ethical challenges of mental health clinicians in rural and frontier areas. Psychiatr Serv 56(3):358–359, 2005c 15746521

Roberts LW, Johnson ME, Brems C, et al: Ethical disparities: challenges encountered by multidisciplinary providers in fulfilling ethical standards in the care of rural and minority people. J Rural Health 23(suppl):89–97, 2007 18237331

Roberts LW, Barry LK, Warner TD: Potential workplace discrimination based on genetic predisposition: views of workers. AJOB Primary Research 2(3):1–12, 2011a

Roberts LW, Warner TD, Moutier C, et al: Are doctors who have been ill more compassionate? Attitudes of resident physicians regarding personal health issues and the expression of compassion in clinical care. Psychosomatics 52(4):367–374, 2011b 21777720

Roberts LW, Warner TD, Erickson JA: A preliminary study of employees' views of genetic research: perceived harm, risk, and willingness to participate. AJOB Primary Research 3(4):72–80, 2012

Roberts LW, Beresin EV, Coverdale JH, et al: Moving beyond community mental health: public mental health as an emerging focus for psychiatry residency training. Acad Psychiatry 38(6):655–660, 2014 25339288

Roberts LW, Reicherter D, Adelsheim S, et al: Partnering in Mental Health: A Guide to Community and Academic Collaboration. New York, Springer Science+Business Media, 2015

Rosato J: The ethics of clinical trials: a child's view. J Law Med Ethics 28(4):362–378, 2000 11317428

Rosen DS, Blum RW, Britto M, et al: Transition to adult health care for adolescents and young adults with chronic conditions: position paper of the Society for Adolescent Medicine. J Adolesc Health 33(4):309–311, 2003 14519573

Rosenbaum L: Understanding bias—the case for careful study. N Engl J Med 372(20):1959–1963, 2015 25970055

Rousseau C, Drapeau A: Premigration exposure to political violence among independent immigrants and its association with emotional distress. J Nerv Ment Dis 192(12):852–856, 2004 15583507

Rubin SB, Zoloth L: Margin of Error: The Ethics of Mistakes in the Practice of Medicine. Hagerstown, MD, University Publishing Group, 2000

Ruiz-Casares M: Mental health: Tailor informed-consent processes. Nature 513(7518):304, 2014 25230633

Runyan C, Robinson P, Gould DA: Ethical issues facing providers in collaborative primary care settings: do current guidelines suffice to guide the future of team based primary care? Fam Syst Health 31(1):1–8, 2013 23566122

Sabin J: Is managed care ethical? in Controversies in Managed Mental Health Care. Edited by Lazarus A. Washington, DC, American Psychiatric Press, 1996, pp 115–128

Sachs GA, Stocking CB, Stern R, et al: Ethical aspects of dementia research: informed consent and proxy consent. Clin Res 42(3):403–412, 1994 7955902

Sadler JZ, Hulgus YF: Clinical problem solving and the biopsychosocial model. Am J Psychiatry 149(10):1315–1323, 1992 1530068

Sargent DA: Preventing physician suicide. JAMA 257(21):2955–2956, 1987 3573296

Schafer S, Nowlis DP: Personality disorders among difficult patients. Arch Fam Med 7(2):126–129, 1998 9519915

Scheidt PC, Lazoritz S, Ebbeling WL, et al: Evaluation of system providing feedback to students on videotaped patient encounters. J Med Educ 61(7):585–590, 1986 3723570

Schernhammer ES, Colditz GA: Suicide rates among physicians: a quantitative and gender assessment (meta-analysis). Am J Psychiatry 161(12):2295–2302, 2004 15569903

Schoenbaum M, Kessler RC, Gilman SE, et al: Predictors of suicide and accident death in the Army Study to Assess Risk and Resilience in Servicemembers (Army STARRS): results from the Army Study to Assess Risk and Resilience in Servicemembers (Army STARRS). JAMA Psychiatry 71(5):493–503, 2014 24590048

Schulz PM, Schulz SC, Dibble E, et al: Patient and family attitudes about schizophrenia: implications for genetic counseling. Schizophr Bull 8(3):504–513, 1982 7134894

Schwartz AC, Kotwicki RJ, McDonald WM: Developing a modern standard to define and assess professionalism in trainees. Acad Psychiatry 33(6):442–450, 2009 19933884

Schwartz HI, Vingiano W, Perez CB: Autonomy and the right to refuse treatment: patients' attitudes after involuntary medication. Hosp Community Psychiatry 39(10):1049–1054, 1988 3229738

Seal KH, Metzler TJ, Gima KS, et al: Trends and risk factors for mental health diagnoses among Iraq and Afghanistan veterans using Department of Veterans Affairs health care, 2002–2008. Am J Public Health 99(9):1651–1658, 2009 19608954

Searight HR, Gafford J: Cultural diversity at the end of life: issues and guidelines for family physicians. Am Fam Physician 71(3):515–522, 2005 15712625

Self DJ, Olivarez M, Baldwin DC Jr: The amount of small-group case-study discussion needed to improve moral reasoning skills of medical students. Acad Med 73(5):521–523, 1998 9609864

Shanafelt TD, Bradley KA, Wipf JE, et al: Burnout and self-reported patient care in an internal medicine residency program. Ann Intern Med 136(5):358–367, 2002 11874308

Shanafelt TD, Balch CM, Dyrbye L, et al: Special report: suicidal ideation among American surgeons. Arch Surg 146(1):54–62, 2011 21242446

Sharp T, Moran E, Kuhn I, et al: Do the elderly have a voice? Advance care planning discussions with frail and older individuals: a systematic literature review and narrative synthesis. Br J Gen Pract 63(615):e657–e668, 2013 24152480

Sharpe M, Mayou R, Seagroatt V, et al: Why do doctors find some patients difficult to help? Q J Med 87(3):187–193, 1994 8208907

Shield KD, Gmel G, Kehoe-Chan T, et al: Mortality and potential years of life lost attributable to alcohol consumption by race and sex in the United States in 2005. PLoS ONE 8(1):e51923, 2013 23300957

Shimm DS, Spece RG Jr: Introduction, in Conflicts of Interest in Clinical Practice and Research. Edited by Spece RG Jr, Shimm DS, Buchanan AE. New York, Oxford University Press, 1996, pp 1–11

Sholevar GP: Cultural child and adolescent psychiatry, in Lewis's Child and Adolescent Psychiatry: A Comprehensive Textbook. Edited by Martin A, Volkmar F. Philadelphia, PA, Lippincott Williams & Wilkins, 2007, pp 57–65

Siegler M: Searching for moral certainty in medicine: a proposal for a new model of the doctor-patient encounter. Bull NY Acad Med 57(1):56–69, 1981 6937229

Siegler M: Sounding boards: confidentiality in medicine—a decrepit concept. N Engl J Med 307(24):1518–1521, 1982 7144818

Siegler M, Rezler AG, Connell KJ: Using simulated case studies to evaluate a clinical ethics course for junior students. J Med Educ 57(5):380–385, 1982 7069760

Silver HK, Glicken AD: Medical student abuse: incidence, severity, and significance. JAMA 263(4):527–532, 1990 2294324

Simon RI, Hales RE: The American Psychiatric Publishing Textbook of Suicide Assessment and Management, 2nd Edition. Washington, DC, American Psychiatric Publishing, 2012

Single E, Rehm J, Robson L, et al: The relative risks and etiologic fractions of different causes of death and disease attributable to alcohol, tobacco and illicit drug use in Canada. CMAJ 162(12):1669–1675, 2000 10870494

Sinha P: Why do doctors commit suicide? The New York Times, September 4, 2014, p A27

Skloot R: The immortal life of Henrietta Lacks. New York, Broadway Books, 2011

Smith LB, Sapers B, Reus VI, et al: Attitudes towards bipolar disorder and predictive genetic testing among patients and providers. J Med Genet 33(7):544–549, 1996 8818938

Smyth B, Hoffman V, Fan J, et al: Years of potential life lost among heroin addicts 33 years after treatment. Prev Med 44(4):369–374, 2007 17291577

Spitzer RL, Kroenke K, Linzer M, et al: Health-related quality of life in primary care patients with mental disorders. Results from the PRIME-MD 1000 Study. JAMA 274(19):1511–1517, 1995 7474219

Stanford Medicine: WellMD. Available at: http://wellmd.stanford.edu. Accessed August 13, 2015.

Steinberg D, Mills D, Romano M: When Did Prisons Become Acceptable Mental Healthcare Facilities? Stanford Law School Three Strikes Project. February 2015. Available at: http://law.stanford.edu/wp-content/uploads/sites/default/files/publication/863745/doc/slspublic/Report_v12.pdf. Accessed January 4, 2016

Stobo JD, Blank LL: Project Professionalism: staying ahead of the wave. Am J Med 97:i–iii, 1994

Sugarman J, McCrory DC, Powell D, et al: Empirical research on informed consent. An annotated bibliography. Hastings Cent Rep 29(1):S1–S42, 1999 10051999

Sulmasy DP, Geller G, Levine DM, et al: Medical house officers' knowledge, attitudes, and confidence regarding medical ethics. Arch Intern Med 150(12):2509–2513, 1990 2244767

Sulmasy DP, Terry PB, Faden RR, et al: Long-term effects of ethics education on the quality of care for patients who have do-not-resuscitate orders. J Gen Intern Med 9(11):622–626, 1994 7853071

Swanson J, Holzer CE 3rd, Ganju VK, et al: Violence and psychiatric disorder in the community: evidence from the Epidemiologic Catchment Area surveys. Hosp Community Psychiatry 41(7):761–770, 1990 2142118

Swanson J, Estroff S, Swartz M, et al: Violence and severe mental disorder in clinical and community populations: the effects of psychotic symptoms, comorbidity, and lack of treatment. Psychiatry 60(1):1–22, 1997 9130311

Swanson J, McGinty EE, Fazel S, et al: Mental illness and reduction of gun violence and suicide: bringing epidemiologic research to policy. Ann Epidemiol 25(5):366–376, 2015 24861430

Sweet MP, Bernat JL: A study of the ethical duty of physicians to disclose errors. J Clin Ethics 8(4):341–348, 1997 9503083

Szasz TS: Involuntary psychiatry. University of Cincinnati Law Review 45(3):347–365, 1976

Tanielian TL, Pincus HA, Olfson M, et al: General hospital discharges of patients with mental and physical disorders. Psychiatr Serv 48(3):311, 1997 9057231

Targum SD, Dibble ED, Davenport YB, et al: The Family Attitudes Questionnaire: patients' and spouses' views of bipolar illness. Arch Gen Psychiatry 38(5):562–568, 1981 7235858

Tarzian AJ, ASBH Core Competencies Update Task Force 1: Health care ethics consultation: an update on core competencies and emerging standards from the American Society for Bioethics and Humanities' core competencies update task force. Am J Bioeth 13(2):3–13, 2013 23391049

Teal CR, Gill AC, Green AR, et al: Helping medical learners recognise and manage unconscious bias toward certain patient groups. Med Educ 46(1):80–88, 2012 22150199

Teel K: The physician's dilemma: a doctor's view—what the law should be. Bayl Law Rev 27(1):6–9, 1975 11660887

Tejada-Vera B: Mortality From Alzheimer's Disease in the United States: Data for 2000 and 2010. NCHS data brief, No 116. Hyattsville, MD, National Center for Health Statistics, 2013. Available at: http://www.cdc.gov/nchs/data/databriefs/db116.htm. Accessed January 4, 2016.

Tomamichel M, Sessa C, Herzig S, et al: Informed consent for phase I studies: evaluation of quantity and quality of information provided to patients. Ann Oncol 6(4):363–369, 1995 7619751

Trippitelli CL, Jamison KR, Folstein MF, et al: Pilot study on patients' and spouses' attitudes toward potential genetic testing for bipolar disorder. Am J Psychiatry 155(7):899–904, 1998 9659854

Trockel M, Karlin BE, Taylor CB, et al: Cognitive behavioral therapy for insomnia with veterans: evaluation of effectiveness and correlates of treatment outcomes. Behav Res Ther 53:41–46, 2014 24412462

Tsai J, Rosenheck RA: Risk factors for homelessness among U.S. veterans. Epidemiol Rev 37:177–195, 2015 25595171

Tseng WS, Streltzer J: Cultural competence in clinical psychiatry. Washington, DC, American Psychiatric Publishing, 2004

Ubel PA, Zell MM, Miller DJ, et al: Elevator talk: observational study of inappropriate comments in a public space. Am J Med 99(2):190–194, 1995 7625424

Ullom-Minnich PD, Kallail KJ: Physicians' strategies for safeguarding confidentiality: the influence of community and practice characteristics. J Fam Pract 37(5):445–448, 1993 8228855

United States Census Bureau: Income, Poverty and Health Insurance Coverage in the United States: 2013. September 16, 2014. Available at http://www.census.gov/newsroom/press-releases/2014/cb14-169.html. Accessed December 18, 2015.

University of New Mexico Health Sciences Center Institute for Ethics: Values History Form. Available at: http://hscethics.unm.edu/common/pdf/values-history.pdf. Accessed December 17, 2015.

U.S. Committee for Refugees and Immigrants: World Refugee Survey 2009: United States. June 17, 2009. Available at http://www.refworld.org/docid/4a40d2b580.html. Accessed February 5, 2016

U.S. Department of Health and Human Services: Trials of War Criminals Before the Nuremberg Military Tribunals Under Control Council Law No 10, Vol 2, pp. 181-182. Washington, D.C., U.S. Government Printing Office, 1949. Available at: http://www.hhs.gov/ohrp/archive/nurcode.html. Accessed November 2, 2015.

U.S. Department of Health and Human Services: Protection of Human Subjects. July 14, 2009. Available at: http://www.hhs.gov/ohrp/humansubjects/guidance/45cfr46.html. Accessed February 1, 2016.

U.S. Department of Health and Human Services, Administration for Children and Families, Administration on Children, Youth, and Families, Children's Bureau: Child Welfare Outcomes 2008–2011: Report to Congress. Washington, DC, U.S. Department of Health and Human Services, Administration for Children and Families, Administration on Children, Youth, and Families, Children's Bureau, August 16, 2013. Available at: http://www.acf.hhs.gov/sites/default/files/cb/cwo08_11.pdf. Accessed August 6, 2015.

U.S. Department of Health and Human Services Office for Civil Rights: Breaches Affecting 500 or More Individuals. Available at: https://ocrportal.hhs.gov/ocr/breach/breach_report.jsf. Accessed January 13, 2016.

U.S. Department of Labor: The employment situation—December 2014, in Bureau of Statistics News Release, January 9, 2015. Available at: http://www.bls.gov/news.release/archives/empsit_01092015.pdf. Accessed January 24, 2015.

U.S. Department of Veterans Affairs: The Veteran Population Projection Model. Washington, DC, National Center for Veterans Analysis and Statistics, 2014. Available at: http://www.va.gov/vetdata/Veteran_Population.asp. Accessed January 21, 2015.

van der Steen JT, Gijsberts MJ, Hertogh CM, et al: Predictors of spiritual care provision for patients with dementia at the end of life as perceived by physicians: a prospective study. BMC Palliat Care 13(1):61, 2014 25589896

van Staa AL, Jedeloo S, van Meeteren J, Latour JM: Crossing the transition chasm: experiences and recommendations for improving transitional care of young adults, parents and providers. Child Care Health Dev 37(6):821–832, 2011 22007982

Vitiello B: Ethical considerations in psychopharmacological research involving children and adolescents. Psychopharmacology (Berl) 171(1):86–91, 2003 12677353

Vogt D: Mental health-related beliefs as a barrier to service use for military personnel and veterans: a review. Psychiatr Serv 62(2):135–142, 2011 21285091

Voss Horrell SC, Holohan DR, Didion LM, et al: Treating traumatized OEF/OIF veterans: how does trauma treatment affect the clinician? Prof Psychol Res Pr 42(1):79–86, 2011

Walker RM, Lane LW, Siegler M: Development of a teaching program in clinical medical ethics at the University of Chicago. Acad Med 64(12):723–729, 1989 2590351

Wallerstein N: Power between evaluator and community: research relationships within New Mexico's healthier communities. Soc Sci Med 49(1):39–53, 1999 10414839

Warren JW, Sobal J, Tenney JH, et al: Informed consent by proxy: an issue in research with elderly patients. N Engl J Med 315(18):1124–1128, 1986 3762630

Weinert C, Long KA: Understanding the health care needs of rural families. Family Relations 36(4):450–455, 1987

Weiss BD: Confidentiality expectations of patients, physicians, and medical students. JAMA 247(19):2695–2697, 1982 7077764

Wells K, Klap R, Koike A, et al: Ethnic disparities in unmet need for alcoholism, drug abuse, and mental health care. Am J Psychiatry 158(12):2027–2032, 2001 11729020

Wertz DC, Fletcher JC, Mulvihill JJ: Medical geneticists confront ethical dilemmas: cross-cultural comparisons among 18 nations. Am J Hum Genet 46(6):1200–1213, 1990 2339711

Wettstein RM: Confidentiality, in American Psychiatric Press Review of Psychiatry, Vol 13. Edited by Oldham JM, Riba MB. Washington, DC, American Psychiatric Press, 1994, pp 343–364

White House Office of National AIDS Policy: National HIV/AIDS Strategy for the United States: Updated to 2020. Washington, DC, White House Office of National AIDS Policy, July 2015. Available at: https://www.whitehouse.gov/sites/default/files/docs/national_hiv_aids_strategy_update_2020.pdf. Accessed September 14, 2015.

Williams D, Tricomi G, Gupta J, et al: Efficacy of burnout interventions in the medical education pipeline. Acad Psychiatry 39(1):47–54, 2015 25034955

Williams ES, Skinner AC: Outcomes of physician job satisfaction: a narrative review, implications, and directions for future research. Health Care Manage Rev 28(2):119–139, 2003 12744449

Wilson LS, Pillay D, Kelly BD, et al: Mental health professionals and information sharing: carer perspectives. Ir J Med Sci 2014 25018144 [Epub ahead of print]

Wittich CM, Burkle CM, Lanier WL: Medication errors: an overview for clinicians. Mayo Clin Proc 89(8):1116–1125, 2014 24981217

Wong BM, Imrie K: Why resident duty hours regulations must address attending physicians' workload. Acad Med 88(9):1209–1211, 2013 23886997

Wong JG, Lieh-Mak F: Genetic discrimination and mental illness: a case report. J Med Ethics 27(6):393–397, 2001 11731603

Woolley D, Clements T: Family medicine residents' and community physicians' concerns about patient truthfulness. Acad Med 72(2):155–157, 1997 9040261

World Health Organization: The Global Burden of Disease: 2004 Update. Geneva, World Health Organization, 2008

Yearwood EL: Microaggression. J Child Adolesc Psychiatr Nurs 26(1):98–99, 2013 23472273

Zuardi AW, Ishara S, Bandeira M: Burden and stress among psychiatry residents and psychiatric healthcare providers. Acad Psychiatry 35(6):404–406, 2011 22193741

Cases for Discussion

Laura Weiss Roberts, M.D., M.A.

CASE 1

A physician sought care informally from his neighbor who was a psychiatrist and a colleague at the nearby community hospital. The physician was having difficulty in his marriage and wanted psychotropic medications but "off the books" because he did not want his patients to lose confidence in his surgical skills. The psychiatrist was sympathetic and tried to clarify what symptoms his neighbor was experiencing. The physician suddenly balked, stating, "Hey, you aren't my doctor just because you give me some pills. You don't need to know anything."

CASE 2

A 16-year-old adolescent with bulimia is engaged in a day treatment program. She has been doing well for 3 weeks, with marked improvement in her symptoms, mood, and observed behavior. Two days before being discharged from the program, the treatment team discovers that she has been sneaking alcohol onto the hospital grounds and has engaged in sex with another patient. She begs the day treatment program director to keep this information from her parents.

CASE 3

A male medical student is rotating on the psychosomatic medicine service, which provides consultation to an outpatient gynecology clinic. The student accompanies the attending physician while interviewing and examining some patients. He notices with surprise that his girlfriend is in the waiting room.

CASE 4

A 56-year-old Hispanic woman with schizoaffective disorder is approached to participate in a 12-week trial of a new medication. She is required to be medication-free to enroll in the trial. She agrees to participate, but while staying at her sister's house before the beginning of the trial, she begins to experience serious symptoms. Her sister objects to her enrolling in the trial.

CASE 5

A middle-aged male complained of ongoing depression, fatigue, and decreased libido. Trials of antidepressants proved ineffective. Ultimately he was found to have extremely low testosterone levels. He enrolled in a clinical trial comparing different hormonal therapies. He felt much better after testosterone replacement therapy was initiated, but he began presenting with recurrent sexually transmitted infections. He agreed to counseling to work on negotiating safer sex practices. Six months after receiving counseling, he presented with genital lesions.

CASE 6

A 20-year-old college student from a traditional Vietnamese family who is active with the local Vietnamese community has been visiting her school's mental health services regularly for problems related to testing anxiety. Initially, the sessions focused on stress management techniques, but lately they have become more like psychotherapy talk sessions. Her psychiatrist believes that there are deeper issues having to do with her relationships with her parents and other relatives that must be addressed through psychotherapy. The student consents to the psychotherapy, but she feels intensely uncomfortable with the sessions. Her community views psychotherapy with great suspicion and disapproval, and she feels that she is betraying her family and community members' trust. She decides to stop seeing the psychiatrist.

CASE 7

A patient demanded discharge 2 days after an emergency appendectomy. He was febrile and tachycardic, had signs of peritonitis, and yet was insistent that he leave the hospital. The medical team was conflicted about discharging the patient against medical advice: the nurses and residents believed the patient had the right to refuse treatment, but the attending clinician did not agree. In the initial psychiatric evaluation, the patient showed irritability and very subtle indications of diminished attention, was oriented except to day of the week, and had no other apparent abnormalities on an abbreviated mental status examination. He was noted to be very tremulous. Within an hour, the patient was frankly agitated, disoriented, and expressed disorganized thoughts. Additional history was then obtained in which it was revealed that the patient had been drinking 1–2 pints of vodka daily prior to admission.

CASE 8

A patient gives informed consent to undergo a course of electroconvulsive therapy (ECT) for treatment of very severe major depression with psychotic features. The patient improves greatly, but after the sixth treatment, the patient refuses further ECT or medication interventions.

CASE 9

A 22-year-old woman has opioid dependence, cocaine and cannabis abuse, and posttraumatic stress disorder (PTSD) resulting from a kidnapping and repeated rape 4 months prior to presentation for treatment. Her PTSD symptoms are severe, and she needs help with case management for her legal problems and unstable housing. She misses most of her psychiatric medication and therapy appointments, however, and also takes her methadone irregularly, and she does not seem to be benefiting from treatment. The treatment team repeatedly states its expectation that she participate more consistently in treatment but is reluctant to discharge her for noncompliance. After 6 months, she drops out of treatment.

CASE 10

A patient with a remote history of substance abuse has recently been diagnosed with very advanced ovarian cancer and is experiencing severe pain but is very reluctant to take medications with any addictive potential.

CASE 11

A 45-year-old man sees an internist for his primary care and a psychiatrist for his mental health needs at a multidisciplinary clinic. The patient has been living with chronic illness for 20 years. As a result, he takes high doses of pain medications prescribed by his internist. He has developed a trusting relationship with his psychiatrist and finally admits that he sells his pain medications to pay his rent and car loan. He takes just enough of the medications to test positive on monthly toxicology screens that the internist requires as part of their pain management contract.

CASE 12

A psychiatrist is caring for a prominent local business owner and philanthropist who has been admitted for observation after sustaining a serious concussion in a bicycling accident. During the hospitalization, the patient becomes disoriented and irritable and develops signs and symptoms highly suggestive of alcohol withdrawal. The psychiatrist provides care according to the standard alcohol withdrawal protocol, and the syndrome resolves. As the hospitalization progresses, the psychiatrist finds various staff people walking by the patient's room apparently to catch a glimpse of the patient. Not all of these individuals are directly involved in the patient's care.

CASE 13

A 36-year-old psychiatrist invests in a small start-up company with friends from college. The start-up links wealthy individuals in need of health services with first-available appointments with physicians who run cash-pay or concierge medical practices. The company charges a significant fee for coordinating the initial visit by the patient and also obtains a steady flow of funding from the medical practices, which are pleased to have access to wealthy patients. The psychiatrist begins to see opportunities for linking wealthy individuals with mental health services.

CASE 14

A 24-year-old college student with very severe anorexia nervosa states that he intends to die and refuses to eat or accept tube feeding. His family admits him to a hospital for psychiatric and medical care and obtains a court order for a feeding tube. The family feels immensely grateful for the care he is receiving and asks if they can make a donation to the hospital.

CASE 15

A psychiatrist's 34-year-old patient committed suicide by overdose and was found by his roommate. The patient used both over-the-counter and prescription medications. Panicking about a potential lawsuit, the psychiatrist wonders whether he should change his treatment notes to suppress the observation that the patient had previously reported suicidal ideation.

CASE 16

A 27-year-old Chinese American woman who is a fourth-year psychiatry resident has been a high achiever all her life. She sets strict standards for herself and can be very self-critical when she fails to meet them. Lately, she has been struggling with strong feelings of worthlessness and shame because her work performance has been declining. Over the past month, she has felt increasingly fatigued and has difficulty concentrating at the hospital. She has called in sick multiple times. When at work, she appears distracted and withdrawn. She spends much of her time off alone at home. Her primary care physician refers her to a psychiatrist for evaluation. The psychiatrist offers an initial diagnosis of depression and begins to discuss treatment options with her. She vehemently denies the diagnosis and resists any forms of treatment. She worries about the response from her family members, who maintain very traditional values, if they learn of her diagnosis.

CASE 17

A psychiatrist receives a phone call from a close friend whose father died after a long and difficult illness 8 months ago. The friend has been having difficulties concentrating at work and problems sleeping. Sleep has been particularly problematic lately, and the friend tearfully asks if the psychiatrist would provide some medication to help with the insomnia and depression.

CASE 18

A 25-year-old single gay man was diagnosed with HIV 1 year ago but does not want to take antiretroviral medications because he has "heard about the side effects." He has a viral load of 5,000 copies per milliliter and an absolute CD4+ T-cell count of 800 cells per milliliter, indicating that he is doing well, but he remains at risk of infecting others if he engages in unprotected sex. His primary care provider explains the treatment-as-prevention model of care and the clinic's policy of starting all HIV-positive patients on antiretroviral medications, but the patient continues to refuse them. The primary care provider refers him to the clinic's psychiatrist for evaluation, but the patient refuses to attend the appointment. He returns for care several months later to be treated for syphilis but continues to reject antiretroviral medications.

CASE 19

A psychiatrist who frequently works as a *locums tenens* physician across several adjacent states receives a social media "friend" request from a patient he saw on one occasion 2 months previously. He thinks, "Why not?"

CASE 20

A 34-year-old African American man with generalized anxiety disorder enrolls in a clinical trial, and 4 weeks after he consents, he asks to leave the experiment. His reasons are unclear, but the research team believes that the other study volunteers are making him feel uncomfortable.

CASE 21

A psychosomatic medicine fellow is on call at the hospital, covering the emergency department. Police bring in an agitated, incoherent, middle-aged patient who was wandering in the parking lot of a nearby shopping mall and appears to have fallen. The patient has no medical record in the system. The fellow searches the patient's name on the Internet, seeking additional information.

CASE 22

A 37-year-old man has a 20-year history of alcohol dependence and a 2-year history of cognitive impairment from a head injury sustained in an assault. Now he is impulsive, emotionally labile, lacking in judgment and planning ability, and chronically suicidal, and he continues to drink alcohol at every opportunity. After several unsuccessful attempts by physicians to have him committed to long-term treatment, a legal guardian is named. The patient leaves the group homes and nursing homes where he is placed, however, and he is eventually found wandering on the street.

CASE 23

A psychosomatic physician gives talks for a pharmaceutical company. He also lectures about psychopharmacology in a psychiatry residency training program and is often invited to speak at grand rounds in various clinical departments in the region. The psychiatrist informs the residents of his relationship with the pharmaceutical company prior to beginning his first lecture.

CASE 24

A 42-year-old man with paranoid schizophrenia and heroin dependence, a long history of nonadherence with medications, and initially no interest in addiction treatment was gradually engaged through his case manager's willingness to work with him on an application for disability. The patient eventually was stabilized on antipsychotic medication and entered a methadone program. He has been living independently and clean from illicit drugs for more than a year.

CASE 25

A woman is brought to the hospital with her husband after being in an automobile crash. She is alert and very distressed. She has internal injuries and a very low hematocrit. The emergency physician recommends immediate blood transfusion. The patient is a devout Jehovah's Witness and does not wish to accept the transfusion. She does accept intravenous fluids and is fully cooperative with her care beyond her decision to decline the transfusion. A psychiatrist is called, as well as the consultant from the patient care ethics service. The patient is found to have sufficient decision-making capability, and her husband confirms both her religion and her refusal to receive blood products. The emergency physician remains very concerned about her condition. Suddenly, her pressure drops, and she is taken for surgery to determine the source of her internal bleeding.

CASE 26

A 39-year-old woman with alcohol dependence and severe panic disorder, who has abstained from alcohol for 4 years but uses marijuana regularly, has been maintained on relatively high doses of clonazepam for panic disorder. After her daughter runs away from home, the woman relapses on alcohol and is hospitalized for detoxification. The patient remains abstinent from alcohol 9 months later but continues to smoke marijuana.

CASE 27

A young man has been meeting other men through a popular smart phone app and decides to start preexposure prophylaxis treatment to reduce his chances of becoming infected with HIV. He has private insurance but understands that he is responsible for a high copay. He learns that the manufacturer sponsors a copay assistance program and also markets the medication for the treatment of HIV/AIDS worldwide, including in resource-poor countries.

CASE 28

A 43-year-old man with cocaine and alcohol dependence, on parole after serving 9 months on felony assault charges, is court-ordered for treatment. He reports that he has been clean and sober in outpatient treatment for the past 4 months but then admits to using cocaine with a girlfriend twice in a week. The counselor recommends intensive outpatient treatment, but the parole officer detects cocaine on a urine drug screen and sends the patient to jail for a week. Upon release, the patient undergoes 12 weeks of intensive outpatient treatment and remains clean and compliant with treatment for the remainder of his 18-month probation.

CASE 29

An adolescent Hispanic female is brought to the hospital after a suicide attempt. The patient is deaf and has limited English language skills. She lip reads and uses sign language to communicate. She is stabilized and transferred to the psychiatry unit. Her aunt, who is fluent in sign language, offers to interpret for the nurses and psychiatrist, but the patient does not want her family involved in her care. Medical translators who are proficient in sign language are available at the hospital.

CASE 30

A 46-year-old psychiatrist is racked with guilt, remembering every mistake and poor outcome from the past 20 years in his clinical research activities. At night he experiences repetitive and intrusive thoughts. Using alcohol occasionally helps him sleep, because he feels "less tortured" by his hard memories. His research assistant often finds that the psychiatrist's research records are incomplete.

CASE 31

An attending psychiatrist asks a resident for a prescription for an antidepressant, stating that he does not want any potentially stigmatizing or damaging information in his electronic medical record.

CASE 32

A 22-year-old immigrant woman without family nearby offers to clean the home of the psychiatrist in trade for a prescription for antidepressants for her and her roommate, both of whom suffer from depression. The psychiatrist states that he cannot accept the trade, but he can enroll the two women into a clinical trial that would provide basic mental health care and would randomize them into two different treatment groups.

CASE 33

An obese woman with schizophrenia is admitted to a psychiatric unit involuntarily. She has severe persecutory delusions and feels very frightened by and untrusting of others. She is refusing all medications but says that she is willing to remain at the hospital. It is discovered that she is 26 weeks pregnant.

CASE 34

A 17-year-old with bipolar disorder and bulimia reports to her psychiatrist that she is in love with a 28-year-old man. They routinely have unprotected sex. She is wondering about birth control and about her medications. She does not want her family to know about the relationship.

Index

Page numbers printed in **boldface** type refer to tables or figures.

Social justice. *See also* Justice
   mental health care services and,
      301, 302
   psychiatric genetics and, 275–276
Social media, and e-innovation in
   psychiatry, 278, 279
Social phobia, 308
Social relationships
   in case examples, 336, 339, 340
   psychotherapeutic relationship and,
      31, 36
   small communities and, 106, **107,**
      110, 116, 168
Society for Adolescent Medicine, 94
Socioeconomic factors, in clinical
   decision making, 22–23. *See also*
   Economic costs; Social
   relationships
Special populations, and psychiatric
   research, 251–252, 255–258.
   See also Addictions; Adolescents;
   Children; Culture and cultural
   issues; Difficult patients; End of
   life; HIV/AIDS; Small
   communities; Veterans
Spinal cord injury, and decisional
   capacity, 40
Stanford Medicine WellMD program,
   235
Stigma
   addiction and, 182, **183**
   against mental health problems and
      treatment in military, 123
   HIV/AIDS and, 153
   psychiatric illness in clinicians and,
      230
Strength, of people with mental illness
   concept of in psychotherapeutic
      work, 58
   ethical use of influence and, 67
Stress
   of clinicians in small communities,
      109, 114–115
   clinical training and, 288

HIV/AIDS and psychosocial, **149**
   psychiatrists and self-sacrifice, 198
Substance use disorders. *See also*
   Addictions; Alcohol abuse and
   alcohol use disorder
   in case examples, 118, 156, 337, 341,
      342
   in DSM-5, 179
   economic costs of, 181, 303
   veterans and, 120
Substituted judgment standard, and
   surrogate decision making, 50, 69
Suicide and suicidal ideation
   in case examples, 72, 118, 145, 236,
      294, 308, 339, 342
   high-risk situations and, 60
   of medical students and residents,
      225, 236
   physician-assisted, 162–163, 164
   prediction of, 62–64
   rate of for physicians, 198, 223, 225
   veterans and, 121, 123, 125
Supervision, strategies for ethics in
   clinical, **294**
Surrogate decision making
   informed consent and, 49–50, 51–52
   treatment refusal and, 69
Systems of care, 297–308. *See also*
   Health care systems
Szasz, Thomas, 69

*Tarasoff v. Regents of the University of
   California* (1974, 1976), 66, 67, 80,
   97
Telemedicine, 115
Tenofovir disoproxil fumarate (TDF),
   154–155
Terminal illness. *See also* Chronic
   illness
   cultural issues and, 137, 139
   end-of-life issues and diagnosis of,
      158
   truth telling issues in diagnosis and
      treatment of, 78